YOUR BEST LIFE

YOUR BEST LIFE

A DOCTOR'S SECRET GUIDE TO RADIANT HEALTH OVER 40

DR LOUISE WISEMAN

The information in this book has been compiled as a way of general guidance to the specific
subjects within it. It in no way replaces medical, healthcare, pharmaceutical, dental, orthodontic,
psychological or other professional advice given by practitioners who know you personally and treat
you clinically based on your medical and family history and their consultation with you. Nothing in
this book constitutes personal medical advice to the reader, nor should it be interpreted as so. Please
consult your GP or family doctor before changing, stopping or starting any medical treatment or
instigating any change in lifestyle. So far as the author and any contributing specialist interviewees
are aware, the information is up to date as of November 2019. Practice, laws and regulations all
change and new research is constantly emerging. The reader should obtain up-to-date advice on any
issues concerning their health. The author, contributors and publisher do not take any responsibility
for any liability arising directly or indirectly from the use or misuse of the information contained
in this book. All information is given following current UK guidelines (always subject to change),
and different countries may have different requirements for healthcare. Any brands mentioned are as
examples given in good faith and there has been no paid advertising within this book.

Matador
9 Priory Business Park,
Wistow Road, Kibworth Beauchamp,
Leicestershire. LE8 0RX
Tel: 0116 279 2299
Email: books@troubador.co.uk
Web: www.troubador.co.uk/matador
Twitter: @matadorbooks

ISBN 978 1838594 350

British Library Cataloguing in Publication Data.
A catalogue record for this book is available from the British Library.

Printed and bound by CPI Group (UK) Ltd, Croydon, CR0 4YY
Typeset in 11pt Bodoni 72 by Troubador Publishing Ltd, Leicester, UK

Matador is an imprint of Troubador Publishing Ltd

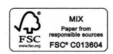

For my children
May you always have a dream, a plan and a smile

CONTENTS

HOW TO USE THIS BOOK FOR YOUR BEST LIFE

I do not expect you to read this book from cover to cover. This is a book filled with information, opinion and anecdotes. After the informative chapters, you will read the stories of fabulous women like you. These will inspire, motivate and ultimately make you realise we are all in this search for the **best life** together.

The book is organised like a journey through your body. I could have written three books as we are incredibly wonderful, complex beings. Here lies the framework for what I believe are the most important areas of mental and physical health, and spiritual wellbeing. These are based on my career as a doctor and then my opinion as a woman. **Nothing in these pages is prescriptive or medical advice and nothing supersedes or replaces a medical consultation and examination by your own doctor who knows you and your medical and family history.** Please read the disclaimer at the front of this book thoroughly and then read it again.

I went through hell and back with an acute illness that motivated my career break and the search for even BETTER health. I want to provoke you to think about yourself differently, to grasp every opportunity in life by looking after your body and mind. I truly believe that the way to get women to do this is to help them *understand how their bodies work*. If I just told you what to do, this book could have been five facts: **eat well, exercise, relax, sleep, love.** However, if you know *why* you need to do those things it might infiltrate your psyche deeper and reflect in the choices you make. Women have come to my talks and then told me later that they have lost their excess weight, started self-care, exercised, and so on. I did not put them on diets or prescribe specific gym classes – I just explained what you need to do to look after your body and hopefully prevent disease or detect it early.

I want this to be a book you keep and refer back to when the relevance of a chapter arises in your life. I want you to share any wisdom with your friends, daughters, nieces and grannies. Any topic that gets women talking about **loving themselves** again is invaluable.

By discussing with specialists on the frontline, this is the most accurate account I can make, but opinions change, medicine moves on and/even doctors differ in opinion. None of the takeaway messages will be rocket science, they will all be things you can do inexpensively at home, whatever your age. The opinions of the specialists and ladies in this book **are their own and not necessarily mine**, so it is like listening in on many conversations and taking from it *what you need.* Have fun on this journey. We start with happiness and end up with sleep – both incredible parts of life. There is a plethora of wondrous female stuff in between.

Just like a family doctor is a gateway to other professions, this book provides a gateway to other books, resources online or avenues for you to privately explore. One book cannot hold all the answers but may spur you on *your own path* to your best life.

Resources are highlighted in bronze.

Good facts in green.

Questions and alarming points in purple.

It is invaluable to me that you have given your hard-earned money and precious time reading my book. I hope these words reach you deeply and encourage you to reach higher for your health and wellbeing.

PRELUDE
TO A BOOK

I am sitting up in bed. My 38th birthday was last month. I cannot breathe. The salt water keeps flooding into my mouth. Coughing barely clears it. I turn my head to the end of the bedroom. There is an elderly lady dressed for a funeral – a neat black veil over her coiffed hair. Am I imagining her? I turn away. I am not ready for her yet. Sleep beckons and I drift off.

I hear the key in the lock downstairs. I hear the giggling sounds of my little daughter as she runs in across the wooden floor. My husband shushes her: "Mummy is sleeping." I manoeuvre myself from my sweat-laden bed and shuffle onto the landing. My heart is pumping manically, whether I sit, lie or stand. I lean my body over the bannister so they can hear me. "I need... I need you to get me to the doctor." My husband has looked concerned for days. The doctor who telephoned yesterday did not understand how I felt; I was mentally begging her to visit. I should have been more clear. Now I have no choice. I *have* to go.

I pull on clothes, my heart pounding relentlessly. I gingerly walk down the stairs. The thumping in my chest, in my ears; and the salt water, it keeps coming – what is that? I hold back from my beloved daughter. My husband puts her pink fluffy coat back on and she looks puzzled that she is going out again. She runs towards me with outstretched starfish hands. "No, no, darling, don't come near!" I can't have my darling girl infected by this beast. I have quarantined myself in the bedroom for days. Not wanting to infect anyone with this flu. Except it's not like any flu I've *ever* had.

I climb into my husband's silver 4 by 4. The daylight stretches my ability to keep my eyes open. My daughter is chattering away, asking me if I am okay. I make reassuring noises with my eyes closed. The car starts and I feel it swing around corners and somehow we are at the GP surgery. I instruct my husband to wait outside with my daughter. He doesn't and they sit near me. I am called straight in. I make jovial greetings with the male doctor. This kind, smiling doctor I have only met once. I play it down. I say I am ill but am not sure. He shoves a pulse oximeter quickly on my right index finger and the numbers flash up 'oxygen saturation 82'.

F**k me, I am ill.

He listens to my heart and chest and looks at the heart rate reading on the monitor. 155 beats per minute. *Bloody hell*, I think, and see the panic in his kind face.

"Get your husband to take you now – no time for an ambulance – to A & E. I will tell them you are coming."

I know those words. I have said them enough. To one or other of my 1,600 patients when they have shown possible signs of a heart attack or breathing difficulties. But this is *me*. I get back in the car. It's such a high step up. I can hardly do it. I slump to the side as I fasten my seatbelt, eyes closed again. "I'm not going to die, am I?" I ask my wonderful non-medical husband.

He drives fast and I close my eyes, the salt water still coming. I cough into another tissue. What is that damn stuff?

We park randomly outside A & E. We walk in. I spot an old colleague, Roger, walking towards me – I have not seen him since I was the junior anaesthetist and he was the wise junior medic. *He is now the consultant in charge of the whole department.* I want to hug him. The low oxygen has made me delirious, like I have had a bottle of wine and no food. I stagger.

"Roger! So nice to see you – I am not looking my best!"

"For God's sake, Louise, sit down; we need to get the oxygen on you."

I relent. I let them. The oxygen is dry blasting onto my mouth and nose. The mask smells of plastic and my old work in anaesthetics. I have put masks upon so many others but the smell is so intense when it's on your own face. This is *my* mask. I breathe it. A drip line is quickly placed in my arm. The oxygen saturation on the machine is 82 again; it worries them – they mutter. The medical gathering around me is enlarging. They shove me quickly into a backless hospital gown and then a wheelchair to X-ray. I manage to stand and breathe for the films to be taken. I go back in the wheelchair, back to the bed. I am the patient now. Helpless. Hopeless. That damn salt water. I am drowning.

A beautiful young medical registrar clip-clops towards me in fancy heels. I tell her I love her shoes. I think I tell her I wear shoes like that at work. I told you – it's like being drunk. She flushes my drip with cold saline and then antibiotic. The nurse and Roger arrive and they all hover.

"You have a very severe pneumonia. Both sides. Full up. We need to get these antibiotics in you really fast and see how we go." Roger looks worried.

The beautiful registrar leans over close. **"I had pneumonia in house jobs, sats 85 – it's frightening. You will be okay, I promise."**

I want to cry. I let a tear fall silently down my cheek. I don't want my daughter to see.

The next 12 hours are a blur. People come to meet me. The physiotherapist, she takes no prisoners, says they will get me better but I *have to work for it*. I have to blow into this and that and lie down while she pummels my chest. It is temporary bliss and the salt water drains into my mouth as she commends me on my coughing. Small wins. The night passes somehow and light comes into the ward. There is someone from my work on the nurses' phone *checking I am alive* – I half smile to myself. I am.

I am moved up to another ward. I have graduated. I am next to someone on high dose chemo and no immune system. I beg her not to come near but over the next few days she will share stories of her life, her illness and her pain. I will try and give comfort constrained by the drip attached to me, a metal pole and the oxygen mask. I will give the junior doctor advice in the night as he tends to her nausea and vomiting. He tries the anti-sickness medicine I recommend and she has peace for a few hours. My first nights are hell for those around me. This cough is the worst. I cannot hold it in. The salt water floods out like molten lava once it starts. The cough is periodic through the night, and the lady opposite, confused by her urine infection, calls me darling and asks me to sit with her. She thinks I am her niece and tells me she can make me better. Then, as my nocturnal coughing irritates her already confused brain, she starts shouting and telling me to shut up. I cannot move. I lie there and look out through the gap in the curtains at the moonlight. I want this coughing to stop, I want rest. This is nothing compared to what my neighbour is going through and I can't bear to keep her awake. The next night I give in to temptation and accept the sleeping tablet that the kind nurse has been trying to persuade me to have every night. I get up in the morning, dragging my drip stand to the bathroom four metres away. Grappling with the other hand to hold my gown shut. I look in the mirror. I look shocking. (I am crying now six years later as I write this.) My face is pale as chalk, my eyes sunken. I look at my stomach as the gown falls to the side and my post-baby tummy is gone. My stomach has shrunk inwards and the skin is dry. The belly above my emergency caesarean scar is just a slight flap of skin. The scar is more visible from eye level. My pounding heart and temperature must have burned the fat away this week. I turn to go to the toilet. Glad of the privacy away from the poor confused lady hurling abuse. Then I see the toilet overflowing with paper and excrement. But I have to go. It took so much energy to get this far from my bed. I can't bear to bother the nurses. I try to flush it and, with the candour of a *Carry On Nurse* sketch, I attempt to unblock the toilet with the plunger next to it, whilst still grappling with my drip stand and retaining sterility around my drip site. With one great effort – all that I have in my infected body – the loo flushes and is clear. I relieve myself, wash my hands like Harry Houdini fighting the flexing plastic drip pulling my skin taut, and I return to the bed. I tell my dear neighbour about what I just did. She looks horrified and we both laugh as the lady opposite says something unrepeatable. We are a team my neighbour and I. We talk more about our lives. She asks about my children. I tell her that I haven't held them for a week now and not seen them for two days. She tells me about her grandchildren and how proud she is of them. We are a team my neighbour and I.

My new medical team sails onto the ward like a royal procession. The consultant addresses me directly. They need a contrast scan to see if I have clots all over my lungs. I plead that I have no risk factors but they insist. My heart rate is so high. They won't give up. The consultant explains that my blood oxygen was so low on the saturation curve that it would have been a few hours at home. That would have been it. DEAD. I swallow the salt water in my mouth and take it all in. Bloody oxygen saturation curves, I know about them. He is probably right. We discuss the physiology. My favourite subject. His juniors stare at me blankly then look to the floor. "*I have been there!*" I want to shout. When you can happily walk away from the bed as you are the healthy doctor and not the patient. My perspective is still skewed by my illness and I have to *phone a friend*. I phone Richard at the surgery where I work. I know he is on duty and will speak sense. The receptionists, whom I love like family, put me straight through to the line in his consulting room. It's not *what* you know but *who* you know. Richard's pragmatic tone, talking to me, like *me*, and not a 'sick person', calms me down. He tells me I *have* to have the scan but I am going to get better and it will *all be okay*. I phone another friend, Hazel – a leading consultant anaesthetist who used to teach me, now my friend. She tells me: "We just want to live to see our children reach adulthood safely." She has said it. I cry to her on the phone and she understands, she doesn't judge.

I lie in the scanner wondering how I got there. The whirring noise starts and I do my best to breathe when instructed, and *not cough*. Somehow the damn salt water has abated for a few minutes. Everyone is kind and efficient. Kindness is queen. I always tried to be kind. I am glad I did.

My darling friend Vicki visits. I am so worried about her seeing me like this. She has just watched her dear father die from lung cancer in a French hospital bed and I don't want to remind her. She doesn't show that she is frightened. She tells me I do not look as bad as she thought! We laugh and for a seconds I feel human. I don't want to keep her long, she has her son to go back to, and I hug her, trying not to breathe near her face. My other friends text to send love and I feel blessed. My parents come to the bedside. They have visited before, but we were never alone. We are alone now and I watch my mummy and daddy cry. They now let me see how worried they are. I seem to be turning a corner. Dad says the memory of this awfulness will fade. I feel their pain and want to take it away. I hold them close. I still haven't held or seen my children. My mum and dad sit there, on the yellow bedspread, holding their only child.

I was lucky enough, with medicine, care and rest, to recover fully from this unfortunate infection and return to my job as a healthy GP four months later. My life and mindset were permanently changed – a brand new respect for good health, and a desire to *become even healthier* than before and stay that way!

Hence the notion for this book was born. A doctor who, prompted by her illness, looked at how to preserve what we *take for granted* – the immense value of *feeling well and strong* to go through midlife and beyond. The result should be glowing radiance to take forward through the exciting second half of life. I want to inspire you on this journey to your **BEST HEALTH** and your **BEST LIFE**. My own path paved the way for my research and the consolidation of remarkable knowledge and wisdom from some of the best health specialists in the world.

Avatar Lou will appear from time to time to summarise my advice!

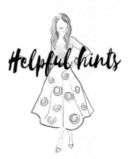

INTRODUCTION

STEP INTO THE SUNSHINE AND FEEL OPTIMISTIC ABOUT WHAT IS TO COME

I am not famous. I am not a celebrity. I am a mother of two children, a 46-year-old former GP, now writer and voracious reader. I am a **woman**. I love life and want to live it with maximum energy and enjoyment. I do not want to feel old before my time. I want to preserve myself as best as I can, without needing a surgeon's knife or a doctor's needle.

There is so much information available to us now and it is invading our lives in so many different ways. Not only do we have our real family and friends, we have contacts far afield on the World Wide Web, some of whom we will *never meet* and yet claim to know. We see ordinary people being lauded as 'celebrities' and we 'follow' them electronically, so information is constantly shared. If we are 'sharing' about eyelashes and shoes, why are we not sharing information about the very essence of our lives – our health?

Take a look in the mirror. Are you your best self right now?

Do you hanker for the face and body you had at 20? Do you feel life is over now you are middle-aged or beyond? Are you constantly comparing yourself to the 'perfect' images of young women who surround us?

OR

Do you see a woman with maturity and wisdom? Do you look and feel better than ever? Do you now know what is best for YOU? Age *can* bring confidence to inspire others – we have one chance and this is it!

You probably have responsibilities; you may even be the sandwich generation caring for those younger and older. How much time do you spend caring for **yourself**?

This book is about trying to work out how to look after *you as you are now*, somewhere between the ages of 40 and 90. It is in having knowledge that we women become strong. In knowing that we are giving ourselves the best chance, the guilt and the negativity have to step aside. **Step into the sunshine and feel optimistic about what is to come.** Do not sit at home firefighting as 'inevitable ageing' just happens to you. If we have knowledge, we have choices. We can elicit change, and the knock-on effect is not just on us but also on those around us: our partners, children and friends. The real friends you see in the café, not the ones on the screen in front of you.

I was a doctor working in the UK NHS for 15 years, then I decided to take time out to be with my children. Whilst working as a GP I was advising women about their health and emotions, but so much of this was dealing with the effects of self-neglect. Little thought is given to the prevention of illness and the preservation of our bodies in their healthy state. Stepping off the career ladder to be a 'stay-at-home writing mum', my questions then came from my friends:

What works? What does this mean? Is this cream good? What will make me feel better? What will make me look better?

There is no single answer. There is nothing that will guarantee full good health, but there is a lot that can be done to increase your own odds and not leave them to the roulette of life. Here, I am going to try and uncover what each field of healthcare is currently saying, to give women a chance to actually have some control and take charge of their bodies. From your bones outwards I want to get under the skin and see how *we can* as women optimise health. Our raw beauty will be allowed to shine out. Some of my advice will be common sense that you hope to glean from chatting with a friend. Some will be similar to what I used to jot down for my patients, things they could do to help themselves in between doctor appointments. I will recommend further books to read. Any new facts will be evidence-based, after my research of contemporary papers and talking to specialists on the frontline.

There is no reason to reach middle age and feel that life is over.

Don't just take my word for it! I have interviewed many prolific women; they all inspire me and have achieved something wonderful in their lives. Many are in a different career to the one they chose in their 20s and are living their lives to the full. I will be looking at where their beliefs in health and beauty originated from. Who were their female role models? How do they manage to 'have it all', or does anyone really 'have it all'? Nearly all of these women have overcome immense obstacles in life in order to succeed – none have had it easy.

Indeed, I want to replace the term 'fighting ageing' with *'graceful ageing'*, as turning back time is not within anyone's reach. I know you will at some point be inspired to look straight at that woman in the mirror and look after her in the manner she deserves. Who knows, you may in turn inspire someone else to live their life to the max!

You are a beautiful woman. Your age only adds to your beauty. Think about that. You will have aged during the time taken to read this book but you should be inspired to now do it well and possibly live longer, happier and more radiantly! What do we have to lose?

BEAUTY
OVER 40

THE IMAGE OF BEAUTY NOW AS A WOMAN IN MIDLIFE

"Ageing is out of your control. How you handle it, though, is in your hands."

Diane Von Furstenberg

As a teenager I would save my pocket money to buy *Vogue*. I would gaze at the photography in awe. I wanted to be THAT GIRL in the magazine. In the present day, girls are influenced by beauty images 24/7, everywhere.

I remember collecting free beauty samples, believing real beauty would seep out of the little sachets and enhance my face! I would go with a boyfriend in the '90s to see moody French films and study the French actresses, raw in their allure with just a dash of red lipstick – so different to the contouring and highlighting of today. Aspiration to beauty seemed more 'simple'. One actress, whom I had adored as a teenager, sat in my consulting room as my patient many years later. She almost mourned the passing of her youthful beauty and the riches it had bestowed upon her. Yet she was still *such a beautiful soul* and I wondered what praise and adulation would do to your psyche once the blooming years had passed. *We identify so much by what we look like on the outside but surely that cannot be all we have to offer?*

So, there is a paradox: I admit to having a massive interest in products and potions and ways of living, to mean I can try and look my best, but I also see the stark reality of what life looks like to women now. If young girls are exposed to marvel created by airbrush and artifice, what are we to tell them? Similarly, as women over 40 we can be vulnerable to what we see and must retain confidence, self-esteem and self-worth.

There is a wealth of treatments promising to restore our youthful visage. How old do you look? *Time* seems to no longer be the determinant, rather the extent of your facial work. If the procedures are out there and performed safely by qualified medical personnel, no one should judge a woman's choice whether or not to partake. That is not an argument for this book.

Most of us admit to some fascination with the 'before and after', or makeover. What I want to bring you in this book is the *before and after you can achieve* by being informed and looking after yourself before you think of a more interventional route. In our fascination with celebrity lifestyle, I will try to strip back and find out the essentials of what **real** people do to look after themselves for the finite time they are on this planet, both in and out of the public eye. Women should **help one another** achieve and gain health. Let us uncover the truth together.

DISPOSABLE, REPLACEABLE, FORGOTTEN BEAUTY

"Maybe she is born with it, maybe it's her plastic surgeon."

Our society has changed immensely in the last decade. We can watch faces on television in high definition. We can compare and contrast wealth, clothes, faces, bodies. We are in a throwaway society. If something does not perform we are quick to replace it. I could be talking about the sofa that your parents saved up to buy, which the puppy chewed, and they fixed it with new material or a throw over the top, so it was still *your* sofa in *your* living room. Fast forward to now and your own sofa is damaged. It's still comfortable to sit on and serves its purpose but it *does not fit with your ideal aesthetic*, so you **trade it in and get a new one**.

Now look at your face. It is the face you were born with, it is similar to your biological parents; this face is genetically *yours*. You grew up with it, you became familiar with the *feel* of it and the recognition of it being *your* face.

You go through adolescence and you watch your face change; you see puppy fat, spots. In your 20s you are in your 'prime'. You learn ways of accentuating your best features or covering your worst.

Then, like the sofa, a few worn patches appear, you approach middle age and you have lived your life! You have seen a few parties, laughter and tears. The wrinkles are rites of passage like pen marks on the sofa, but heaven forbid a rip appears! A furrow in your brow that you cannot bear to study.

What do you do? Do you look around for ways to fix your face, like your sofa? Is the patching-up actually a new beauty regime and time taken to put on sunscreen and moisturiser?

Or do you want a trade-in, a quick fix, new plush pillows plumped up with filler and new material smoothed by Botox?

Neither is wrong and it is not my intention to dictate. I just want to ensure that your choice is informed so you know what can be done naturally *before* you call the aesthetician. We cannot turn back time, it has passed while you have read these very words, but we can influence how we embrace ageing that is entirely beautiful in so many ways.

HEALTH
OVER 40

 "Live less out of habit and more out of intent."
Amy Rubin Flett

While working as a family doctor, many women would present themselves to me asking for simple advice at various natural stages in their life. In a short consultation, I often felt frustrated that I could not give enough information within the minutes available. Apart from talking incredibly fast and (as my colleagues would vouch for) running incredibly late, the best method for me was to also give the patient some kind of scribble to take away. This could be a few top tips or some literature references for them to seek out.

A problem with worrying about our health in any way is the feel of *loss of control*. Similar to my own spell of ill-health, this lack of control in making yourself better can lead to a downward spiral of despair. Of course, there are many dire situations where this is unavoidable – at times of extreme illness, or when you are blighted by excruciating pain. However, for most situations of mild illness, unknown symptoms, or in disease prevention, it is possible to regain some power over it.

During my pneumonia the physiotherapist was the one to power me up with some control. I was to walk up some stairs. No trouble to me normally – I had been a long-distance runner, a cyclist; I never sat down at home until the illness struck. So I walked and walked up and down countless hospital stairs, feeling somewhat valiant in my plight. I tried to march purposefully, eyes ahead past the night staff at the nurses' station so they wouldn't stop me and tell me to go back to bed!

This was the *only control* I had. I had no control over the doctor giving me the correct medicine or the nurse coming at the right time to give me a painkiller. I had been struck down and humbled by illness and no amount of knowledge or medical degrees could change that.

However, had I been more careful of my health, managing stress and my life/work balance, would the infection have been so severe?

It is important that every woman understands that she has to feel *some control* over her health. By being informed around possibilities for improvement in later life, you can regain more steer over your own path.

MY PERSONAL REALISATIONS ABOUT HEALTH

Is disease inevitable?

Working as a GP I realised many of our patients were there due to STRESS, directly or indirectly. In medical school we studied 'Pathology' – *the science of the causes and effects of diseases, especially the branch of medicine that deals with the laboratory examination of samples of body tissue for diagnostic or forensic purposes* – and would look at slides of cancer, infection, progressive disease, and see the havoc they played on the body. If I knew someone who had suffered the disease it gave it meaning. If not, I just looked in horror at how healthy tissue could morph into something very different. This was on a laboratory plate; in reality that disease was *massively impacting a person's life, hopes and dreams.*

I was seeing at a microscopic level how the human body *could go wrong* and how you could stage the disease from the extent of change. Sometimes there was **cause and effect** – 'this is what happens to your gut if you catch the bug campylobacter' – but sometimes it seemed to just **happen** within that patient's body.

My maternal grandparents died in close succession from cancer when I was ten years old. They had lived a 'healthy' lifestyle, so there was a sense of **Why them? Why so young?** I was mature enough to comprehend the loss, and sensitive enough to see how it destroyed my mother. Our grief was interspersed with great anger at the *cancer* word, and I took that with me throughout my teenage years. So there I was, studying the plates, thinking about my grandparents. What was this? **The inevitability and passive acquirement of disease?** Awful things happen to wonderful people, and I have stood at the bedside of many patients and pondered this.

There is an obvious connection – for example, if someone smokes they are *more likely* to get lung cancer – but there is a large grey area about less dramatic lifestyle choices that may be having a serious impact on our future health. There is medical evidence that your lifestyle can have a **direct effect on your body**. There is also the knowledge of early signs of disease that if not missed will give you a warning and may mean the illness can be halted or cured. **It is those facts that I want to present in this book so that you have them in your mind as you go making your life choices.**

There is also a switch that only **you** can manipulate on or off... motivation!

"Oh, just one more glass of wine – it's Friday!"

"Another four biscuits – I deserve them!"

I have been there, done that and bought the T-shirt. I can be the least accountable to myself. The last thing you want to read is a book written by someone who is the epitome of virtue. There is the concept of balance and living a real, achievable life, not one of deprivation.

How about you hand yourself back a little more control as to the cards you are going to be dealt? There are no guarantees, some diseases are inevitable; there is no magic answer or the medical profession would have nailed it; but SURELY if you are holding this book you have an inkling that you could improve your energy, health, mood for the *better* by how you treat yourself?

Back to the Pathology exam time. My body reflected the stress it was under mentally. After the exam I was very underweight despite not calorie restricting myself. My parents were shocked when I returned home. I had elicited *change in my body by my mental state* and my handling of the pressures I was put under. Here was a first example to me of the **mind controlling the body**. **Could the mind also control or prevent disease?** The anxiety that makes your heart pump in a stressful situation is a potent example of the mental state affecting the physical. On a day-to-day basis how can we manipulate this quality to help us achieve better physical health? How can we regain control of our powerful mind–body connection in middle age and use it to our advantage? With stress-reduction techniques we now have evidence that we can reduce our biological age and may even look younger in the process. I will teach you to meditate if you have not done it before, and I will remind you why you need to do it if you have.

You need to know how and why to care for your eyes, teeth, skin, breasts and gut. You need to know the signs of disease of the feminine mystery that is gynaecology. In being educated about the natural state that is menopause, you can decide what will help you flow through this change (no pun intended) and when you need to ask your doctor's advice. You need to strengthen and maintain your muscles and bones to work against the natural decline with age. You need to be aware of how to protect your mind and reduce the chance of debilitating diseases, alongside harnessing the power of your brain to improve your experience of life and your level of joy in this great phase of life. **Nothing will replace you seeing your doctor** but you might be able to follow a path of self-help before getting to the point of needing medical opinion.

Hence, the goal for this book is to return control into the hands of the beautiful wise woman holding it. I want to inspire you about healthcare in all the amazing systems of your body and step up your life to a greater level of fulfilment, nourishment and fitness. **Your best life is to come**...

NATURE DOES
NOT HURRY, YET
EVERYTHING IS
ACCOMPLISHED

LAO TZU

CHAPTER 1: HAPPINESS

MEDITATION, MINDFULNESS AND AWARENESS
OF THE SENSATIONS OF THE WORLD AROUND YOU

A decade ago, I would have needed to explain these terms, but now they are part of our vernacular. In so being, they are easy to dismiss: "Oh yes, I am mindful." Are you really? Do you understand that it is a way of BEING and not just a phrase for thought processes as you chew your food?

Stress is the health epidemic of our time. Technology means that we are in the fortunate position of being able to work anywhere. The downside is we can be on call for our social and work lives 24/7, unless we set boundaries. Do you set boundaries? Are these powered by feelings of guilt, not helpful to self-esteem? Do you feel you are omnipresent but not actually 100% present, at home or at work, as you waft in the internet 'ether' between the two? I hear you.

You may be like the women who follow me on social media who requested that a priority for the book be 'managing stress'. You may have ongoing concerns for the younger people in your family and parents. Daily life can be drenched in worry. I cannot write away problems, but there are coping mechanisms that can help.

You protect your phone by recharging and, similarly, your mind must 'recalibrate' away from a constant bleep of notifications. You are allowed to just BE. Meditation is the antidote to the hyperactive mind, teaching you patience and less compulsion. We are the generation which demands everything yesterday, but waiting and 'boredom' create a healthy mindset of being quietly happy with oneself.

MEDITATION AND MINDFULNESS

Mindfulness is observing the present moment with non-judgemental awareness. Not judging your thoughts. Intentionally focussing on the here and now. Can you train your brain to observe rather than immediately react to stress?

Meditation is the practice of controlling your mind and focussing on the present moment; in that sense it is mindful. All meditation is mindful but not all mindfulness is meditation.

Let that sink in for a moment.

Take a deep breath.

Hence you can see why we talk about the two words in tandem.

THE SCIENCE BEHIND MEDITATION

Experienced regular meditators show changes in brain activity. The adult brain can undergo changes through a process called 'neuroplasticity', which may include development of new circuits (like rewiring) and often new neurones. Two decades of scientific studies at more than 20 universities have identified the effects of meditation on the brain.

Many of the studies looked at very experienced meditators (more than 10,000 hours of meditating experience). One cannot assume that all meditation will have the same effect. In regular committed meditators the following assessments have been made:

- *Reduced reactivity of the AMYGDALA.* This is the area that is responsible for the 'fight or flight' response. In cavewoman times this would have been an appropriate reaction. We would have felt stressed by an oncoming bear, adrenaline (epinephrine) and cortisol would have been released and we would have needed to run!
- In the 21st century the amygdala is stimulated by traffic jams, text notifications and arguments. The result is uncensored adrenaline and cortisol on overdrive, leading to us having a higher chance of high blood pressure, ischaemic heart disease, diabetes and obesity. This '21st century amygdala' needs careful handling. So, if you reduce activity in the amygdala, then the higher areas of the brain function to appropriately handle 'stress', contrasted with the cavewoman scenario.
- *Increased activity of the prefrontal cortex.* This area regulates emotions and reduces stress.
- *Compassion increase.* Areas linked with empathy work better.
- *Memory loss may be reduced/prevented*

- *Focus and concentration increase*
- *Anxiety reduces*
- *You are more capable of regulating thoughts about yourself*
- *Sleep improves*

With meditation the prefrontal cortex is stimulated to produce dopamine. This makes us happier and more content. All of the physiological changes are more likely if you have 20 minutes' meditation once or twice a day, but START EASY – anything is better than nothing. Just like exercise, short episodes can be effective.

THE UBIQUITY OF MEDITATION AND MINDFULNESS

Meditation does not require money, only time. It is being carried out in schools, prisons and hospitals. Programmes of **mindfulness-based stress reduction** (MBSR) are now used in the management of chronic disease and in hospital departments where patients are dealing with intractable pain or the opacity of terminal ill-health. If something can make the experience more 'liveable' then it has to be an essential consideration, but there are limitations and it is not going to cure illness per se. It is not a reason to put medicine away.

Studies show it may be as potent as medication in preventing a relapse in *some cases* of depression, and further studies will show the expanse of conditions to which meditation can be applied in the future. We really need more detailed studies of how meditation works – investigators are quick to state that we cannot direct unwell patients just to meditation, but use it as an **adjunct** to other treatments. There is a vast variation in the quality of teachers and uniformity of therapy. **Again, don't throw away your medications.**

The process causes a downplaying of our sympathetic nervous system (the fight or flight response) by reducing the signals of stress to the hypothalamic pituitary axis (which is like a stress response centre, taking messages from the brain and sending them to the body) so the endocrine system does not release as much cortisol from the adrenal glands. This is why obesity, heart disease and pain can all be theoretically reduced, as cortisol is a driver for many of these processes.

The mainstay of any advice regarding cardiovascular disease will be conventional national guidelines; but, due to low cost and risk, meditation may be considered a *reasonable adjunct* to management for those motivated in lifestyle change. More research is needed.

Studies have suggested that regular meditators may have reduced incidence or severity of acute respiratory infections (colds and flu). Those who meditate regularly show a similar pattern in having reduced severity of colds to those who exercise regularly. It seems meditation may promote even more improvements in the 'perceived symptom severity' of a cold by improved function generally. **Maybe a future point is that meditation helps our baseline quality of life and thus experience of illness.**

A large review of trials examining the effect of 'mindfulness-based meditation' on the immune system found it did have a dosage-dependent effect on some immune parameters but not necessarily on all immune cells in the body. Again, more research is needed.

A variety of neurodegenerative diseases are accompanied by grey matter atrophy (or shrinkage) such as seen in Alzheimer's disease. A large review has corroborated the idea that there is a significant increase in preserved grey matter volume in those who consistently meditate, albeit in assorted regions of the brain. Maybe meditation offsets grey matter atrophy? Grey matter density has been found to be greater in the brainstem regions associated with the autonomic nervous system and cardiorespiratory control areas in committed meditators.

Various doctors integrate mindfulness and meditation into conventional advice for patients, e.g. after breast cancer treatment or orthopaedic surgery. In some cases, this is by phone apps for pain control – a placebo effect exists but there is also evidence of change in chemical cascades in immune and pain systems. Whatever the process, most clinicians would support giving back the patient some control and not causing harm. Yoga, tai chi and meditation promote deep mental and physical relaxation. The practice of mindfulness and being 'in the present' can also mentally strengthen patients dealing with the implications of disease or pain.

Cognitive behavioural therapy (CBT) is well established for anxiety based problems, but mindfulness-based stress reduction can also help improve mood, functionality and quality of life alongside this. In my genetics chapter you will see how the protective caps on our chromosomes (telomeres) are preserved better in those who meditate regularly.

Phew that's a lot of science over!

HISTORY OF MEDITATION

Despite the trendy label, meditation is steeped in history, with roots in ancient practices as far back as 5000 BC. References to meditation can be found in Buddhism, Hinduism, Christianity, Judaism and Islam. However, much of meditation practised now is free from religious associations.

I have not got time for this! I hear you.

Most advocates suggest starting with the aim of *quality over quantity*. The ideal practice of at least 20 minutes a day may not be possible and we may give up! Try three times a week for five minutes at a time and build up slowly. Don't abandon the practice before you begin. All you have to do is try!

We are naturally social beings and we are unique in the empathy we feel for one another. It is what defines us as humans, and our interaction is quite essential. However, we sometimes have to learn 'to be alone'. Accept that our thoughts can still be chaotic and constant but for that moment be absorbed in the present moment.

If you are going through hormonal change then this could be a time to consider starting meditation to improve your capacity to cope with symptoms should they arise, and this may also improve sleep quality.

HOW DO YOU DO IT?

There are many types of meditation and I want to lay the seed for those of you motivated to investigate further. My writing is based on my own readings, talking to those who practise and my basic experience.

There is no single way. You must find the best for you. This was a lightbulb moment for me.

You can meditate at home, on an aeroplane, a train... The more practised you are, the more integrated into everyday it can become and provides a great tool in panic type scenarios. You may want to set the tone with an aromatherapy diffuser gently wafting your favourite oil into the room or you may want to just get on and do it straight off.

Meditation can be guided with a teacher, in a class or by yourself. It can be online or using apps (see resources). If you have never meditated just try this quick sample...

AN EASY INTRODUCTION TO BREATH MEDITATION

Similar to how Terrence the Teacher introduced me to meditation, just consider for now this easy practice. *Read it through then think about it before trying.*

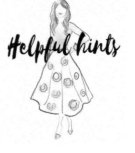

1. Find yourself a comfortable chair and sit upright, hands in lap.
2. Close your eyes.
3. Note the sensation of your breath as your lungs fill and release.
4. Feel the placement of your feet on the floor, your body in the seat and make sure your shoulders are relaxed.
5. Now focus further on your breath. You can count slowly the breaths themselves (one breath in and out is one) as you take slow deep breaths. Maybe count one to ten then restart, always coming back to the breath. Allow yourself to focus on the breath for a couple of minutes. Thoughts may come in; let them drift out and come back to your breath. **Try to step back from those thoughts; don't engage with them.** When you are ready, open your eyes. That was a meditation.

In addition to this you can focus on breathing out for longer than breathing in.

An example of this is 7/11 breathing. Breathing in for a count of 7 and out for 11. If this feels too long, try in for 3 and out for 5. By making the outbreath longer we blow off more carbon dioxide from our lungs, and deep breathing also stimulates the vagus nerve to slow the heart. This has a calming effect on the body. A secret tool!

When you are distracted from meditation by everyday thoughts (like a parent distracted from conversation by a child), return to the meditation **with no concern about having drifted off**. **You have not done anything wrong.**

That was another lightbulb moment for me – you cannot do it wrong.

Breath meditation is one of many types – in this sense tai chi and yoga come under this umbrella as breathing may be focussed upon.

A FEW NAMES OF TYPES OF MEDITATION SHOW THE DIVERSITY OF PRACTICE

Breath	(focussing on breathing)
Physical movement	(walking a short distance outside, focussing on the sensation of walking)
Language	(talking kindly to oneself)
Inner smile	(we smile inwardly to each of the major organs of our body, activating energy of loving kindness within us)
Gratitude	(listing what you are grateful for – many people do this in the early morning along with their morning stretches, starting the day in a positive way)
Loving kindness	(imagining loved ones near to you and giving out feelings of love and kindness to them. One then imagines those given these thoughts then spreading the good wishes back. If undergoing emotional difficulty with someone this can trigger a spiral of emotions and obviously sadness at those lost, so choose only if it works for you)
Visualisations	(guided imagery to imagine, e.g. beach scene)
Repetition of affirmations	(repeating phrases in your mind which are positive and empowering)
Repetition of mantras	(single words which are repeated many times) Transcendental meditation (learned from a teacher) involves mantras. These can be helpful in stress insomniacs and for many who find that thoughts intrude too much in other forms of meditation. There are various resources online for choosing a mantra which should feel right for you.
Body scan	(you focus in turn on different areas of the body and make sure they are relaxed)

| **Sound meditation** | (you become bathed in sound) This can be from a gong/tuning fork/sound bowl – many report a sense of peace and wellbeing for a few days afterwards. |

Online resources
www.terrencetheteacher.com
www.leocosendai.com
www.tm.org

Apps
Insight Timer, Breathe with Terrence, Calm, Headspace, Silatha

Book resources
Mindfulness for beginners by Jon Kabat-Zinn
The Art of Stillness by Pico Lyer
Full catastrophe living by Jon Kabat-Zinn

EATING AND MINDFULNESS

Eating is essential, so habits should be healthy as the repetition of behaviours is cumulative. Put phones away and use dining to reconnect with loved ones or yourself. Prioritise this time, don't rush. You will always get the best stories of the day as you chew unrushed, aiding digestion. Savour and enjoy food. The preparation of food can also be a great mindful pursuit, one I now relish.

MINDFUL TOUCH

We crave touch from birth and we are designed to get a sense of energy and reassurance from it as we grow. This may be reduced due to upbringing and social beliefs. Re-embrace this. A teenager still needs hugs even if they appear to be transiently floating in the room! A shoulder rub is a loving gift to the busy large and little people in your life.

Touch can also apply to our environment. In good weather, go outside and put your bare feet on the grass and note the sensations around you. Walk on the sand of a beach and feel everything. *You did not need a doctor to tell you that, but it is far better than a scroll through photos of people you barely know on your telephone feed.*

THE POWER OF SCENT

Scent can evoke nostalgia, memories and emotions in a second. After 30 years, I remembered my late granny's scent as my husband gifted me the same for Christmas. There is an 'ancient' part of the brain called the limbic system which does not speak a language as such but communicates in emotions. This is triggered by primitive mechanisms when we smell something.

After a respiratory virus three years ago, I have never fully regained (maybe 60 per cent) my previous excellent sense of smell. It can help in this kind of situation (if your doctor has ruled our any obvious other cause) to do your own 'smell training' which might require smelling, for example, essential oils or coffee regularly to try to retrain your senses. More information can be found at https://abscent.org/smell-training

Here I have the privilege of quoting words by renowned perfumer ROJA DOVE:

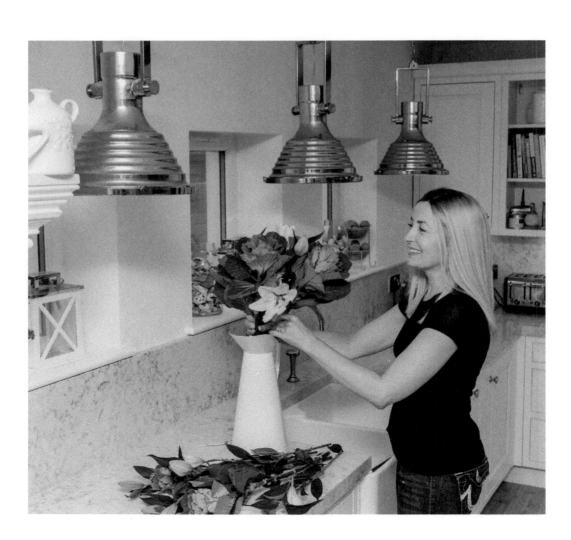

OVERVIEW OF PERFUME

It is often said that our eyes are the windows to our soul. I believe them merely to be observers, whereas our nose absorbs the world's life essences. Since the dawn of civilisation, perfume has been with us, evolving within the complex fabric of the human psyche and culture. Scent is intangible. It can touch us, move us, and inspire our very being. It can transform us into seducers or seductresses, elevating and transporting us to an ethereal realm of memories and sensations.

Unlike fashion and nature, fragrance disregards age, colour and vantage. As we age, and our bodies start their slow inevitable decay, our skin starts to shout the truth, however hard we try to silence it. Our clothes begin to show the lumps and bumps we wish we didn't have but, like a true friend, fragrance is loyal, non-judgemental and kind. Sit with someone and breathe in their scent and they give you one of the most beautiful of all gifts – the gift of memory. You may not have seen someone for years but, with one breath of their scent, the memories come flooding back, dreams are revived, love is rekindled.

A photograph is cold, two-dimensional and, in time, will fade; a perfume brings back moments in our lives in vivid, glorious technicolour. Nothing but perfume, in my opinion, is able to transport us in this way – a single drop of scent can take us from the mundane to a temporal world of fantasy and escapism.

There is a revival in creative perfumery, shifting the craft back to the genius of the Master Perfumers. The art of perfumery is once again in the hands of the gifted. As the saying goes, 'without marketing you have creativity, without creativity you have nothing'.

THE SENSE OF SMELL

I have often seen people in perfumeries spray a fragrance and physically recoil, pulling their head away from the scent in a violent manner. The obvious reason they do this is because they do not like the smell, and yet a dress or a lipstick in the wrong shade would surely not bring about such an extreme reaction. Such a response is deeply rooted in a person's psychology and illustrates the profound effect a recalled negative olfactory memory can have.

To understand this process better, imagine you are going to visit your grandmother. She has baked a cake as a treat for you. When you enter her house, all that greets you is the smell of the cake and the vanilla which it contains. It is the first time you have encountered vanilla and so the smell for you is positive. A friend of yours also visited a relative who had baked a vanilla cake. They took a piece and ate it, but the cake was not made for them, and when they were caught taking a bite of it, they were given a swift smack – so the smell for them is negative.

As adults, they go into a perfumery and are both sprayed with the same fragrance, one of whose olfactory components is vanilla. It might bring about warm loving memories for one, and a disturbing association for the other. It is, therefore, easy to understand the importance of olfactory experiences throughout childhood in relation to our responses to them in adulthood; they form the foundation on which a lifetime's odour response is based.

By our early teens, the bulk of our olfactory 'fingerprint' is formed. This is not a definitive pallet, as there are still many odours to be encountered of differing intensity throughout the rest of our lives. As we develop, we begin to understand varying degrees of subtlety and sophistication in smells. Our life's experiences will add nuances, light, and shade, to our olfactory fingerprint.

I have always used the simile that odour molecules work like a cat-burglar – they intrude unannounced into our mind and soul. When revisited, they unlock the floodgates of memories and emotions, leaving a profound imprint. Smell is, arguably, the most intimate of our senses. If we can marry the maximum number of positive associations in a fragrance to its wearer, we will have found a fragrance which not only reflects their personality but will contribute to a profound sense of wellbeing.

SCENT AND AGE

Scent is always a reflection of the time it was created. Scents send subliminal messages that sum up moments in time, makeup changes, hairstyles change, as does fashion. Unlike fashion, fragrance disregards age, colour and vantage.

Certain floral notes can take years off a fragrance and its wearer. Freesia, peony, lily of the valley and orange blossom, in small quantities, give a wonderful vivaciousness to a scent. They are used in abundance in perfumes targeted at the youth market. But, like fruity notes, they are quite volatile, which creates a feeling of movement and energy.

The most important thing is that the skin becomes drier with age – especially after menopause – the oil production affects the acidity of the skin. It also affects the holding power, so just as with the face, the older we get, the more you need to apply cream...

Could you please give a brief summary of notes that encapsulate key age groups for women, including: 20s, 30s, 40s, 50s, 60s+?

20s: Look for something uncomplicated. Women in their 20s usually like a scent that is sweet and easy, not deep and complex. Fresh citrus notes and understated white florals are good choices.

30s: By now you may have settled into your career and entered a serious relationship, life changes that will be reflected in the scent you choose. You will likely prefer a fragrance with a more centred feel now. Woody, dry notes such as sandalwood, vetiver and musk became important.

40s: The woman in her 40s is established in her career but still wants life to be quite fun. For this sexy and very confident person is recommended sultry gourmand and oriental notes.

50s: This age is all about re-establishing life on your own terms. Powerful chypré fragrances, characterised by their woody, mossy and spicy notes, will suit this highly sophisticated woman.

60s: Menopause often causes the skin to lose moisture, and because the oil in perfume sticks to the oil in skin it won't last as long.

70s: The sophistication and grace of someone who has reached this time in her life is often illustrated by her choice of fragrance. Many women will pick something very tender, or perhaps something that reminds them of another time or an important person.

How do our scent palettes evolve as we age? How does that correlate to our fragrance-buying habits?

I do not think it appropriate for a woman to buy the latest thing. I do however believe this is the time for her to discover the woman she really is. It is essential therefore to allow yourself time when fragrance shopping. Do not go with a friend as they will inflict their tastes and presumptions about you and your style on you. Spray a few fragrances on blotter cards, turn them over to conceal the brand, and then smell them away from the perfumery department. Maybe take yourself to a smart little bar and slowly sniff and deliberate alongside a glass of well chilled champagne. After all, this could become a long-term love affair and it needs to be approached like a game of seduction – slowly and with pleasure. Smell one at a time, comparing each one to the next, eliminating to find the one which has seduced you.

WELLBEING

Fragrance is one of the best things you can buy to make you feel good as each ingredient works on our subconscious, releasing hormones, which amongst other things give us energy, lift us from glumness, or enhance sensations of pleasure.

Give yourself a boost: Vanilla is a psychogenic aphrodisiac which enhances positive sensations; sandalwood has been proven in scientific trials to increase positive feelings; and citrus notes are instantly uplifting.

Increase happiness: For those needing a psychological boost, fragrances with aldehydic top notes lift the spirits – aldehydes add a sparkling effect which can give a tremendous boost to the psyche.

Promote relaxation and sleep: Lavender, chamomile, bergamot, jasmine, rose and sandalwood all have soothing, calming qualities that help encourage sleep and relaxation.

Citrus notes can *boost creativity* and give an uplift but are often short-lived so spritz regularly!

Thank you so much, Roja!
www.Rojaparfums.com

JOURNALING

You may not have kept a diary since you were a teenager! Mindfulness helps us turn the volume down on our crazy, modern life, and journaling may be a channel to direct our focus and achieve inner peace. I have written in my sleep chapter about journaling to leave mental space for a calm evening routine. Journaling might help you halt panic (and shut down fear centres) as you approach life with a more 'observer' attitude and you may end up making better decisions as a result.

In journaling you can address the past, the present and the future. You can use this to focus onto the paper your:

Thoughts

Fears and worries

Aspirations, hopes and dreams

Memories

Long-term goals

I recommend paper and pen, far more tactile and symbolic and possibly more effective in conveying emotion than electronic notes. Journaling amplifies the mind–body connection, makes goals more real and possibly creates a plan/mental route to achieve them. In journaling you are acknowledging thoughts. This can be positive and negative so try to end upbeat each time.

While writing to yourself you are in a safe and secure environment, so you may feel more free than, say, talking to loved ones. Set the time to journal. I would have to separate this from organisational list writing as it must feel much more **self-indulgent**.

Two minutes may suffice or words may flow for thirty!

JOURNAL IDEAS

Write about your negatives

- what upset you
- what worried you
- what made you angry

Write about your positives

- what you enjoyed
- what was unexpectedly good or surprised you
- what made you happy

Write about your gratitude

- (a good point to discuss with children who are too fast-paced to consider)

Write about your memories

- a guidance letter to you as a child
- a loving motivational or guidance letter to yourself at 20

Write about your future

- what you want to do/where you want to be in one year (health, happiness, career, family)
- your five-year goals (when, how, planning)

Then write about connection

- who you treasure but have not made time for/how you can change this

Then write about general observations

- I want more...
- I want less...

None of this refers to possessions or accumulation of material wealth. It refers to satisfaction in daily life, reassurance, happiness and accomplished endeavours. **It is highly personal and does not need to look clever or perfect.** It is a thought picture from your deepest places. You may want to complete a picture over a week or write short notes daily. Treasure the paper it is written on. My own journaling and prioritising led to me reuniting with dear friends whom I had not seen for more than a decade. I addressed my priorities and worked to achieve them. Go on, make that call – it will be worth it!

I DECIDED TO MAKE MY OWN PLAN FOR SELF-CARE...

Life is busy if you are living it. The conveyer belt of day to day can be hectic, feeling out of your control. You don't realise until a cog in the system breaks and everything falls down around you. You must contemplate ways of helping yourself before you are pushed to the limit. If you don't look for help and ways to survive *before* the boat sinks, you will drown with it.

There are ongoing worries in life that cannot be eradicated by positive thinking. These all add up to a brain that usually has 'too many tabs open at once'.

I have met patients and friends who exude calm and serenity. I have read motivational books by celebrities and experts who convey a sense of being at peace. There is a lot of valuable motivation out there if you can see it amongst the glitz. Let's be real, most of us do not have an unlimited bank account and staff to 'do' for us, so making time to even think of one's own needs can be perceived as a luxury you cannot afford. Stop now and rethink that. You have time. Somehow, with a little restructure, time can be made free.

I am a complete control freak. Whether it is with work or home, I have always been a 'micromanager'. As a doctor my need for this attention to detail probably kept me in good stead, but when it comes to everyday life not all the same rules apply. As you mature you realise some things cannot be controlled and you must learn to let some things go.

There are lots of ongoing pressures on women over 40. One thing I found myself repeatedly saying to my patients was for them to 'take back' just some little time for themselves, guilt free. Working, and caring for a family/home/pet, or even a window box, are pursuits that can drain the battery. We manage to recharge our phones every night, so why not our brains and emotions?

Self-care is now a popular phrase. It encompasses a range of activities and attitudes and is used in social media and regular speech, and all aspects of health seem to have 'self-care' advice potential. A science paper from the 1980s describes self-care in health so it is probably not such a novel idea. This paper uses the definition 'activities are undertaken by individuals in promoting their own health, preventing their own disease, limiting their own illness and restoring their own health'. We now use the phrase to describe anything from taking the time for a bath to visiting our pharmacy early on in a viral illness. All doctors would want to see their patients in improved health without medical intervention. I am not talking about taking serious matters into your own hands or just using an app when you should be seeing a medical professional. We still should **not** let technology totally overtake the power of human-to-human interface. Let us go back to basics and look at some non-science, practical approaches. Whatever self-care is, let us look at the 'easy to achieve' parts that can give you back confidence and a feeling of control and calm.

There is a new field in the last decade – positive psychology – and this is really aimed at focussing on things that MAKE LIFE WORTH LIVING. Not for fixing problems but to help us maximise our potential and improve our happiness. This exciting area not only looks at the individual but also at a community level what the impact of more positive change could be.

Stepping back from that science and just writing as a woman in the world of today, a world dominated by tech and demands, a basic pattern has emerged to me over the years of my writing. Through my layman's eyes I see we need to nurture ourselves in more ways than one. I have written about the power of meditation, mindfulness and the evidence behind them in a clinical and non-clinical setting. On a personal level though, I feel we need to be doing things that care for three aspects of our lives, and I have summarised them into three words: MIND BODY CREATE.

WHAT DO I MEAN?

- Do activities to nourish your **mind**, your **body** and also **create** something.
- Cover two of these or even all three with one activity.
- See how it makes you feel.

However cynical you are, you will probably agree that you could benefit by looking after all these aspects of yourself. What would help you personally? What can you work into your life? Maybe in creating something and looking after your mind and body you are also looking after your soul. Keep it simple: just think of what you do every week to look after mind and body and what of that is also creative. You don't need to tick all three boxes. Random examples that spring to mind:

- Yoga will look after mind and body; if you teach it you are probably being creative too!
- Learning a new recipe and trying it out on others will cover all three.
- A walk will help mind and body; take your camera with you and you might create something!
- Exercising – body ticked, and the chemical changes make us happier so mind is covered too.
- Gardening will give you a workout while you create something.
- Making journal entries to organise or offload your thoughts will help calm your mind and may create a joyful, honest read for a later date.

This is so, so basic. It is just suggestions for a starting point to prioritise yourself and your own wellbeing. This is the least medical of all my writing but it is related to both perceived and real health. The pure scientists amongst you may deride me for writing such a basic piece. Never mind them. We talk about being thankful or getting our children to talk about the best parts of their day at night-time – we adults need a little of this reflective TLC as well. Even if you started just taking time for one or two of these activities over the week and booking time for you, it could enrich your life. Let me know how you get on.

Now for a laugh…

THE UNDERESTIMATED POTENCY OF LAUGHTER

My endeavour is to inform you and make you think but more importantly get you out there to laugh with others. We know that laughter causes changes in the heart itself. Endorphins (chemicals) released cause blood vessel receptors to release nitric oxide and this lowers blood pressure, reduces inflammation and make clots less likely to form. Endorphins make us feel great too!

When we are stressed long term, cortisol is chronically high and this causes changes which can affect the hippocampus, which is where our short-term memory is consolidated. If laughter reduces our stress and reduces our cortisol it will have a protective effect here.

There are different types of laughter:

- Spontaneous: This is genuine laughter from an external stimulus, whether it's your friends or a TV show.
- Self-induced: Spontaneous from a thought or making yourself laugh.

- Stimulated: By tickling or physical stimulus.
- Induced: By drugs, alcohol or other substances.

Only spontaneous and self-induced laughter have the real health benefits. It also provides a bonding experience if we laugh together, and a study has shown that the degree of shared laughter with a partner predicts the healthiness and strength of the relationship. So, keep laughing with or at each other! Neuroimmune parameters are altered in our body when we laugh, giving the immune system a boost.

Anyone who has read *Twelve Patients* by Dr Eric Manheimer will remember the chemo patient support group set up and run by patients themselves – a large part of the support was from the laughing 'at and with each other' as a kind of therapy.

Laughter is medicine. It will help the brain stay active for longer, and the bonding hormonal effect amongst women in particular is linked to greater survival and recovery from disease, and potentially longer lives. See my chapter on friendship.

"Always laugh when you can; it is cheap medicine."
Lord Byron

Book resources
The Self-Care Revolution and *The Little Book of Self-Care* by Suzy Reading
The Self-Care Project by Jane Hardy

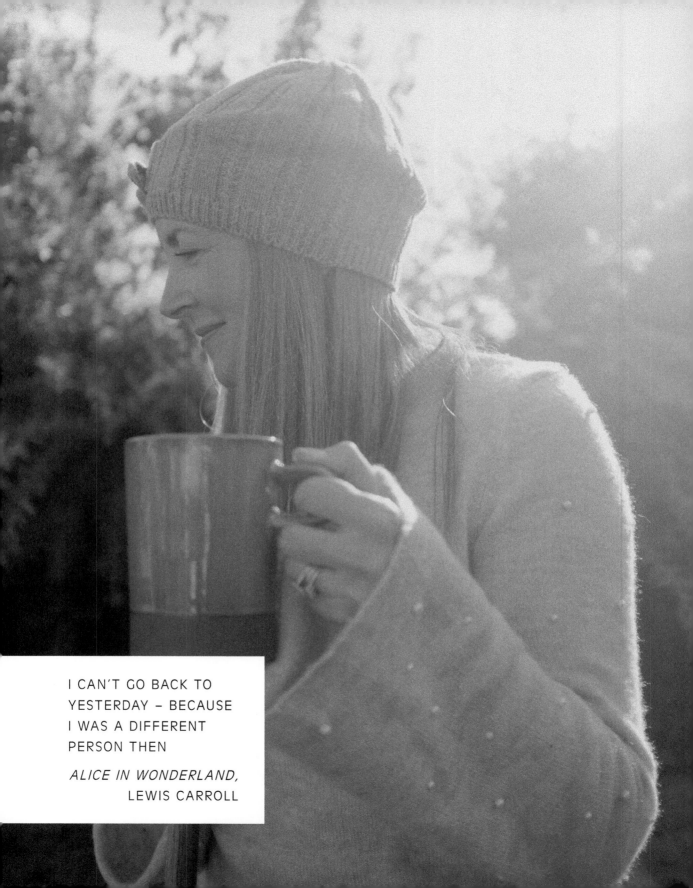

I CAN'T GO BACK TO
YESTERDAY – BECAUSE
I WAS A DIFFERENT
PERSON THEN

ALICE IN WONDERLAND,
LEWIS CARROLL

CHAPTER 2:
THE PSYCHOLOGY
OF AGEING

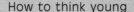

How to think young

Whatever age you are, your knowledge is related to that particular age. When you are 20 you are an expert at being 20; when you are four that is all you have ever known. As you age your perception of ageing may change, but there has been much research over the years about our attitude to ageing and our attitude to older people. We are living longer; and in an age where beauty and youth are prizes, it is no surprise we are studying the process with great enthusiasm.

The fact is, we have an increasing ageing population, but this does not seem to mean that we have lost the concept of old age as being a 'negative' state to be dreaded. Stereotypes of old age can be derogatory – the old person grumbling in the corner, criticising the young – but the reality is that this is often far from the truth. In generations past, elders were revered and respected – that era is no more for many 'advanced' societies. With the passing of the respect, so also the benefits of spending time with multiple generations has been lost. My parents' friend can only get the attention of his visiting teenage grandsons by turning the mains electricity off at the fuse box to interrupt the Wi-Fi! As an adult woman though, would you not agree that the *most fascinating person in the room will likely be the oldest*?

IF YOU ARE GOING TO LIVE LONGER, MAKE IT FUN

As a society, we have to prepare ourselves for ageing and this must happen early on, with education in schools, our homes and our communities. Someone whom I class as one of my closest friends, not a relative, originally came into my life as a neighbour. She is more than 20 years my senior but that is no barrier to our friendship. We are cut from similar cloth with views about lifestyle and ageing. She also worked in the healthcare field but it is of constant surprise to me how our views on being a woman are *identical*. Younger people are inherently arrogant in their belief that they are pioneers but often our predecessors have been there long before us!

I share these intense intimate beliefs with my own mother who is of a similar age to my neighbour but I assumed that was genetic, she is of course 'my mum'.

My surprise at the depth of this friendship with a lady who has far more life experience than me suggests I also have some biased attitudes to ageing.

When I talk to teenagers I am intensely aware of trying not to be boring. I clearly remember that age and what it felt like. However, a teenage girl may really be *looking for* maternal figures alongside their mothers to bounce ideas off.

ARE YOU VISITING GRANNY THIS WEEKEND?

There is such a massive place in our society that needs to be filled by each generation helping the other and teaching them. There have been many studies looking at the effects of intergenerational interaction, and results show that the state of mind of the elderly improves when interacting regularly with the young and that **both generations** dispel their preconceived ideas of the other age group. The young gain a more positive view of ageing.[*] One of the reasons for this type of contact having such a beneficial effect is that the elderly people in these studies feel *useful*.[**] If you have worked all of your life in a fulfilling career or raising a family, when it suddenly stops this is more than empty nest syndrome.

Feeling useful is incredibly important. I have seen how my own father has flourished in a voluntary role in the community. It has given him purpose and mental stimulation. In this role as an elder he is consulted not only for professional advice but is also seen as a guiding figure for the younger folk. This is something we tend to ignore these days. We feel we know it all, or at least Google does, but we cannot dispense with the knowledge that our elders can impart – if only we would listen.

[*]/[**] Read more in my Blue Zones chapter

As quoted in The Telomere Effect **by Dr Elizabeth Blackburn and Dr Elissa Epel,** your opinion of ageing may be shaped by your life experience. If your parents died young of illness, you will naturally have a tainted view of old age. If you want a life sitting in a reclining chair watching TV, that may be all you end up with at 65. Do you really want to settle for this? As these wise authors quote: **"if you can form a clear positive picture of how you'd like to age, you suddenly have a goal to work towards while ageing".**

YOU ARE AS YOUNG AS THE WOMAN YOU FEEL

Another study showed that there are really two ages we have: *ideal* age and *felt* age. Felt age is obviously how old we feel we are. If this is younger than our real age it is associated with enhanced wellbeing and positive developmental assessments. If, however, you always focus on wanting to be younger (your ideal age) and feel negative about where you are now, your perception of ageing will be less beneficial.

Can we manipulate this?

If you think of ageing in a positive way, odds are you'll live seven and a half years longer than someone who doesn't.

Alternatively...

"The knowledge of the inevitability of death is the underlying sense from which all other fears are ultimately derived"

(MCCOY et al. 2000)

If you transfer this sentiment to ageing you have a powerful combination. We all know people who when you tell a story reply:

"Oh, I know someone with a worse cancer than that."

"Oh, I had that and nearly died!"

How does that attitude affect our everyday thinking? In concrete terms, affecting our chromosomes and in turn our lifespan? You will read later on how your genetics only account for a small part of how long you may live, and how lifestyle and the way you think is far more important. Look how these lifestyle factors can add years...

Factor	Survival advantage
Healthy blood pressure	4 years
Lower cholesterol	4 years
Lower body mass index	1 to 3 years
Non-smoker	1 to 3 years
Tendency to exercise	1 to 3 years

SO, WHAT WOULD BE MY CONCLUSION FROM THIS?

Working as a general practitioner, it was always achingly apparent that illness scares all of us, whatever age we are. However, you can be 60 with the outlook of a young person, and you can be 30 already digging your grave with negativity. This tends to show on peoples' faces and general demeanour, and having love and support and family is obviously a great help. Some of us may not have that as a given *so need to integrate into society* to build up a network. Remember, you can choose your friends…!

- Visit your elderly and younger relatives – it will do you both good!
- Volunteer; check on neighbours.
- Chat to your colleagues of different ages.
- Think positively about each life stage and ignore the horror stories!
- Surround yourself with 'expert ager' role models!

Helpful hints

CHAPTER 3: THE GENETICS OF AGEING

 Look after your chromosomes and they will look after you

Once you get into your 30s/40s, the self-obsession of youth alters. We start to look around and value our friendships with other women who have survived the tumultuous years. Where once you discussed clothes and toddler tantrums, you may now compare the first signs of 'middle age'.

When you look around at your peers it is clearly evident that people of the actual same age can look a completely different age. Putting aside cosmetic treatments, why do some people look younger than others?

The answer may lie in their chromosomes.

Our body is made up of cells.

The nucleus is like the **control centre of the cell**.

Within the nucleus, DNA (strand-like material) is packaged into thread-like structures called chromosomes that look like big Xs, to put it basically.

At the end regions of these chromosomes (big Xs) the DNA proteins are coated with a protective 'sheath' of proteins called **telomeres**. These are like plastic tips on a shoelace. They are actually a series of proteins at the end of a chromosome **protecting** it from shortening.

The essence is: **the longer the telomere, generally the better health and lifespan.** Shortening indicates more chance of the 'ageing' diseases – cardiovascular, diabetes, cancer, and so on, although some of it is not always so clear-cut where cancer is concerned.

In general, scientists have proved that **preservation of telomere length leads to a higher chance of longevity, 'delaying' the time until we stop becoming disease free and in that sense 'age'.** They studied tens of thousands of people, not just from a genetic point of view but also from the point of view of what could be done to preserve or lengthen the telomeres so preserving longevity and health.

One of the main findings was that a sense of feeling safe *in your neighbourhood or community* had a massive part to play in how your telomeres could be preserved. **Social support** is also massively important in life. If you do not feel safe and feel threatened, biochemical signals in the form of free radicals (that can attack our body inside) are abundant and this can shorten the telomeres. The community you live in – the degree of violence, rubbish around you, aesthetics, trust, feeling of safety – can actually affect your telomere length and thus health.

Short-term **intense stress** in life is not so bad. But a state of **chronic inflammation** (maybe from chronic stresses) leads to the release of pro-inflammatory proteins in the body and this makes the telomere DNA susceptible to oxidative stress. *In simple terms, short-term stress may not age us but long-term stress can lead to inflammation and age us faster than necessary.*

What is even more profound is their studies on children and the effects of pregnancy on the foetus. Mothers' levels of folate (folic acid), oestradiol (oestrogen), and their mental state even could have an effect on the telomere length in the foetus. Rather frighteningly, toddlers at the age of three who were having fizzy sweetened drinks four times a week would have a discernible shortening of their telomeres. Also, if the mother had drunk soda regularly in pregnancy this was seen to have an effect.

I found this literally staggering as I read it.

If a child at three years was found to have shortened telomeres (for whatever reason), by the age of eight years – still a child – there was evidence in their carotid arteries (blood supply to the brain) of greater build-up in the wall. We would naturally equate these changes later on to increased risks of stroke, and so on. Childhood adversity, such as exposure to poverty, violence, and so on, had an effect on telomere length later on. Doesn't this all seem immensely shocking? Factors that we already knew had a 'bad effect' on us actually have now been **proven scientifically** to have a tangible detriment on our bodies at the very core – our chromosomes.

Now, here is the exciting part. Don't give up if you don't think you would score high for telomere health. You can actually reverse this!

Prominent scientists in this field are keen to state from their research that much can be done to nurture and even *improve* our telomere length. They say, as would anyone, that there is no secret to a long life. However, making changes that improve our telomere length can hopefully

increase our chances of living a longer life (YAY!) before we naturally fall prey to the diseases of ageing like cardiovascular disease, diabetes, and so on. We tend to think these are automatic and *inevitable* with getting older but in effect they are suggesting that we can manipulate the paths our bodies are taking.

Regular exercise, yoga, meditation, mindfulness and relaxation all help protect telomeres.

We cannot alter our personalities, but being positive and not pessimistic is protective. Set aside some time for encouraging your own positive thinking and self-awareness. Having some quality time with your friends and family is more potent in preserving your health than we even used to imagine. Making your environment feel safe and like home to you could be immensely valuable.

Reading resources
The Telomere Effect by Dr Elizabeth Blackburn and Dr Elissa Epel
Prime Time by Jane Fonda

CHAPTER 4: EYE HEALTH – SEEING THE WORLD IN COLOUR

"The eyes are the window to the soul"

William Shakespeare

Eyes are immensely important to every human being. They give us an understanding and interpretation of the world, and if they are not functioning the world becomes a blend of only sound, touch and smell. **Light is life-giving**, and what our eyes see is simply light reflecting from objects. It is a sense that we assume to always have, until our eyes fail us, and the devastation this can potentially cause is reason enough to look after our sight.

I have many friends who claim to have perfect vision and have never required glasses. They will proudly tell me that they don't need to see an optician, and I can understand the principle of *'if it ain't broke, don't fix it'*. However, there is a lot more to an optician's appointment than just looking for a new pair of glass frames. A comprehensive eye check gives a great snapshot of your general health. Similarly, when a trainee doctor learns to examine a patient, looking at the patient's eyes is one of the first essentials before you even feel their pulse!

In general terms, we are all used to saying "You look bright" or "You look tired", and often this will be from looking at our eyes and the skin surrounding them. Of course, a doctor will look at the white of the eye for signs of jaundice or liver disease, the eyelids for signs of thyroid disease or innervation problems, and so on. The optician and the doctor both examine inside the eye and this can show things that are *not quite so obvious*…

WHAT YOUR OPTICIAN LOOKS FOR IN AN APPOINTMENT

Within the eye there can be signs of **raised pressure in the brain** which could need a hospital referral for a scan and consultant opinion, or simply signs of **generally raised blood pressure**. The optician will be able to detect certain signs of **diabetes** if the raised blood sugar has been allowed to go on too long. There is a simple test with a puff of air to the front of the eye that allows measurement of eye pressure and can detect **early glaucoma**. The optician will do sight testing and examination to look at the lens of the eye and find **cataracts**. By testing your **visual field** (as in how much of a full picture of vision you have from each eye), conditions that may *initially* only lose partial sight can be detected early. The way our brains work is that they adapt to the current conditions, and you may lose part of your vision or have a blind spot, but your brain works so cleverly to adapt that you would not notice. By very specific testing with a special light box, the optician will be able to catch you out and find out if part of the vision is missing.

WHY YOU MIGHT VISIT YOUR DOCTOR CONCERNED FOR YOUR EYES

Red eye – painless or painful

Sometimes, very high peaks of blood pressure or even a bout of heavy coughing mean that the pressure in the blood vessels of the eye is so high that the vessel ruptures and there is an obvious, often quite painful-*looking* **red eye** – this is not *actually* painful but usually alarms us so much that we do visit the doctor. Amongst other investigations the doctor will routinely take your blood pressure to check that undiagnosed high pressure is not the cause. If you have a **painful** or **painless red eye** you should see your doctor. Pharmacists will often advise with obvious cases of **irritated, watery eyes** from **conjunctivitis** due to allergy or infection and give you appropriate eye drops, but anything more involved and they have to refer you to a doctor.

Flashing lights or floaters

Some conditions, such as suspected **detached retina** where a patient often describes **flashing lights** or seeing **'floaters'** in their vision or **blurring like a curtain** across their sight, mean the general doctor will refer urgently to a specialised doctor – an ophthalmologist – for potential urgent treatment.

Sudden loss of vision

Any sudden **loss of vision** and you would be urgently referred to hospital for investigation and treatment.

Injury and viral infection

Injuries or abrasions to the eye can be examined in Accident & Emergency and in severe cases need specialist treatment. **Foreign bodies** are often removed in A & E or by specialists. Sometimes **shingles or the herpes simplex virus** can affect the eye area and this needs to be treated very carefully and very promptly to preserve the sight.

Dry eyes

There are certain conditions that affect women especially in later life – **dry eye and dry mouth syndrome**, also called **Sjogren's**. This can be quite debilitating and will need replacement drops as you can imagine how the wet surface of our eyes naturally imparts comfort and protection against infection.

So, as you can see, the eyes are complex in the conditions they can suffer from – some of which you would notice if they happened to you, but some might go undetected if you are not having your annual check.

BUT WHY DO PEOPLE LOSE SIGHT AS THEY AGE?

Presbyopia or short-sightedness

We all joke about having to take one pair of glasses off and put another on as we get older. Mobile phones are a good test of our near vision. It is the normal loss of ability to 'near focus' that occurs with age, otherwise known as why you have to extend your arm to read. Presbyopia can also be called the 'ageing eye condition'. Now, how thrilling does that sound?!

As we age, the natural soft lens in our eye hardens gradually and the muscle fibres around the lens do not function so well, so focussing does not happen so easily for close objects.

When you are young the lens is soft and flexible, allowing the tiny muscles to easily reshape the lens to focus the light on the back of the eye. It is thought that presbyopia is more likely over the age of 35 years. Some people notice this more than others. You might find you have some of these symptoms:

- headaches
- eye strain
- hard to read small print
- hold paper more than arm's distance away to read
- problems seeing close-up objects

The natural tendency of many people is to then buy some glasses off the peg in the chemist to help them read and sew. These do not require a prescription and will help with close vision only. Of course, this may be all that is needed, but a proper eye check is recommended and a prescription for the correct reading glasses, to prevent headaches and eye strain. Glasses that are 'bifocal' have the lens you need for distance and then the lower half of the lens only is for reading or focussing on near objects. These can take some getting used to at the beginning as you may feel dizzy walking down the stairs and so on! My mother used to hang on desperately to our bannisters when her glasses were changed. There are bifocal lenses available these days that can be well tolerated by many, and also bifocal contact lenses.

Cataracts

Some of the changes in the eye lens are inevitable with age but we can maybe try to prevent them. The lens, as you would imagine, is usually clear and refracts (bends) the light onto the retina, and the electrical signal then passes to the optic nerve so the message can get to our brain. Over time, as we age, this clear disc can become cloudy or misty and is said to form a cataract. There is a change in the layout of the cells and how much water they contain.

Who gets cataracts?

Cataracts can be caused by diabetes, medicines such as steroids, other eye surgery or trauma but the majority are just related to the changes with ageing. There is still a lot of research about the direct causes of cataracts but theoretical causes are smoking, having a poor diet with scarce antioxidant vitamins, and lifelong exposure to sunlight. My reaction to this would be to:

WEAR SUNGLASSES OUT IN BRIGHT DAYLIGHT/DRIVING/SUNLIGHT AND LOOK FOR WAYS TO IMPROVE YOUR DIET'S VITAMIN AND MINERAL CONTENT. As always throughout this book, stop smoking!

There is much debate as to whether cataracts are inevitable or whether healthy foods can help prevent them. It is thought that if you have a very healthy diet full of coloured fruit and vegetables and wholegrains you *may* have a decreased risk of cataracts.

Vitamins thought to be helpful are A, C and E, lutein and zeaxanthin.

Fish with its high omega-3 content *may* reduce the risk of cataracts or their progression. Some studies think they have shown links and other studies have found no benefit. It is something worth discussing with your optician or ophthalmologist. Sometimes taking an excess of one vitamin or nutrient can be harmful, so it's a complicated issue. Of course, eating well has no risks so that is probably the best route. Supplements for eyes can also be quite expensive so care should be taken in choosing the right one. **See my interview with a consultant ophthalmologist at the end of this chapter.**

Ideally you should be eating good quantities of fruit and vegetables, wholegrains and fish within your diet! Dark green and colourful fruit and veg are great for eye antioxidants and they contain folic acid and calcium that should be included in a healthy diet anyway. Some researchers in Australia found evidence that high salt intake increased the risk of cataracts.

The onset of cataracts can be quite insidious – you may feel like your glasses are dirty or you just cannot see clearly. You may need more light to see smaller print and may find you have problems seeing things when out walking. Colour may appear more yellow and the headlights of a car, when you are driving at night, may dazzle you more than normal.

Surgery can replace the opaque lens with a lens implant. I used to help anaesthetise patients for this in my Anaesthetic years and it was one of the most rewarding operations. The patients would arrive with their glasses and visual aids and wake up with better vision before an eye patch was put on to go home. Sometimes the vision is not at its best until a few days afterwards when any swelling has gone down and you have fully recovered. The decision of when to have surgery is something to discuss with the ophthalmologist or eye surgeon. If the cataract is there, there are rules the optometrist follows to assess your safety for driving.

Age-related macular degeneration (ARMD)

The macula is the tiny bit at the back of the eye – a part of the retina that helps you with your central vision. If you develop ARMD this can lead to the loss of part of your vision – usually this is the central part from where you are looking straight at something. It can become distorted or blurry over time. If you have ever had a focal migraine you will know what it is like to have a blind spot in your vision and how disconcerting it can be. This would obviously affect you daily.

Who gets ARMD?

It is more common over 65 but possible in the 40s and 50s. More women have ARMD but this might be because they live longer. It is not thought to be definitely all inherited but there may be some genetic patterns in some families. Smoking is a massive risk factor for ARMD – presumably because of the blood supply to the back of the eye being compromised. It is not totally proven but it is thought that exposure to ultraviolet from sunlight *may* contribute – another reason to wear sunglasses and protect your eyes from sunlight in life. Because the causes are not completely well known, one may develop ARMD without these causes sadly.

Signs of early ARMD

Detail becomes harder to see. Sensitivity to bright light may be noticed or you may find that you have a blurry or wavy part to your vision. If these things happen, you should see the optician/

optometrist quickly. Then you will be seen if necessary by the GP and possibly referred straight away to the eye doctors.

The cells that are affected in the macula (back of the eye) are called 'cone cells' and are responsible for seeing colour and detail. Side vision and seeing in dim light will not be affected by ARMD.

Once you are referred you may be given the diagnosis of wet or dry ARMD. Dry ARMD is the most common and is gradually developing, causing the loss of your central vision. Wet ARMD occurs when blood vessels grow in the eye to try to fix the problem. This causes swelling and bleeding in the area. This can cause scarring and a complete blank patch in the central part of the vision. This wet ARMD can develop very rapidly. If you have dry ARMD and it is mild you may just be monitored with retinal photographs for a while. There are further involved tests to look at the back of the eye and the blood vessels.

How do you treat dry ARMD?

There is no real treatment. It is thought that vitamins A, C, E and zinc and copper minerals within the diet can help slow it down, along with the antioxidant nutrient lutein. **There is no evidence yet that taking these can prevent the disease**. However, we would never doubt the virtues of a good diet with plenty of fruit and vegetables.

How do you treat wet ARMD?

There are injections into the eye that can stop further blood vessels growing at the back of the eye and thus stop the sight deteriorating, and there are rare risks associated with this that will be outlined by the specialist doctors.

The ROYAL NATIONAL INSTITUTE FOR THE BLIND has a helpline on 03031239999 for this condition and the eye clinic will have staff to give you support and counselling. The macular society www.macularsociety.org may also support you. You can learn to read without using the central area of the vision and there is help available with this from the society. Driving ability needs to be discussed with your optician and the DVLA.

THE IMPORTANCE OF SUNGLASSES

There is a recurring theme in my writing here regarding preventing eye disease in that the eye must be **protected from sunlight** to continue to function healthily. We are far more aware of this now than in previous decades. The ubiquitous nature of sunglasses and choice means there really is no excuse; sunnies should be a daily habit in bright sun.

Choose your sunglasses with care. Lens colour is not a predictor of ultraviolet protection and you want to block both UVA and UVB from your eyes (see skin chapter). Some dark lenses, those without adequate ultraviolet protection, will actually allow your pupil to dilate and allow more ultraviolet into the eye to potentially cause damage, so make sure dark glasses have the proper rating from a reputable manufacturer. You can look for the CE sign which says they should be up to European standards; or in some cases, such as Boots Optician UK, their glasses meet the British Standard EN 12312-1:2013. Then look at the rating:

Category 0   no tint or very light (for aesthetic/fashion/comfort and offer no protection)

Category 1   light tint for weak sunlight (and who can predict?!)

Category 2   medium tint for average sunlight

Category 3   dark tint for strong sunlight including reflected light off water and snow (most good glasses are this)

Category 4   very dark tint – not safe for driving or road users as blocks too much light! The kind of lenses that react to light (Reactolite and similar) can be great for all-round protection; but sometimes, as the glass of a car window blocks some UV light, the glasses themselves *may not respond within a car* and give you as much protection. Wraparound styles of glasses obviously protect the delicate skin around the eyes and many studies show that people miss this area out when applying sunscreen so try to remember to protect it.

A cloudy day will shockingly only take away 10% of ultraviolet exposure. Remember, **scratched glasses are useless** as the light will get in. Red and orange fashion lenses may distort colours – important to know when you are driving and looking at traffic lights!

So, as you can see, sunglasses are not just a fashion statement, they are an essential in your bag when leaving the house and to be worn when driving, whilst in the sunshine or even on a bright cloudy day. They are not just for vanity!

Some contact lenses offer some ultraviolet protection these days (especially silicon-based lenses) but only protect the area they cover – this is not enough. The rest of the eye and surrounding tissue is very delicate.

ARE CONTACT LENSES SAFE?

I didn't have to wear glasses until I was about 23 when I needed them for distance when driving. Then, by the time I got married at about 26, I decided I did not want to walk down the aisle in my glasses, or not be able to see everyone, so I went to try lenses. I have used soft daily disposable lenses since. Of course, there are many different types and the type that is suitable for you will depend on many factors (I like the fact that they are disposable as I spent many an hour looking for one of my friend's long-term contact lenses at university whenever she dropped them). The optician will decide what is required to correct your eyesight, whether you have an astigmatism and so on and what will fit in with your lifestyle.

You can order contact lenses from the internet if you have your prescription but don't let that mean you skip appointments with a qualified optician. Usually the contract to supply your lenses through the optician **includes the eye check every year or two years** so is a far preferable method. As I mentioned above, all of the checks to your eyes are imperative, and even more so the checks to the actual structure of the eye to check it is not being damaged or scratched by the lenses themselves during the process of putting them in and taking them out. If you wear lenses long term, there are changes in the eye. Most of these reverse on stopping wearing lenses. Any risks are obviously assessed by you and your optician against the optical, cosmetic and sheer convenience values of wearing lenses. You should be aware of the infection risks so that you continue to take impeccable care of your eyes. Dramatic infections are often reported in the popular press but in fact the majority wear lenses with no problems if they are careful. Read more in the expert interview at the end of this chapter. Here are some helpful hints.

- Wear correct sunglasses
- Annual optician check
- Report any changes in vision
- Eat plenty of wholegrains, leafy greens, vegetables, fish
- Cleanse make-up thoroughly from eyes at night
- Be meticulous about contact lens hygiene
- If doing computer work, every 20 minutes look 20 yards into distance and blink 20 times to help keep eyes lubricated

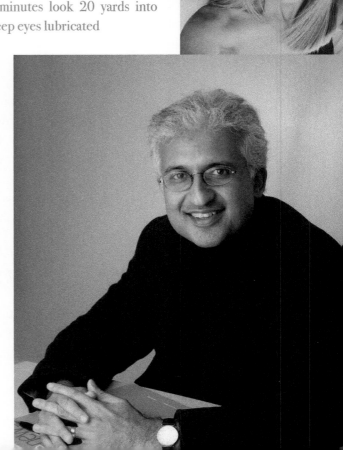

To get the real future science and the care of eyes from an expert, I interviewed Mr Raman Malhotra, internationally renowned consultant eye surgeon and ophthalmologist.

This information is like gold dust for anyone concerned for their eye health. If you are not too worried now you might want to refer to it in the future. The dietary and common sense advice really applies to us all and is invaluable. Some of this advice is very specialised, referring to specific eye conditions.

Do you think individuals who seemingly still have perfect vision should still have an annual check with an optician anyway to check for other eye signs/signs of disease? What age do you suggest this becomes routine?

Yes. Annual checks form part of screening and there are a number of indications for this. The most obvious would be those with diabetes, particularly late onset where the presence of diabetic retinopathy may exist even on diagnosis. This should, therefore, be annually initially and ideally with photographic screening. Other examples would be:

- Intraocular pressure (IOP) for **glaucoma**, especially with a family history. The NHS advocates annual screening above the age of 40 or for those with a family history. It is useful perhaps two-yearly for individuals without a family history. Certain ocular conditions such as **pseudoexfoliation** syndrome (can lead to glaucoma) can be detected without having any symptoms. **Pigment dispersion syndrome** can cause spikes of pressure with exercise, etc. and therefore subtle symptoms of mild ache, blurring of vision or even halos with bright lights which may be ignored as being normal can reflect undetected spikes of raised IOP.
- **Cataracts**. Especially the type known as posterior subcapsular cataract (PSCLO) which can often cause more symptoms of glare rather than reduced vision. Again this can be put down to natural ageing. More common with certain medications, steroids being a common culprit. Individuals often ignore the fact that inhaled steroids or even steroid creams have a systemic absorption and can cause PSCLO if used long term.
- Certain medication can cause **irreversible retinal disorders**. Hydroxychloroquine for example, used in treating inflammatory immune disorders, can cause macular disorders, and screening is advised for individuals that reach a certain cumulative dose. Drugs such as Roaccutane (isotretinoin) can cause visual problems that may initially be undetected, such as reduced peripheral vision that can progress to tunnel vision. It can also result in increased dry eye. It is therefore important to monitor visual function and at least alert individuals as to symptoms to look out for whilst on this medication. Changes may be reversible in some cases.
- **Age related macular degeneration**. It is advisable over the age of 60 to be examined for signs of early ARMD, especially if there is a family history. Individuals can then consider changing their lifestyle to help reduce risks: stop smoking and consider supplements.

Tell me about the complex topic of supplements for ARMD.

This is a more contentious issue as the evidence for supplementation reducing the risk of wet ARMD is based upon some famous trials that were carried out a number of years ago. Most evidence for the benefit of nutritional supplements has been based on four types of supplements:

1. **AREDS or AREDS-like formulas**, the **age related eye disease study (AREDS),** was designed to investigate whether active supplements would reduce the risk of advanced ARMD. The main components of their formula were vitamin A as beta-carotene, vitamin C, vitamin E and zinc. The formula was a type of active treatment therefore doses were *much higher than the dietary reference intake outlined by the Institute of Medicine of the USA National Academy.* For example, the amount of vitamin C included in the AREDS formula was 500mg per day whereas the DRI for an adult is only 90mg per day, therefore one has to eat almost seven or eight oranges to obtain 500mg of vitamin C. This clearly has a huge sugar load and impact to consider if an individual wishes to meet these intakes with a normal diet. Dosage of the AREDS formulas can be obtained online. The results showed a 25% reduction in risk of progression to advanced ARMD, however this was only seen in two categories, probably because of the higher natural risk of progression to advanced ARMD, and was not seen in individuals with small drusen only (the five-year risk of progression in these individuals was up to 1.3% or less). It has been shown in the USA that 80% of people over the age of 74 fall into this latter category and *hence most people would not benefit from the AREDS formula.* **Potential risks for the AREDS formula would include kidney stones from vitamin C, fatigue, muscle weakness, decreased thyroid function and increased haemorrhagic stroke risk from vitamin E, increased lung cancer risk in smokers, yellow discolouration of skin from beta-carotene, anaemia, decreased serum high density lipoprotein cholesterol and stomach upset from zinc, and there is a reference (**Klein R. et al., American Journal of Ophthalmology 2004**).**

   Instead of an active supplementation formula some have proposed an enriched diet alone. The Rotterdam Study investigated the effect of a vitamin and mineral rich diet alone in comparison to the AREDS with no active interventions given. This study found that an **above median intake of vitamins C and E, beta carotene and zinc was associated with a striking 35% decrease in incidents of ARMD and concluded that such a diet should be recommended for those with early signs of ARMD and a strong family history.**

   A recent Cochrane review suggested these conclusions to be sound but reiterated the potential harmful effects, particularly for those who smoke or have vascular diseases.

2. **Lutein and zeaxanthin** are also of great interest. They exist in high concentration in the macula hence its yellowish colour. They act in the biological system as an important structural molecule in cell membranes, as a short wavelength light filter, a keeper of the redox balance and a modulator in signal transduction pathways. However, the human body is not capable of lutein synthesis and it can only be obtained from diet. There have been studies showing these as very favourable and one that was equivocal.

   Many manufacturers have begun including lutein and zeaxanthin in their over the counter supplements. The only documented side effect is yellow discolouration of skin characterised by high dermal carotenoid levels. This is reversible and benign and I understand there to be no other adverse effects. **A daily lutein upper level of supplementation of 20mg carries benefits with minimal side effects** and those who are keen or at risk of ARMD may gain some protection by this.

3. **Omega-3 fatty acids.** The role of omega-3 fatty acids in reducing incidents of cardiovascular disease and strokes is well established. The evidence for its benefit in ARMD is inconsistent and not randomised. A recent US twin study found that fish consumption and omega-3 fatty acid intake reduced the risk of ARMD by an estimated 22% if omega-3 was high, however this study was not randomised and hence its impact is limited. Clinical studies, however, have demonstrated that even in individuals already on warfarin and aspirin, a high dose of fish oil does not significantly increase the risk of bleeding. The potential for contaminates such as mercury, commonly found in fish, still poses a health risk to a high oily fish diet, however I myself am very happy to recommend a high oily fish diet, largely because industrial purification processes eliminate these toxins.

4. **Berry extracts.** The interest in berry extracts grew from their antioxidant properties, probably the most notable being blueberry. As far as ophthalmology is concerned this can help reduce the risk of ARMD and improve night vision. Many berry extracts claim to protect eyes from ARMD, e.g. wolfberry known as goji berry which has been long used in traditional Chinese medicine. However, at the moment laboratory evidence is limited, as is precise dosage and frequency, and therefore berry extracts are not recommended based upon a strong evidence base.

The main aspects that identifying ARMD early would perhaps prompt are the main modifications such as smoking cessation, reduction of body mass index and reduction of UV light exposure.

Tell me about the value of protecting our eyes from bright light.

Regarding exposure of UV light and retinal damage, as the human crystalline lens ages and develops a nuclear sclerotic cataract it turns more **yellow** with age. This provides an additional protection to the retina from harmful UV blue or blue/green phototoxicity. When the crystalline lens is removed during cataract surgery and an intraocular lens (IOL) is implanted this additional benefit is lost. Traditional IOLs lacked any UV filter and therefore elderly individuals post-cataract surgery were always advised to wear UV protection following cataract surgery when in sunlight. Modern lens implants now provide some form of UV filtering protection; however, this varies due to lack of firm evidence. My preference for lens implant has always been a yellow filtered lens implant for this very reason, but due to lack of strong evidence many of my colleagues do not consider this a necessary requirement for an IOL. In the Chesapeake Bay Watermen

Study a significant correlation between blue or visible light exposure and ARMD was found. In fact, they concluded that after cataract extraction blue light exposure is greater than at any other point in life. Yellow filter IOLs are able to block all of this light. Concern has been raised that these yellow filter IOLs may affect visual performance under scotopic conditions (defined as light levels on a moonless night) because blue light is more informative in this environment. However, again the evidence for this is not strong. Individuals who have undergone bilateral yellow filter IOL implantation have found no significant changes in terms of colour perception. Hence yellow filter IOLs may still offer a theoretical protection from ARMD.

Do you believe that a nutrient-rich diet with plenty of antioxidant vitamins (coloured fruit and veg and wholegrains) can reduce the incidence of cataracts, or is this a misnomer?

This is a complex matter. Certainly severe nutritional deficiency is well established as a cause of cataract, however it is uncertain as to whether nutritional supplementation certainly in a European population affects progression of cataract. This has been studied extensively. Basic science research does show that vitamin C supplementation as well as lutein and zeaxanthin reduces the risk of cataract formation but a large interventional trial with high dose vitamin C versus placebo did not replicate these findings. An FDA review concluded insufficient evidence to suggest supplementation with carotenoids lowered the risk of cataract formation. The conclusion of a number of reviews and meta-analysis is that supplementation with vitamin C, lutein and zeaxanthin or a multivitamin may help certain populations but is unlikely to affect the progression of cataracts in most patients.

What about eye supplements generally?

One of my family members has signs of dry macular degeneration with multiple soft drusen (this has the potential for progression to wet ARMD) and, having discussed this with retinal colleagues, I and my colleagues have suggested supplementation with MacuShield or something similar. To my knowledge, this is available over the counter. It does not contain beta carotene so is not a risk for smokers. That said, I would certainly support a nutrient rich diet with plenty of antioxidant vitamins, not necessarily to reduce the incidence of cataract but certainly to ensure that individuals are not deficient in these key nutrients and therefore unwittingly placing themselves at risk of preventable progression.

Tell me about dry eye problems.

Dry eyes is classified as either aqueous deficiency type (classic burning, sore, uncomfortable symptoms) or evaporative type (more common type the majority of which is due to meibomian gland dysfunction which is highly prevalent in individuals above the age of 40). Individuals with evaporative type dry eye often have symptoms of reflex tearing when in cold, windy weather and simply attribute this to a normal finding. Either causes may have predisposing factors that can be treated, e.g. features of rosacea, a lifestyle of a low clear water intake, high red meat intake, moderate to high intake of alcohol or caffeine.

Dry eye symptoms can often be troublesome but not enough to warrant seeing a doctor and can be easily treated with lifestyle changes before resorting to medication or ophthalmic consults.

How often do you see severe damage or infection from chronic contact lens use or incorrect usage? What kind of problems?

Thankfully over the last 20 years, contact lens related corneal damage or infections have become less common due to education. Individuals **do not use tap water to wash lenses** (particularly water that is stored in loft based tanks). Through epidemiology studies this was found to be the greatest risk factor for acanthamoeba contact lens related infections. Individuals now are careful about not sleeping with contact lenses in and minimising lens time. We do still see cases of acanthamoeba type keratitis though, but reduced as there is a greater tendency for monthly and even daily disposable contact lens usage. The main problems nowadays are of evaporative dry eye that is exacerbated by contact lens use.

The meibomian glands are the tiny glands along the rim of the eyelid. When these get blocked they can cause problems; what are the remedies?

Meibomian gland dysfunction is where the glands are inflamed or obstructed. **Blepharitis** is when there is an apparent overgrowth of staphylococcus epidermidis (bacteria) with crusting involving the lash roots. Meibomian gland dysfunction is the more common cause for dry eye related symptoms which may include reflex tearing. Blepharitis is a finding that can exacerbate symptoms of ocular discomfort in individuals with dry eyes.

For individuals with **blepharitis**, lid hygiene is invaluable, we now recommend lid wipes which do not irritate the eye and are effective in removing debris from the lash root.

For **meibomian gland dysfunction**, treatment has got to be directed at underlying general health to reduce risk factors, and these can be considered similar risk factors to those for rosacea. The best local treatment would be hot compresses to help maintain pores to stay open and immediately after this to carry out some form of lid massage to express out meibum within the gland in order to encourage a higher turnover of gland secretions and less stagnation. The Eyebag Company mask that is usually placed in the microwave and stays warm has been recommended. I would always advocate lifestyle changes and simple measures be considered.

Thank you to Raman, for his extremely helpful and highly informed advice.
Neither Raman nor Louise benefit financially from any of the brands mentioned.

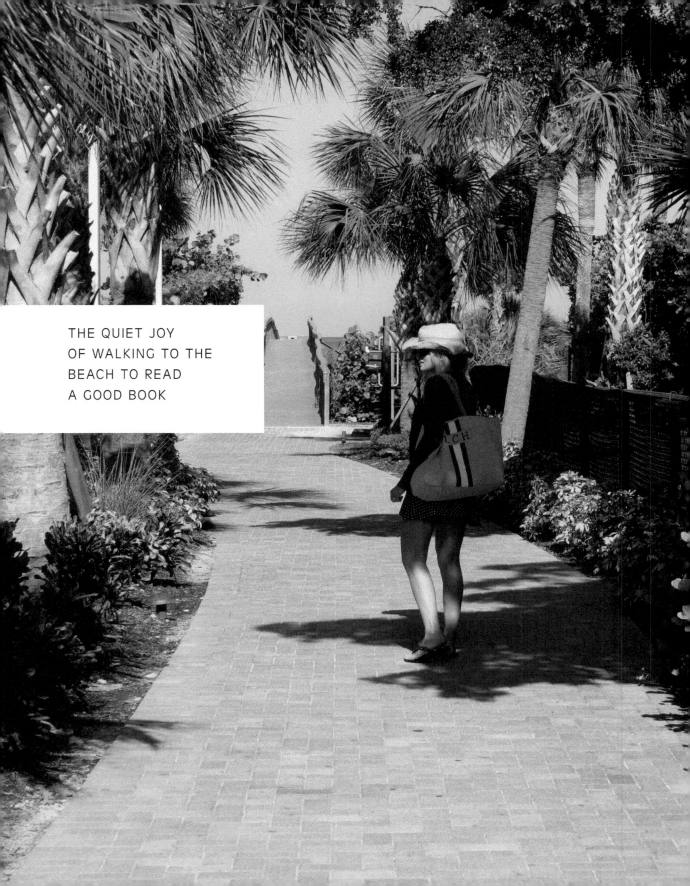

THE QUIET JOY
OF WALKING TO THE
BEACH TO READ
A GOOD BOOK

CHAPTER 5: PROTECTING MENTAL HEALTH AND MEMORY

A prime concern as we age is the possibility of losing memory, cognition and function. Any state that can take away our independence and autonomy brings with it a large amount of fear, and any doctor or nurse will have seen the devastating effect a dementia diagnosis can have on patients and their families. I know of three close female friends who are coping with their parents' diagnoses.

It is beyond the scope of this book to talk in great detail about dementia but it is of relevance here to look at evidence for what *may* prevent the illness in terms of lifestyle. There are no guarantees, this is only trying to manipulate the odds.

Due to the fact that so many factors are at play in the development of dementia it is difficult to find good studies. Doctors like 'randomised controlled trials' where one group of people, say, have certain food added to the diet and they are compared to a control group who don't, but of course life is not 'unifactorial' like that. Dementia research is rapidly increasing.

WHAT IS DEMENTIA?

Dementia describes a range of cognitive (thought-related), behavioural and psychological symptoms that include memory loss, problems with reasoning and communication and change in personality. This can impair the ability to carry out daily activities. We know that in the UK alone there are nearly a **million people** living with dementia (1 in 14 people over 65 years old) and this is increasing. However, maybe a third of people with established dementia are not recognised and many people might be feeling they are not getting enough support.

WHAT IS ALZHEIMER'S DISEASE?

This is the most common cause of dementia. More than half a million people in the UK have this kind of dementia. It is just one type of dementia. In this, proteins build up in the brain and cause 'plaques' and 'tangles' so that nerve cells die and brain tissue is lost. Some of the messengers or chemicals in the brain are also depleted and this is what some medicine works on. Here is a summary of all the main types of dementia. You will see how in some cases there could be overlap.

- **Vascular dementia** (related to interrupted blood supply to the brain, e.g. small strokes)
- **Dementia with Lewy bodies** (tiny deposits of a protein can lead to dementia or Parkinson's disease or a combination of both)
- **Frontotemporal dementia** (refers to the area affected in the brain and there are abnormal proteins inside cells)
- **Mixed dementia** (this is often from Alzheimer's and Vascular combined)
- **Young onset dementia**
- **Creutzfeldt-Jakob disease** (prions – abnormally shaped proteins – affect the brain)
- **Alcohol-related brain damage**
- **HIV-related cognitive impairment**

How does Alzheimer's disease present?

- Mild memory loss
- Difficulty recalling events
- Difficulty learning new information
- Hard to find the right words
- Hard to solve problems and make decisions or perceive things in 3D

Other forms of dementia can present in similar ways but, for example, if the dementia is vascular and being caused by small strokes you tend to see a slightly more dramatic step-wise presentation of symptoms. We all go through phases of forgetting things – usually if our minds are anxious or preoccupied. These symptoms in dementia become more regular.

The doctors and nurses will look at the whole picture and perform investigations. In some cases, medication will be given to help with certain symptoms (depression, psychoses, agitation, aggression), although there is no specific cure. Dementia can often be successfully managed without medication. A great resource in the UK is www.alzheimers.org.uk.

If you are reading this book you are very likely to have at least a modicum of interest in your health, or maybe you just wanted to look younger?! Oh shucks, sorry, that may happen but is not the sole priority of this book! I digress – you probably would like to do things that *should help protect your health* even if it is still a little bit of a gamble **as long as it does not do any harm.** There is encouraging but not conclusive evidence that there may be positive effects in preventing dementia by:

- **Cognitive training**
- **Blood pressure management for those with high blood pressure**
- **Increased physical activity**

So, Sudoku is a thing? Let us look a little more closely.

Cognitive training

- Enhance reasoning by problem-solving, e.g. playing bridge, doing crossword puzzles
- Enhance memory, e.g. learn a new language
- Enhance speed of processing, e.g. identifying visual information on a screen

What is more difficult to evaluate is whether or not any advantage, say, in memory from the above, persists if the skill is stopped, and does improving your memory actually enhance your reasoning and speed of processing and vice versa? Would this then help one live independently for longer? Would you be more likely to remember to take your medicines? Many of the good studies did not involve computer-based training but *more social activities*, so one can question whether the social side was an important factor in this. Having fun with friends playing bridge surely has to be good for your soul and that in turn may light up your brain a little?

Blood pressure management
Of course this is paramount for our general health!

Researchers think it may be important to control blood pressure during the midlife years (35 to 65) as there is encouraging evidence that this may help *prevent or slow progress* of some dementia. It would be unethical to not treat those with high blood pressure, so studies are not really conclusive, but it makes sense that reducing our risk for strokes and heart attacks will in turn reduce our risk for brain-related change.

Physical activity

We know exercise is good for us and it stands to reason it would protect our brain. Again, the evidence is not clear-cut but is encouraging that physical activity may work by indirect measures such as *reducing high blood pressure, the chance of stroke, reducing obesity and depression*, which will in turn protect our brain health.

With all of these approaches we need more studies for longer to know the real facts. These three factors have been highlighted as needing further evidence. **I say, as they are beneficial to wellbeing anyway we have nothing to lose and maybe some memory to retain.**

Other factors are treating diabetes and depression better, lipid-lowering treatments like statins and their effect on dementia, sleep studies, social studies, and b12 and folate supplements where needed.

Along similar lines, in 2017 a major review by the *Lancet* identified nine possible risk factors that we could modify to reduce our risk of dementia:

- **Education (lack of a secondary education)**
- **Hearing loss**
- **Physical inactivity**
- **High BP**
- **Non insulin dependent diabetes**
- **Obesity**
- **Smoking**
- **Depression**
- **Social isolation**

This will all only account for just over a third of a person's risk of getting dementia. If you see any of these that you personally can improve (too late to go back to school), work out how you can go about it now to future protect your brain. There are bits we can't control, like age and genetics (but we think environmental factors are needed with the genetic risk to make it real).

FOOD AND DEMENTIA

There is some evidence that eating a Mediterranean-style diet can reduce the risks of developing problems with memory and thinking. This is explained in more detail in the food is life chapter. Fruit and vegetables are high in antioxidants and this may help to protect the brain cells from damage in Alzheimer's. The diet can also reduce the brain inflammation and lower cholesterol to improve memory and thinking problems by aiding circulation. Studies are varied in their results, and those who follow the Mediterranean way of eating may be healthier generally, accounting for some of the effects.

We know that a good balance of vitamins and minerals is essential for body and brain function. Vitamin b12 in particular if deficient can cause memory and cognition problems. This can especially be a problem for vegans or vegetarians and will often be tested alongside tests such as thyroid function when a patient presents with memory problems. Fortified cereals and nutritional yeast products like marmite contain B12.

It is easy to see how not just one factor but a combination results in dementia. The same message is that you will be knocking off more than a few birds with one very powerful stone if you start improving these aspects of your health.

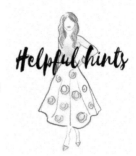

- Stop smoking
- Drink within guidelines or less
- Mediterranean diet, low saturated fat, avoid excess sugar or salt
- Regular exercise (will also help with diabetes, obesity and high BP)
- Socially active lives
- Keep blood pressure and cholesterol within healthy margins

SEASONAL AFFECTIVE DISORDER (SAD)

I recall, around age six, looking across sun-bleached playing fields at school, overjoyed that this heralded the long summer holiday ahead. We learn association with weather and the seasons early, but what if, as an adult, you learn to dread a season? Duvet days are fabulous – not so much if there is more 'down' in your *day* than your duvet.

We all move fluidly along a mood spectrum and we are complex creatures. **Seasonal affective disorder** (SAD) is a name given to those suffering 'recurrent major depressive episodes with a seasonal pattern'. This *can* happen in summer, but usually autumn ignites a heart sink, winter dread; described as having your own 'portable cloud'. No mere melancholy, it is a helplessness and low mood not to be dismissed. While you may not have the disorder, you may identify with some aspects of it.

We also associate different times of year with certain events, like bereavement, that trigger similar emotions. For some, simply a 'fear of cold' saddens them.

There was evolutionary advantage to 'hibernation' behaviour in our predecessors. Winter could be for procreation, creating summer babies. Doing less with our days conserved resources and required maintaining a layer of fat to provide nutrition. Pointless now if shorter days leave you craving carbs to see you retain more fat in a centrally heated home, with no motivation *whatsoever* to exercise.

We joke about loving going 'out out'! Well, feel like this and you won't even want to venture 'out' for milk.

Why do some of us feel this more than others?

In the 1920s, a psychiatrist noted that some patients elicited 'moodiness in autumn', then passed over to spring in 'excitement'. It wasn't until the 1980s that scientists started to formalise the theory of 'SAD'. There are many suggested reasons why it occurs as the days shorten in seasonal areas. If you live nearer the equator, the difference in seasonal light is less, so there is less effect. If you start life nearer the equator and move further from it, north or south, you may be more at risk of SAD. Those living at higher latitude, such as those with Icelandic genes, are more resistant to these mood changes. Similarly, a genetic tendency towards SAD symptoms can occur.

It is no coincidence that we hanker for second homes on Greek islands. The light hits our retinas and we behave differently. Not just stripping off to swimsuits, we may LAUGH more as we engage with life amongst sparkling seas! But why? More light in your eye and increased happy chemical (serotonin) in your brain... Studies have shown that those suffering with SAD have less stability in their serotonin levels comparing seasons, possibly less ability to cope with lower amounts.

Long winter nights can throw off our circadian rhythm – the pattern in our brains and bodies that gets us into, then out of, bed. Some of us may find our melatonin (sleep hormone) and sleep cycle starts at a different time of day in winter. Some may oversleep; some lie awake, listless.

Surely it's because all of us spend too much time watching screens and staying indoors, not working the fields and seeing the light? Well, sort of. Put us in the bright light of summer and the melatonin levels decrease and we have more get up and go. Our libido soars and we feel ALIVE.

About 6% of UK dwellers are affected severely. In the fertile years SAD is *40% more likely in women than in men.* Maybe us gals are just more in touch with our surroundings? If you recognise yourself in this, even partly, it is important to take action or you could be missing out on a good part of your year.

What to do if the seasons aren't cheering you

- Get outside – *20 to 30 minutes (ideally with some exercise) five or six days a week can alter your brain chemistry. Outdoor light can be 2 to 20 times brighter than that inside!*

  The vitamin D *from sunlight will also reduce your chance of SAD symptoms and Public Health England recommends 10 micrograms vitamin D per day from October to March for many adults (cloudy UK dwellers). Better still, fill your plates with* omega-3 *and* vitamin D *rich goodies to help your brain stay above water – oily fish, red meat, liver, egg yolks, fortified cereals – choose what fits in with your choices. Avoid excess caffeine, alcohol and simple sugars; it is not enough to lament the winter weight gain in June when nothing fits – address it now! The* Mediterranean diet *(see the food is life chapter) gives you a fix of fruit, veg and wholegrains better than a speed-dialled pizza.*

  Getting into green spaces *and* socialising, *aka laughing, will create self-care that tackles problems rather than 'marinating' in them indoors.*

- Dance/exercise *class. We know* music *has mood elevating effects, so shake off the blues by shaking that booty. Music at home can make us focus and relax.*
- Relax *and enjoy the confines of winter. Try knitting. Not a joke. It could make you laugh. Try painting – no one need see the result. Start a book club +/- wine.*
- Open the curtains. *Not rocket science; light works through a window! If you have the means, visit a friend in sunnier climes – now your new BFF – she doesn't need to know why!*
- Set boundaries. *If entertaining your extended family, twice removed, annually coincides with your lowest ebb in January, then delegate it to someone who sings the joys of icy winters. Know your limits.*

Getting help

If it gets serious and you cannot shrug this off, you must seek help from your doctor. A professional may formally diagnose you if you have had two seasonal episodes of depression. What distinguishes it from other depressive diagnoses is the resolution as the seasons revert. Assessment may involve completing a 'Seasonal Pattern Assessment Questionnaire'.

The bright fact is that many people only suffer once and you may not suffer annually. SAD rarely leads to suicidal behaviour or extreme loss of function but MUST be taken seriously if present. It may naturally resolve after a few years.

Difficulty recognising the huge implications of this condition means that many just rumble on – if nothing else, productivity at work declines in winter and so does enthusiasm. All the more reason to plan a good office Christmas party. If you are like most, slightly affected by the season and not officially SAD, then try the lifestyle changes mentioned.

Toolbox against SAD in more severe cases

- Moonlight provides 0.2 lux (measurement of light intensity)
- Winter light 20,000 lux
- Sunny summer day is 100,000 lux

Studies of **light lamps** (these give about 10,000 lux) have not clearly established *why* they may work. *There might be a placebo effect because you know you are looking at... a lamp!*

No 'double blind' trial here!

However, the general impression is that *light actually helps many*. This can be a **light box**, **visor** or even a **dawn simulation alarm** that gently wakes you with some low-level light. All have been shown effective in *some* patients – many perceive light boxes as more effective. Others prefer the convenience of dawn simulation as they can get on with their day. These are not provided by the NHS so you have to research. You have to follow careful instructions and use a light box for at least 30 minutes a day. Many users describe a feeling of 'peace'. Side effects include eye strain/visual disturbance but these often resolve as you become 'acclimatised'.

Cognitive behavioural therapy can be very effective. Therapy may force you to do things like socialise if my motivation here hasn't succeeded!

Medication may be an important option in severe cases – ideally the *less sedating* antidepressants. All to be discussed with your doctor.

You may need a combination of treatments, or mild cases may simply resolve with some self-care approaches.

Joy at the changing of the seasons

As we mature we become more appreciative of nature, more connected and grounded. The changing of the seasons emphasises the wonder of life. We may recall previous HAPPY events. Pumpkins and Christmas wreaths. This feeling of 'healthy nostalgia' increases as we get older. We feel a gratitude to our life experience that brought us to this point, and we might appropriately downplay the negative of some memories *but not forget them as they shaped us*. There is great quality in being present in each moment and this is supported by reflecting on the past. In the same way we are less likely to engage in conflict as we age, we also may become more sentimental. This is the time to create new memories for our winters ahead, because without them our future will not have an identity.

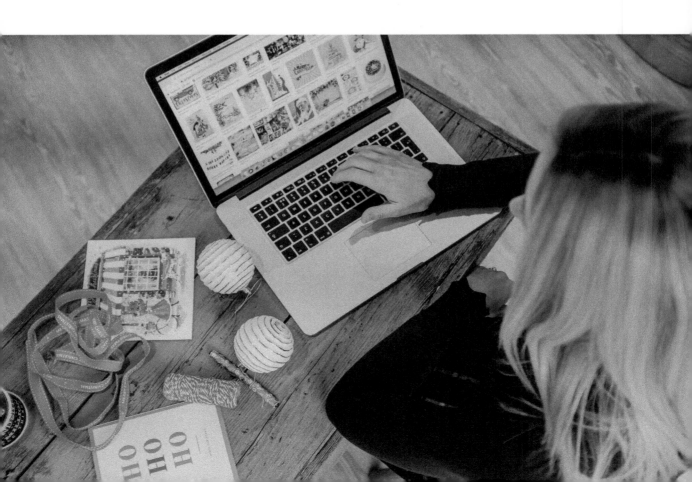

CHAPTER 6: DENTAL CARE AND WHY IT CAN CHANGE YOUR LIFE

Teeth are one of the first things we see on connection with others. Pearly whites may not be the teeth we were born with, such is the scope of dental replacement. Let us look at what you can do to make sure your *own teeth stay healthy*.

Teeth are teeth, why bother?

Our mouths are full of bacteria – something taught to me as an anaesthetist and vaguely mentioned at medical school. Got an upset stomach or a cold? The bug will have entered via your mouth or airways. A lot of the bacteria endemic to your mouth are harmless. The wash of saliva

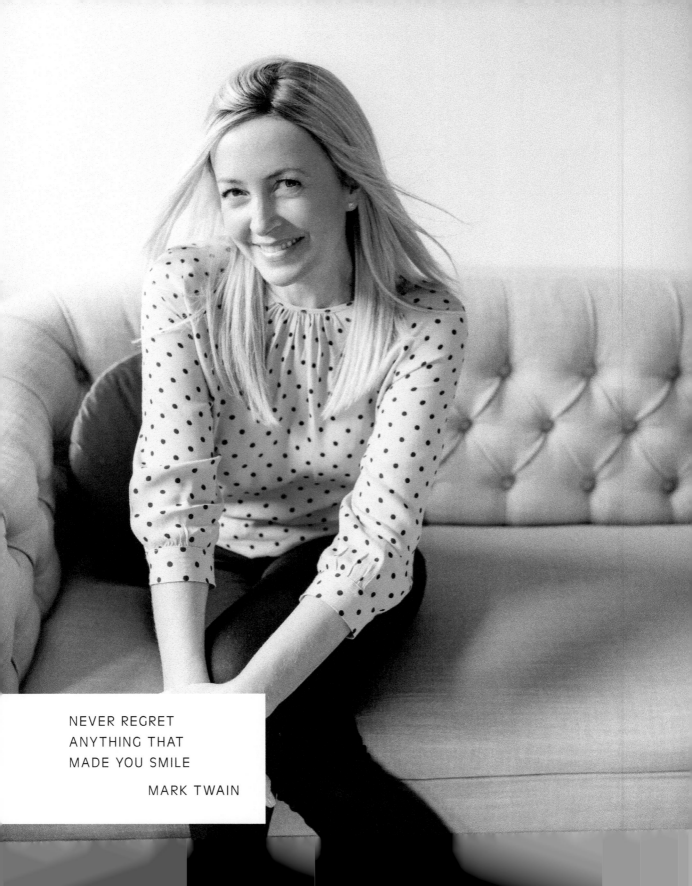

NEVER REGRET
ANYTHING THAT
MADE YOU SMILE

MARK TWAIN

keeps everything moving, along with the pH (acid base balance) that stays healthy, until you have an onslaught of sugar then things quickly change.

Why is 'what and when' we eat important?

We all have something called dental **bio-film,** not a movie of our lives but the natural layer of millions of bacteria which builds up on the teeth, especially at the gum margin where it meets the tooth. You feel it when your teeth haven't been cleaned. As soon as you clean them it starts to build up again.

When we drink or eat sugar this is changed into acid by the bio-film bacteria and this can then attack the enamel. Left unhindered this would form a hole and need filling.

If you **graze** on food and **constantly dip the pH** in your mouth, making it acidic, you risk your dental health. If you don't clean plaque off your teeth correctly this adds to the chance of decay. We also need the fluoride from our toothpaste to help strengthen enamel.

What about gums?

If oral bacteria over multiply, this can lead to tooth decay *and gum disease*. Poor dental health can put you at risk of certain diseases. People with gum disease are *more likely to have coronary heart disease*! This may not be a direct effect but due to shared factors like smoking and poor diet. Some scientists postulate that bacteria from the mouth are thought to enter the bloodstream and produce protein that can cause the platelets (cells that help us clot) to stick together in blood vessels. Blood clots can then of course restrict blood flow and this can have serious consequences.

Gum disease can increase chances of infection and elevate blood sugar in those with diabetes and increases the number of bacteria in the mouth. This can then increase the likelihood of lung infections. Already I can see you reaching for your toothbrush...

Signs of gum disease

- Red, swollen, bleeding gums
- Unpleasant taste
- Bad breath
- Loose teeth
- Regular mouth infections

There can be an inherited tendency to gum disease but the primary cause is plaque. Cleaning carefully and flossing regularly with proper technique (ask the dental hygienist to show you how to get both angles of gum between teeth) reduces the amount of plaque build-up. Be honest with your dentist and see a hygienist if you don't regularly already – the investment is worth it for oral and GENERAL health. None of us can be perfect brushers all the time. Most of us do one side better according to our dominant hand. A hygienist or your dentist may show you exactly where you are missing. My life-changing moment was realising you don't need to drag an electric toothbrush around your mouth but **concentrate on doing one tooth at a time** so each quarter of your mouth takes up 30 seconds. Don't rush and don't push hard.

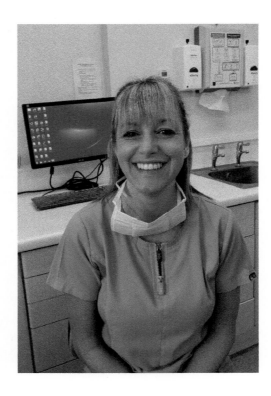

- When you eat food sugars, or anything acidic, the enamel temporarily softens – give it 30 minutes or more before you brush and allow your saliva to neutralise the acid or it may damage your enamel in its weakened state when you brush.
- After acidic food have some water to flush your teeth over. If you are on the run, eating something not acidic and low in carbs like a piece of cheddar cheese may help the teeth.
- Limit snacking between meals as your teeth never get a break from constant acid attack!
- Similarly, don't eat straight after brushing. Allow the fluoride to work on your teeth.
- Daily habits add up over the years and nothing lifts you up like a good laugh with friends, so make those pearly whites something to be proud of.

Let me hand over to another expert specialist, my lovely dental hygienist Nicky.

NICOLA GOUGH CEB Dip Dent Hygiene
BSc (Hons) Primary Dental Care

Dental hygienist cofounder of: www.cpd4dentalnurses.co.uk and www.cpd4dentalhygienists. co.uk, websites offering continuing professional development to dental care professionals.

This information is primarily anecdotal and subjective, based upon 28 years of experience in the dental industry.

What proportion of dental patients do you think visit the hygienist?

This varies, depending on the ethos of the dental practice. The practice in which I currently work has a preventative and maintenance ethos. As such, approximately 80% of patients over the age of 25 are referred to the dental hygienist.

What is the minimum age of patients that you see if referred by their dentist?

Again, this varies from practice to practice. I generally see patients over the age of 25, unless their periodontal risk assessment indicates that they may be at risk of periodontal disease. We have an oral health educator in the practice who sees patients of all ages for oral health advice. When I worked with an orthodontist I saw many children.

Can you see improvements long term when you are seeing people regularly?

Regular hygienist appointments keep patients on track with their oral health. In addition to carrying out scaling, polishing and root surface debridement where required, regular visits enable me to re-motivate the patient and reinforce important messages. However, care of teeth at home with healthy habits is still the most important factor.

What are the mistakes that most people make with their brushing technique?

- Not brushing for long enough.
- Not brushing twice daily (teeth should be brushed before bed and at least on one other occasion, according to the Department of Health).
- Not angling the brush into the gingival margin.
- Not replacing brushes or electric toothbrush heads regularly enough.
- Forgetting to brush the tongue.
- Not looking in the mirror when brushing.
- Rinsing out toothpaste. Toothpaste should be spat out, not rinsed out, to maintain fluoride concentration.

What kind of toothbrush do you recommend?

Department of Health recommendations are to use a manual or powered toothbrush with a small toothbrush head and medium texture. For most I recommend a powered toothbrush with a rotation, oscillation action (Braun Oral B) with a small, round head as there is some evidence to suggest that these can be more effective than manual tooth brushing (Cochrane Reviews). I also notice improvements in my patients' oral health when these toothbrushes are used. However, the most important factor is that the patient brushes for the correct length of time twice daily and that the correct technique is used to ensure plaque removal. A powered toothbrush is not a substitute for an incorrect technique.

Can you explain the importance of flossing?

Unfortunately, the evidence to evaluate the benefits of flossing has been unreliable. However, I *personally* see a huge difference in the oral health of patients who use interdental cleaning methods to reach where the brush misses. I aim to encourage my patients to use aids such as small brushes or interspace brushes, and floss for anywhere these do not fit.

Do you think if teeth are looked after there will still be a decline in dental health over the age of 60 onwards or do you perceive this can be prevented with excellent oral hygiene and nutrition?

The decline in dental health is dependent upon many factors. Achieving optimal oral hygiene, attending regularly for dental appointments and being aware of the importance of good nutrition are all an essential part in maintaining a stable and healthy dentition. However, there are many other factors involved that mean there could potentially still be a decline in dental health. There are certain risk factors for periodontal disease which, among others, include genetics, stress, smoking and diabetes. These risk factors, along with other factors such as the patient's general health and medication, can all affect how the teeth and soft tissues respond as we age.

Can you tell me about different types of floss/devices for cleaning between the teeth?

Interdental brushes come in a variety of makes and sizes and it is possible that an individual may be required to use several different sizes depending on the size of the interdental space. A single tufted brush may also be advised for patients with periodontitis.

Dental floss or tape can be used in smaller interdental spaces and these come waxed or unwaxed. There is a special floss that can be used for cleaning under bridges and around implants. Floss is also available on a stick to aid patients with access to posterior teeth.

There are a variety of toothpicks. I base my recommendations to patients on their disease status whilst considering their personal preference, dexterity and potential levels of compliance.

Have you seen many smiles transformed from all your experience working with dentists?

I have seen some amazing changes in women's lives. The primary aim is to take patients to a state of oral health and stability which does not necessarily involve any cosmetic treatment. Even without cosmetic work, a healthy smile is an attractive smile. I have seen women who have been unable to eat due to toothache or who have gums that are red, swollen and bleed profusely. Their lives have been transformed with restorative care, periodontal treatment and oral health education carried out by members of the dental team. Additionally, a lot of women have had cosmetic treatments – for example, whitening treatments or veneers – which have led to improved confidence. Many of my patients have undergone orthodontic treatment which has led not only to improved appearance but also facilitates easier cleaning and has therefore led to improved periodontal status.

Are there any dental secrets I may have missed that you can impart?

The most important part of maintaining a healthy dentition is HOME CARE. What you do at home is the MOST important part in maintaining a stable and healthy dentition.

Thank you so much, Nicky, I am sure so many readers will find that invaluable.

Wonky teeth anyone?

At around 40 I noticed my bottom teeth, which had always been perfectly straight, were doing their own dance and were a bit uneven.

Fast forward five years and I noticed in a few photos that a top tooth was looking odd. On closer inspection the bottom ones must have moved the top one! Was it vain that I wanted my straight teeth back? After discussion with my dentist, I researched and found the best orthodontist in my area and ended up in Dr Alastair's clinic. After checks and an X-ray/3D scan of what my teeth could look like, I took the plunge. I had never spent this much money on myself but I opted for 'Invisalign', clear plastic brace trays that you replace every week or two until your teeth are straight. I will not write more but in a quick seven months (my teeth were relatively straight already) I now have the smile I used to have, and with wire retainers behind my teeth and a night-time retainer it should not budge. I hope this keeps my bite and eating healthy as I age. Total vanity? Or not? Let's find out why teeth 'keep on moving'.

Let's hand over to the wonderful **Dr Alastair Smith BDS (Bris), MSc, MFDS RCS (Eng), MOrth RCS (Eng) www.pallantorthodontics.co.uk**

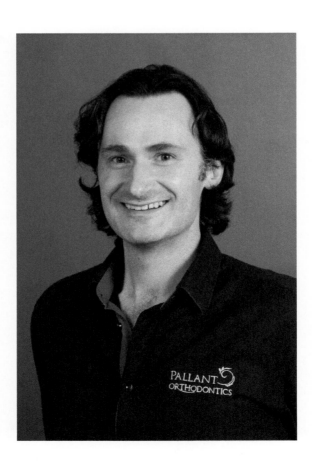

Is the demographic of your female patients in the bracket aged 40 to 60 years expanding?

In recent years there has been a significant increase in the number of adult women seeking orthodontic treatment. One significant change in recent decades is that the incidence of decay has reduced. This means that the dental focus has shifted from filling teeth or replacing missing teeth, to enhancing the long-term health and appearance of the teeth and smile. This has coincided with a general change in the way society views age and the desire to maintain a youthful appearance. Another factor that has contributed to the rise in adult orthodontics is the development of more aesthetically acceptable types of orthodontic appliances such as clear aligners (e.g. Invisalign) and tooth-coloured fixed braces.

Has the era of the 'selfie culture' affected your work generally?

More people are aware of their teeth and smile. Patients seeking treatment often state that they dislike their teeth in photos. The advent of smartphones and social media platforms has caused an explosion in photos that are often then shared with friends. Another way in which 'selfies' have affected our work is that patients are far more likely to record and share their orthodontic journey on social media platforms.

Do you think people are surprised that their teeth continue to move beyond childhood? Can you explain why this happens?

Our body is in a constant state of change and the supporting structures of the teeth are no different. Given this, small movements of the teeth should be considered normal and an inevitable part of ageing. The underlying reasons for age-related tooth movement are multi-factorial. Continued jaw growth in the late teens and early adulthood can play a part. Wisdom teeth usually erupt in the late teens and it was once thought that these teeth played a significant role in crowding. Studies have however revealed this not to be the case. It is also likely that (over the long-term) biting forces gradually move the teeth, resulting in increased crowding of the front teeth. Gum disease or the loss of teeth can result in drifting of teeth near the space. The only way to prevent tooth movement is by wearing some form of orthodontic retainer long-term.

Can you give us an idea of what types of problems adults are referred to you with?

The majority of adult patients are referred simply to resolve the crowding of their teeth and to improve the overall position and appearance. However, there are many other reasons for referrals, including people who have suffered from gum disease as above. Other patients require significant dental rehabilitation, and orthodontics is just one aspect of their treatment. The orthodontist will work closely with the restorative dentist who may be placing implants where teeth are missing or restoring worn teeth with crowns.

Do you take patients who self-refer along with those recommended by their dentist?

Patients are far more empowered now than they ever were. Healthcare is now less paternalistic. Many patients take it upon themselves to research their concerns online and find a clinic they like or even a type of treatment they want! It is incumbent on us to recognise this societal change and provide a pathway for self-referral.

How do you think what is done in orthodontics in the UK compares to the rest of the developed world? Which are the pioneering countries in this?

There is no doubt that the delivery of orthodontics in the UK is largely influenced by the way in which it is funded. This is certainly true for the majority of treatment undertaken for under 18s, which is funded by the NHS. With any state-based system (particularly where there has been limited funding) the emphasis is to make a limited budget stretch as far as possible. This has meant that NHS dentistry has focussed on providing a basic but adequate standard. Outside of this system there are some practices in the UK that have embraced more modern techniques and invested in technology. These clinics are providing orthodontics that can rival treatment done anywhere else in the world. The countries that are leading the field in pioneering and adopting new advances in orthodontic treatments are currently the USA, Japan and Australia.

You were one of the first practices in the UK to use remote monitoring to watch your patient's progress. I was able to upload pictures from my phone app to you, so you could check my teeth without visiting the clinic each time. Can you tell me a little more about this and its potential applications?

Dental Monitoring is an innovative way of monitoring orthodontic treatment remotely. It is an absolute game changer in orthodontics. It works by the patient using an app on their smartphone to take a scan of their teeth. This is uploaded, processed and analysed by artificial intelligence to identify a huge number of parameters related to the position of the teeth and the state of the orthodontic appliance. This is fed back to the practice and enables the clinical team to identify how well the teeth are moving and whether there are any potential problems. It allows the clinician to view the teeth at a pixel-level and with an accuracy of 0.05mm. This is a totally different level of monitoring to what has previously been possible with the naked eye. The patient typically takes a scan every seven days, so in effect has a virtual weekly check-up with the orthodontist. The traditional way of seeing patients is a physical visit to the practice every six to eight weeks. In the case of Invisalign we can, say, personalise the rate at which the client passes through different retainer stages. There are great implications for this type of monitoring in dental care generally.

What is the rough range of time taken for straightening treatments?

Simple cases can take as little as six to nine months, whilst more complex cases can take over three years.

Why the importance of having an X-ray prior to orthodontic treatment?

X-rays are taken prior to orthodontic treatment for a variety of reasons. One reason is to check on the general health of the teeth and supporting structures such as the surrounding bone and jaw joints. It is important to exclude the possibility of pathology of these structures such as decay or reduced bone support as a result of gum disease. X-rays help to provide information about the presence and position of unerupted teeth. Other X-ray findings that frequently influence treatment planning include developmentally missing teeth, impacted teeth or even extra teeth. X-rays can also help provide valuable information about the angulation of teeth and the way in which the jaws have grown, which can be important factors influencing someone's treatment.

What are the best and worst aspects of your job?!

Undoubtedly the best aspect of my job is seeing how orthodontic treatment can transform someone's life by improving their confidence. Many of our patients seek treatment stating that they hate their teeth and smile. Often, they do not like smiling and cover their mouth to hide their teeth. To be able to change this makes the job very rewarding. In orthodontics we may not be saving lives but we are positively changing them.

One of the most frustrating aspects of the job is seeing people's teeth move again following treatment. This can be prevented, or at least minimised, with good retainers and a compliant patient. However, human nature being what it is means that some of our teenage patients do not always remember or feel the need to wear their retainers – as a result their teeth move!

Thank you, Alastair. That will be so helpful to so many women.

My hope is that now you have a new-found, heightened respect for your teeth and are going to go out and get some floss, change your toothbrush head and get those pearly whites shining, alongside booking any outstanding dental appointments. One set of natural adult teeth should be enough to last a long and happy life; make that smile a healthy one inside and out.

Any brands of tooth care equipment used for cleaning mentioned in this chapter are by honest recommendation and neither Alastair, Nicky or I have any financial affiliation with those names mentioned.

CHAPTER 7: HEALTH SCREENING AND BREAST HEALTH

HEALTH SCREENING

Why go to the doctors for screening tests?

Life is all about chances and choices. No two bodies are identical. Medicine is about trying to piece a puzzle together and achieve the best outcome overall. It is not always an exact science and different health professionals will deal with a situation with slightly varying approaches. Guidelines and education aim to ensure that the final outcome is the best for the patient's interest and their long-term health and quality of life.

Health screening, used for **breast** and **cervical** health in the UK, is a complicated science that is thought about and perfected before it is introduced to the population.

People are only screened for a disease if:

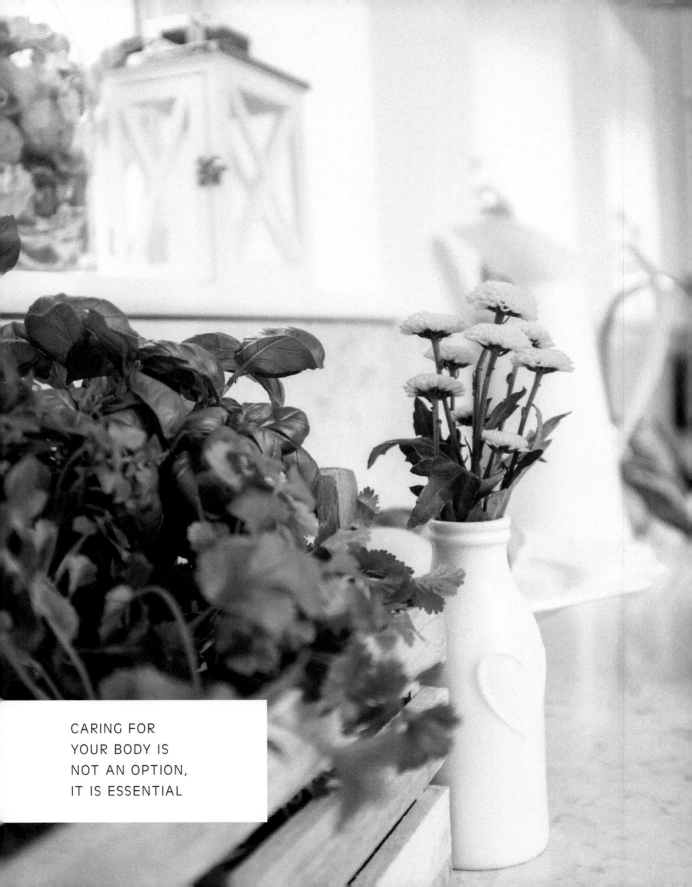

CARING FOR
YOUR BODY IS
NOT AN OPTION,
IT IS ESSENTIAL

- There is an accurate, sensitive and specific screening test
- A sensitive test is one that picks up disease or the beginning of disease easily; a specific test means the test is specific to what you are looking for and does not pick up lots of other things. This is a complex problem when you are designing a screening process. You want to pick up what you are looking for and not miss it, but do not want to unnecessarily alarm healthy people as well. Rarely is a screening process perfect.
- A treatment can be offered if a disease or pre-disease state is detected
- The screening is safe
- By intervening and catching the illness, disease can be prevented/treated or even lives extended or their quality improved.

You may look at this and say: *"But why me? I feel fine. I hate going to the doctors, let alone them putting something in me/on me/looking at me."*

This book is not to bamboozle you with facts and figures. We do, however, live in a developed world where we have the 'luxury' of tests that can detect illness at a point before it affects the quality of your everyday life. It is worth taking advantage of this.

BREAST HEALTH

A woman is most beautiful when she is confident in her own body and most happy when she gives herself the care she deserves

Breasts are a subject for public discussion. Real, implanted, reconstructed, they have become 'newsworthy'. Everyone feels entitled to comment. Let us now reclaim our breasts *for us* and make sure we look after them. Many women reading this book will have never given a second thought to their breasts. Some of you have suffered disease and undergone a treatment regime that changed your life and outlook forever. Some of you have breast implants because you were unhappy with your natural breasts. Some of you may have developed on one side only and have a unilateral implant. Some of you have breastfed; some of you may never have tried, or wished to…

I expect we *all have an opinion about our own breasts.*

Anatomy of the breast

Women's breasts overlie the pectoral chest muscles and are made of fatty tissue and glandular tissue that can produce milk. The amount of fat determines the breast size. There are 15 to 20 sections in the glandular tissue called lobes. Each lobe is divided into lobules where milk is

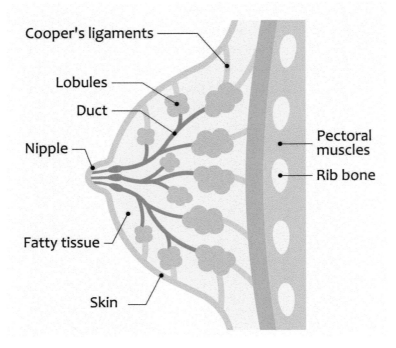

Cooper's ligaments

Lobules

Duct

Nipple

Pectoral muscles

Rib bone

Fatty tissue

Skin

produced. These drain via a network of ducts and ductules to the nipple. The areola is the dark area of skin around the nipple.

Protect your breasts

Have supportive well-fitting bras (worth getting professionally fitted). A bra should start off on the loosest setting so there is leeway to tighten when it stretches through use or washing; chuck it if it hurts. Do not wear bras that dig into your shoulders as this may affect posture. A bra should fit flat at the breastplate and not pull up. No surgeon I spoke to genuinely believed that wire bras cause harm; just make sure whichever bra type you use is comfortable, as ill-fitting bras can cause pain.

In exercise wear a good sports bra. The Cooper's ligaments (the connective tissue in the breast that maintains structure) are under strain with exercise, especially against gravity, and need supporting. Women's breasts **are all different** in terms of the proportion of fat and glandular tissue. At a younger age glandular tissue is normally more 'dense' (this is why mammograms can be inaccurate if there is a lot of dense glandular tissue). When we run, breasts can move up and down, and sideways in other sports. There is less vertical movement as we age. When choosing a sports bra there are two main types and some combinations. **Encapsulation bras** use a defined cup structure to encapsulate each breast so you keep a feminine shape with maximal support. **Compression bras** push the breast tissue close to the body so there is minimal movement. Anyone who has pulled these on knows they can be tricky, but once in place work better than a conventional bra.

Bras are often labelled in terms of low (walking, yoga), medium (cycling, dancing) or high (running, aerobics) impact and, though this may refer to the exercise, really, you have to also take into account the size of your breasts. One of my larger-breasted relatives wears two sports bras to help. Brands such as Boobydoo, Sweaty Betty, Victoria's Secret, Lululemon, Fabletics, New Balance and Under Armour all perform well under different circumstances in research. Ideally, try on and decide which is best for you. Remember, it not only has to stabilise your breasts but also fit close and comfortably around your rib cage.

Sagging can be genetic but worsened by lack of care. Scientists at Portsmouth University are currently studying the different proportions of tissue found in women and whether this determines which of us are more likely to experience sagging. They are also looking at how the breast moves in exercise. These studies could potentially help with different bra designs in the future. Breasts can get heavier as we age and sleeping on our front can also affect their shape. Try a soft non-wired bra at night for support if needed. Yoga or other exercise to strengthen the muscular support beneath may help.

Getting to know your breasts

It is essential that we are all breast aware.

Being breast aware

Take a look in a full-length mirror while standing with your top half undressed at comfortable room temperature. Look at the skin of your breasts and the nipples.

Are there unusual changes in the skin? Is it puckered or drawn in? Are there any red patches or crusting around the nipples that keep recurring? Are the nipples changing in their direction or positioning relative to your breast? Is there any discharge which may or may not be bloodstained from the nipples?

Then examine yourself. There are many ways to do this (you may have been taught by your doctor or nurse) and the most important is to find a method you are happy with. Remember that the upper outer area of your breast nearer your armpit tends to be lumpier as this is where we have more of our glandular tissue. Get to know what is normal FOR YOU and then if a new lump or changes occur you will be aware. Don't forget to feel in your armpit for any lumpiness or tenderness. It is almost like you develop a mental map of what your breasts feel like.

It would be a good idea at this point to watch a video to help you understand how to examine your breasts rather than reading about it. Here we go. The lovely ladies at www.coppafeel.org have kindly allowed me to link to their video:

Coppafeel.org/your-boobs/boob-check-101/

or

https://vimeo.com/298985447

CoppaFeel! also runs a free text reminder service to remind you to check, which you can have by texting BOOBS to 70300. There is more on their website.

If you find something new, or that you are not sure about, and it doesn't disappear after two to four weeks then **please go and see your GP**. They will examine you and, unless they strongly believe it is a hormonally related change that may pass in the next cycle, they will refer you to the local breast clinic. While you wait, try and be reassured that *most lumps that a doctor sees are not cancer*. Breast cancer is also rarely painful and the majority of lumps in the breast will be one of the following:

Breast lumps

- **Normal monthly change** – at least 50% of women have some lumpiness when having cycles.
- **Fibroadenoma** – fibrous non-cancerous (benign) lump. Usually this is in women under 40 or in your 20s. It is the most common benign breast lump. It is from excessive growth of glands and connective tissue in the breasts. They are described as firm and rubbery, or 'breast mice' because they move around. They can be removed if causing a problem but may spontaneously disappear after menopause.
- **Breast cyst** – a fluid-filled cyst that more often occurs nearer menopause. These feel round or oval and smooth and quite firm. They can move when pressed a little and can sometimes resolve with the next cycle. The cyst may still reform or may disappear completely. If it is a 'simple cyst' on a scan with no solid contents, this may be drained by the radiologist or surgeon with a needle under ultrasound control. More complicated cysts are investigated further.
- **Infection** – such as in mastitis when breastfeeding.
- **Fat necrosis** – from trauma to the breast a fatty lump may develop. These are only really removed if very large or causing a lot of discomfort by their size.
- **Lipoma** – fatty non-cancerous (benign) tumour of the breast.

Breast Pain

This can be **cyclical** – worse before a period – or **non-cyclical**, and can actually be from the breast or the chest wall. Women often feel it more in the upper outer area of the breast (nearer the armpit) where there is more glandular tissue. It is thought that up to 70% of women have this at some time.

Speaking to Dr Liz O'Riordan, she explained that many women whose breast pain is on both sides and often going up to the arm actually have musculoskeletal pain, and when you think that a size B cup breast can weigh around 500 grams this is not surprising. Many women are helped by wearing a comfortable soft bra at night-time, as above. When you think of how pendulous our breasts can be when turning it is no surprise that this has a pulling effect on the chest wall and ligaments and so on. Evening primrose oil is often advised for breast pain and can help some women but often has to be taken for up to three months to have discernible effect and the dose needed may be prohibitory in terms of expense.

A large review study looked at breast pain and, although a third of women find their cyclical pain simply goes away, in up to 2/3^{rds} of women it recurs. Rubbing anti-inflammatory gel into the area helped in some studies. There was not enough evidence to advocate taking tablets of anti-inflammatories (ibuprofen). Caffeine use has been associated with breast pain – something I personally find to be true – but there is little research evidence about caffeine restriction. Some women find this and other components of chocolate and sometimes alcohol make breast pain worse, especially if they tend towards cystic breasts. It is worth trying elimination for yourself. There is also not enough evidence to definitely advise evening primrose oil, but still in my experience some women find this helpful. Generally reducing processed foods, especially unhealthy fats, and making sure you follow a high fibre diet with reduced or no alcohol can help reduce excessive oestrogen levels (more common premenopausally) and promote healthy breast tissue.

Breast Cancer

Breast cancer is the most common cancer in the UK and the lifetime risk for women is 13% or one in eight. There were approximately 55,000 new cases in 2014 and screening is offered to those who do not have symptoms. Eighty per cent of cases are diagnosed in women over 50 years. There are 12,000 deaths per annum in the UK from breast cancer.

Symptoms and signs of breast cancer

- *lump in breast*
- *swelling/lump in armpit*
- *nipple discharge/nipple inversion that is new*
- *rash around nipple*
- *change in size or shape of breast*
- *dimpling or thickening of skin in breast.*
- *there may be no lump or change that you can feel in some cases.*

What are the risk factors and protective factors for breast cancer?
What about if you have a family history of breast cancer?

It is always appropriate to first discuss your situation with your GP and they will work out whether a referral is needed. It will depend eventually on whether you meet certain criteria as to whether you are referred to a genetics clinic from your local breast clinic.

Genetic risk factors, as in the BRCA1 or BRCA2 or TP53 mutation, only account for 3% of breast cancers. Those with a family history in a first-degree relative (mother, sister, daughter) or second-degree relative (maternal or paternal aunt, grandmother) may come under the group of these genes or there may be genes that we do not yet know about that are related to breast cancer risk. In those with a family history of breast cancer in the UK there is a clear protocol for doctors to follow. There is usually a regional centre that collates all the information from local clinics and this will include relevant information relating to genetics. These genetics centres will often work out the advice for an individual patient with specific genetic abnormalities and then they will advise the local hospital. Counselling and advice will be given at this stage, before any operative treatment or so on.

Further risk factors are:

- early onset menstruation (before 12) and/or late menopause (over 55) – more cycles means more lifetime hormone exposure
- first child born when you were over 30
- no pregnancies full-term (having children and breastfeeding are protective)
- significant weight gain after menopause and obesity
- regular alcohol consumption
- low levels vitamin D
- high-dose radiation to the chest area
- not enough sleep (melatonin is protective – see sleep chapter)
- long-term hormone therapy
- the combined contraceptive pill – this is not normally prescribed after the age of 40
- hormone replacement therapy.

Please see the menopause chapter. We know that the risk of combined (oestrogen and progesterone) HRT is higher than that of oestrogen alone HRT. If you have your womb you need the progesterone component as well (see menopause chapter). *The risks of hormone treatments decrease back down after the medication is stopped* and recent studies are disputing the time this takes so may be out of date by the time you read this. It is very difficult within a book to inform the reader properly. Each woman's case, the severity of her symptoms for menopause and her quality of life need to be weighed up against potential risk which MUST be discussed with numbers and rates of risk with your doctor. **Keep in perspective that the actual risk of alcohol or obesity can be more than the risk of HRT in breast cancer so it has to be a balanced choice (see menopause chapter) and many newer formulations have reduced risk.**

One could easily feel despondent looking at the list as many of these factors we cannot control and of course sometimes disease arises purely through apparent 'bad luck'. Better to look at what you *can change and no point worrying about what you can't.*

It is important at this moment to reflect on alcohol and smoking being risk factors for breast disease. We associate smoking with lung cancer and alcohol with liver problems but it is actually often very emotive for women to also consider their breast health when making lifestyle changes. It is also mainly only smokers who suffer with something called periductal mastitis. In women who aren't breastfeeding, mastitis is often caused by a bacterial infection. This can occur as a result of bacteria getting into the milk ducts through a cracked or sore nipple, or a nipple piercing. Periductal mastitis is a benign condition and does not increase your chance of developing breast cancer.

Duct ectasia of the breast, mammary duct ectasia or plasma cell mastitis is a condition that is also more common in smokers and occurs when a milk duct beneath the nipple widens, the duct walls thicken and the duct fills with fluid. This is the most common cause of greenish discharge. Mammary duct ectasia can mimic breast cancer.

Reduce your risk of breast disease by keeping your BMI low and by getting exercise.

UK screening programme

In the UK women are first called for breast screening between their 50th and 53rd birthdays (some may be called earlier by the way the system works). They have three-yearly mammography between the ages of 50 and 70 years. Above the upper age limit screening can be requested individually. There have also been various trials where women were called for screening as early as 45 or as late as 75.

Breast screening reduces the relative risk of dying of breast cancer by 20%. **That is one-fifth**. It is thought to prevent 1,300 deaths per year in the UK. On the other side, just under a third of women recalled are over-investigated.

What happens at a mammogram?

The radiographer will examine each breast individually. You will be undressed from the waist up and the breast placed between metal plates. This will be done in two different directions to get two X-ray views of each breast. It is less painful than having a blood test, and the radiographers are very experienced and used to dealing with women having this done.

Once the mammogram has been done the results will be analysed and if abnormal you will have a clinical review with a doctor and possible further imaging (maybe ultrasound) and if appropriate a biopsy. If the biopsy is a small needle (such as if a cyst is seen) you may not need local anaesthetic; if a larger biopsy is taken you will have a small amount of local anaesthetic first in the skin.

Sometimes women may receive a letter after screening that there are small 'white dot areas' which are actually non-invasive breast cancers or micro-calcification. Not all areas of micro-calcification become invasive breast cancer. By catching these changes **early**, treatment can be given and disease progression prevented, which is why women are encouraged to go for screening.

What about breast screening if you have breast implants?

In theory, physical examination of patients with implants could be easier if breast tissue is pushed forward by an implant, and again women are advised to be breast aware. Women are usually advised at the time of their breast implant operation that this may make mammography slightly more difficult but there are special views called Eklund views that can be used, and ultrasound and MRI scans are not affected by breast implants and tend to be the imaging of choice if, say, the implant is ruptured.

It is important to note that, asking an experienced breast surgeon, the majority of recalls after mammogram do not actually have a sinister disease.

In all cases, early diagnosis promotes better outcomes. Whether this be from attending regular screening or routinely examining yourself at home and reporting early changes, it is important to be mindful of breast care. If a diagnosis is made, the surgeon and oncologist will give you a clear plan of treatment, and the breast and oncology nurses will provide information and overall support.

Treatment can include more than one of surgery, chemotherapy, radiotherapy, hormone therapy (this may be long term) and biological therapy. The NHS website, Macmillan Cancer Care, Breast Cancer Care and Cancer Research UK have a wealth of information. Depending upon the surgery there will be chances for reconstruction if wanted at a later date and the nurses will give you information regarding prostheses and swimwear. We know from specific studies that exercise and healthy lifestyle choices, even good friendship support, helps in recovery and longevity after treatment. If you have had armpit (axillary) surgery it is often overlooked that you must protect your arms and hands when, for example, gardening. I used to tell my patients to wear two pairs of gloves when gardening as, if they had an infection from a thorn or similar, reduced lymphatic drainage could cause problems. Lymphoedema (swelling of the limb) can be an uncomfortable complication, especially if infected.

Resources for breast prostheses, mastectomy swimwear and accessories are available at www.breastcancercare.co.uk.

As detailed in my meditation chapter, studies in the USA have shown how meditation practice helps greatly with women after diagnosis. One study was led by a consultant who was a sufferer of the disease herself. The idea is that with Mindfulness Based Stress Reduction women can have techniques to implement when they feel overwhelmed in any way.

Here is an appropriate time to hand over to a **wonderful real expert…**

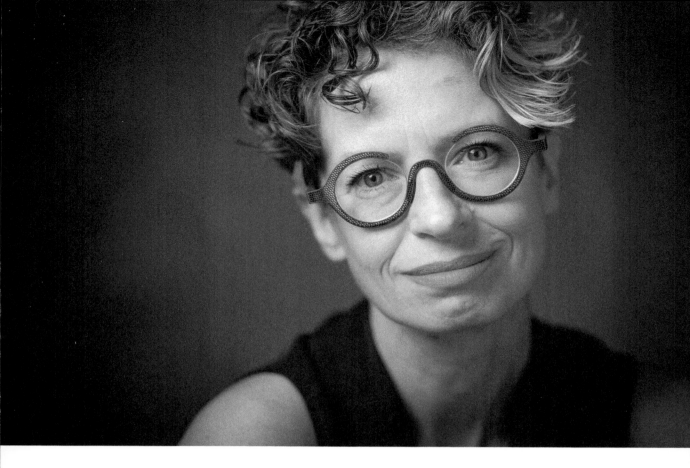

Liz O'Riordan

http://liz.oriordan.co.uk
www.cancerfit.me
Twitter @Liz_ORiordan
Instagram @oriordanliz
PhD Molecular Oncology, Consultant Breast Surgeon

"In 2015 I was diagnosed with breast cancer, and in February 2019 I retired due to the side effects of treatment for a recurrence on my chest wall. I now work as a Consultant in Public Health Medicine one day a week reviewing the notes of people who have died in hospital and sharing the learning from those cases so we can improve the care of dying patients in hospital."

Liz is an accomplished writer in the popular press and medical field and most recently co-author with Professor Trisha Greenhalgh of The Complete Guide to Breast Cancer: How to Feel Empowered and Take Control **(Vermillion 2018). This is an absolute essential for anyone diagnosed or close to anyone with a breast cancer diagnosis.**

Please tell me, Liz, what you would call your 'top myths' about breast cancer that you would like to dispel.

1. What you eat causes breast cancer

   There is no single foodstuff that has been proven to cause breast cancer. It is safe to eat anything and everything *in moderation*, and that includes soy and dairy products. What has been proven, however, is that being overweight does increase your risk of breast cancer. Certain foods like processed red meat may increase your risk, but this is only a very small effect and you would have to eat a lot of bacon for this to happen.

2. If you make it to five years after a cancer diagnosis, then you're cured

   Breast cancer comes back in 30% of patients and this can happen 10 or even 20 years after a diagnosis. Many patients don't realise this, and doctors and nurses don't always tell you what the symptoms and signs of a recurrence are. It's important to find out what to look out for and what to do if you're worried. You could ask your doctor or look on a website, e.g. Breast Cancer Now.

3. Breast cancer always forms a lump

   Finding a breast lump is the commonest way most women are diagnosed with cancer but there are other signs. That's why it's important not only to check your breasts but to look in the mirror as well. Bleeding or a rash around the nipple, a dent or dimple in your breast when you raise your arms, a change in shape or size and a hot red breast (like mastitis) can all be signs of breast cancer. If you have any of these symptoms for more than a week or two, you should get them checked by your GP.

4. Wearing an underwired bra causes cancer

   This is definitely wrong. Wearing a bra is safe and does not cause cancer. It is also safe to wear an underwired bra after breast cancer surgery (once your surgeon is happy that the wounds have healed). Most women wear the wrong bra size and wear bras that are well past their sell-by date. If you haven't been measured for a few years and your body shape has changed, it's worth getting refitted.

5. Exercising and eating a healthy diet will stop you getting breast cancer

   Anyone can get breast cancer – young or old, healthy or unhealthy. There are things you can do to lower your risk, but **the two biggest reasons that women get breast cancer – being a woman and getting older – are out of your control.**

All readers take note...

One of your recommendations to me was that alongside checking their breasts midcycle, women should make a routine of checking other areas, e.g. their vulva, surrounding region and wee and poo being a good start. Do you think there is a gap in education of women who could be helped by different disciplines in medicine 'uniting together' on this, rather than women randomly being aware when a particular condition is in the media spotlight that month?

It's not enough just to check your breasts when you remember. You should also take the time to explore all of your body and know what's normal. You should check your neck and armpits for lumps that might be enlarged lymph nodes. Get out a mirror and look at your labia and vulva. Check the colour of your urine and poo. You have to know what's normal for you. If you do this regularly, you might pick up something serious at a much earlier stage. Ideally youngsters would be educated about checking their bodies at schools, reinforced at universities. When you see your GP, they should remind you to do it. Different branches of medicine could unite behind a campaign telling everyone to check their bits – all the time, instead of highlighting poo in bowel cancer month for example; bowel cancer is diagnosed all year around. When the clocks go back and forward could be a start?

Being propelled into a sudden early menopause by your treatment, what have you learned as a patient that you can impart to other women that doctors who have no personal experience may not realise?

As a doctor I had no idea how to treat the symptoms of an early menopause. I assumed and hoped that GPs would know. I was lucky that oncologists I met through Twitter told me what drugs might help – and I shared that information in my book so patients can go to their own GPs and tell them what to prescribe.

It really has ruined my quality of life. Hot flushes and night sweats make me feel physically ill. The lack of concentration and memory mean I can no longer think as clearly or as quickly. The loss of libido and the associated vaginal dryness can destroy relationships. Joint pain, leg cramps, fluid retention and insidious weight gain do nothing to help women deal with their already altered body image after cancer surgery.

It's not 'just a few hot flushes'. The side effects of hormonal therapy can be crippling, and there are a lot of women who don't take their tablets because of this, even though they know it might mean their cancer comes back.

You are vocal about changes to our sex life after surgery, menopause, medically induced menopause or after any event that changes how we see ourselves. What would you like to see more of in women's discussions? I strongly believe there is still a great stigma in us discussing these issues, which leads to women suffering in silence.

We need the medical profession to talk to every patient with an illness about their sex life. To ask the question. They may not be able to help them or may not be the person who that woman wants to open up to, but they've at least started the discussion. Patients and advocates on social media are helping to make it normal to talk about sex and share the tips and tricks they've learned. It's hard to talk about your own experiences as that involves sharing your partner's experiences, and they may not want to be public about their sex life. I think if we can get more people talking about it in the media and TV it will give patients the courage to come forward and ask for help.

Tell me about your experience as a tri-athlete and how exercise can help prognosis with breast cancer. For you personally, what does exercise provide on a physical and mental basis and how soon after initial treatment was complete did you return to exercise?

When I got married I became a cycling widow and soon realised if I didn't ride a bike I'd never see my husband at the weekends! One thing led to another and I started doing triathlons. I was diagnosed with cancer nine months after my first one. Exercise for me was a way to feel normal, to forget for a while that I was having chemo or was bald. I walked for an hour every day. I started doing my local park run and rode to chemo on my bike in the summer. Some local park runs are now hosting '5 k your way' on the last Saturday of every month, where they encourage cancer patients to run, jog or walk with their friends and family. No matter how slow you are, you are never last as there is always someone bringing up the rear, and it's a great community to get involved with.

I did a sprint-triathlon halfway through chemo, very slowly, and did a half-ironman, again, very slowly, one year after finishing treatment. It got harder to keep going as my treatment progressed, and radiotherapy drained me, but the bare minimum was a walk every day with the dog. I strongly believe that it helped me recover faster, and it made a difference to my mood. I felt I'd earned the right to sit on the sofa all day if I'd had my morning walk.

There is now a huge body of evidence showing that exercise before, during and after a cancer diagnosis can reduce the side effects and complications of treatment, help with fatigue, mental health and reduce the risk of recurrence. It should be the fourth cancer treatment prescribed to everybody. That's why I'm setting up a charity called CancerFit (www.cancerfit.me) to help inspire and encourage patients to exercise.

Thank you, Liz, those points and your book are such a wonderful resource for so many women.

Further resources
Books
The Royal Marsden Cancer Cookbook: Nutritious recipes for during and after cancer treatment, to share with friends and family.
Apps
Couch to 5k, Macmillan
Websites
https://www.parkrun.org.uk/
https://5kyourway.org
http://www.tickingoffbreastcancer.com/

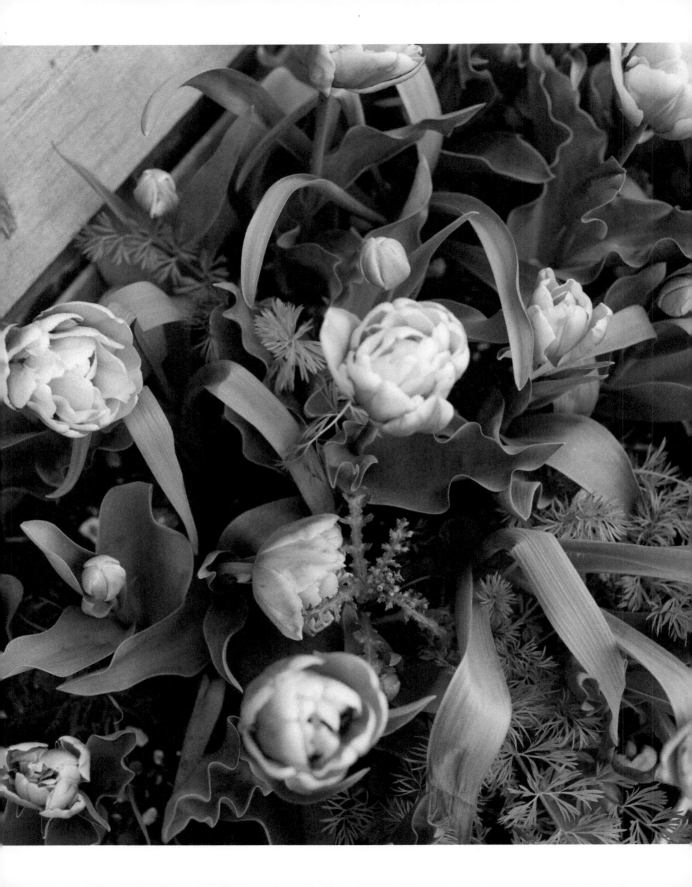

CHAPTER 8:
WISDOM IN OUR
FEMININITY

MENOPAUSE

An interesting fact is that 'menopause is a normal event'. It can have very negative connotations. In my first years as a young GP, when I looked after patients having a tough time, I developed a slight fear of my own menopause. I am going to try to dispel myths here and also help you work out when you *do* need to see a doctor for help *which is vitally important.* If you are fortunate enough to live beyond your fourth decade, menopause is going to happen.

THE MENOPAUSE AND THE WORDS USED

The average age for menopause is 51 years in the UK but there is a whole spectrum either side of this. For some women it can occur much younger...

Premature ovarian failure (POF) or primary ovarian insufficiency (POI)
This is a loss of ovarian function before the age of 40.

One in 100 women will undergo menopause naturally before 40 years (POF or POI) and many are given a medically or surgically induced *earlier menopause* from treatments they are given.

It is suggested that a **menopause is early** if it occurs between 40-45 years old. This again can be natural; or induced by surgery, where ovaries are removed; or by medication that stops the ovaries working.

POF occurs when there have been no periods for four months or so, the follicle-stimulating hormone (FSH) – the hormone that naturally rises in menopause to try to stimulate the ovaries – is raised and oestrogen reduces. This is not the same as temporary, often reversible, stopping of periods that may occur e.g. with stress, anorexia. POF can occur due to many things – infection, metabolic disease, autoimmune disorders or causes such as radiation, chemotherapy or physical damage to the ovary. It can also be linked to syndromes but many cases occur out of the blue and have a substantial genetic factor. There is a strong pattern in mother–daughter heredity in just the same way that many women can follow the menstrual pattern of their mothers. The change in POI is often more sudden over one to three years and often requires hormonal treatment and careful consideration of bone protection.

Surgical or medically induced menopause at any age can also be a shock to the system. Immediate changes often call for hormonal treatments to alleviate the physical symptoms. Sometimes after hysterectomy women *may* (**not always**) undergo hormonal changes even when the ovaries are left behind. Any procedure affecting ovarian blood supply can potentially have an impact. Women undergoing treatment for breast cancer can have dramatic debilitating changes and symptoms (see breast chapter).

WHAT IS THE MENOPAUSE?

The MENOPAUSE is the time at which menstrual periods stop.

I like the analogy 'ME NO PAUSE', and in an ideal world of perfection that would be most women's experience, but there is often no prediction of the path you are going to take.

We say you are POSTMENOPAUSAL from one year after your last period. Of course, you will not know when until it actually happens!

PERIMENOPAUSE is a term used to describe the time from the start of menstrual cycle changes until one year after the final menstrual period. In some women this can be up to ten years, in others incredibly brief. What each woman experiences and describes is highly variable. It cannot be ignored that many may also be dealing with younger children or teenagers when they start experiencing symptoms.

What tends to happen naturally to periods in this perimenopausal time?

When we are born we have ovaries containing a finite number of egg cells and, IN THEORY, from the time of menarche (starting periods) the eggs are released until they are all used up. It is often said that a woman will follow the same pattern as her mother – start periods at a similar age and complete the menopause similarly. There are of course exceptions to this. Children are often better nourished now and start periods earlier as they reach a threshold weight for the start of periods (around 45 kg). Illness and nutrition can affect the woman's path in terms of her menopause.

When a young girl is starting to menstruate, the cycles can be a little 'hit and miss' as her body becomes more efficient at ovulating. When she does release an egg, the cycle is said to be ovulatory. In some cases, they can be painful or erratic. Sometimes her body does not release an egg every month (we say she has an anovulatory cycle) hence they can be irregular at the beginning.

Why can periods become irregular and heavy before menopause, I thought they were stopping?
Similarly to that rocky time at the beginning of periods, at the end of the menstruating life the routine can become disordered and some cycles are anovulatory (no egg is released) and bleeds become further apart. Initially they may actually become closer together and **sometimes heavier**. Two to eight years prior to menopause most women begin skipping ovulations. A substance called inhibin (produced by the ovaries) decreases, decreasing our follicle-stimulating hormone levels that cause egg release. With less frequent ovulations, the lining of the womb can just build up SO thick that it eventually has to be shed (despite there being no egg released) causing a heavier bleed. This carries with it the risk of draining your iron stores or you becoming anaemic. It can lead to tiredness and **lacking in joie de vivre** at a time when you probably have a very busy life! It might be making work difficult or affecting daily tasks.

Ensure at this time that you are having a healthy balanced diet with plenty of iron and mineral rich foods and protein/healthy fats/vegetables for energy and reserve.

Any **lengthening or shortening of your usual bleed** can be downright inconvenient, although some women simply stop their periods straight off to nothing.

Suffering with heavy bleeding? See your GP.
Prioritise and emphasise your symptoms; write them down in chronological order. The GP *may* refer you for a blood test (to check for anaemia and thyroid and other tests) and possibly a scan. See my recommendations for a menopausal consultation later in this chapter. One option for treatment of heavy bleeding is to have a Mirena intrauterine system placed within the womb. This is a plastic T-shaped inert device that can be fitted by a trained GP or gynaecologist. It is passed through the cervix to sit in the womb but releases a small amount of **progesterone** locally to keep the lining of the womb quiet. Women often still ovulate with the Mirena and you may still notice the natural change of your mucous at this time every month, but the **lining of the womb will not build up** (your body detects the presence of the device and believes you are pregnant) and you will often not have bleeds once your body settles with the Mirena. It acts as an effective contraceptive, and if you have it sited around the time of menopause it can also act as

the **progesterone component** of your HRT if that is the route you choose.

It is important as with any hormonal therapy or procedure that you discuss this thoroughly with your GP/gynae or practice nurse to be aware of side effects, contraindications and risks. The Mirena is generally kept in for five years before needing to be removed and sometimes replaced; there are cases when over the menopause time it can be kept in for longer after discussion with the doctor.

If other types of HRT are being given for the bleeding, and indeed they may be helpful, other causes of the erratic bleeding need to be identified or excluded first.

What actually happens to hormones during the time LEADING UP to a natural menopause?

1. Gradually progesterone levels decline.
2. Oestrogen remains normal or increases temporarily.
3. This leads to relative excess of oestrogen (oestrogen dominance) and this will be worsened with high insulin or stress hormones.
4. Then progesterone levels start to decline more.
5. There may be swings of oestrogen up and down as some cycles are anovulatory.
6. FSH and LH levels can become erratic, with skipped ovulations, and then eventually these stabilise.
7. If oestrogen is not counterbalanced with progesterone it can block the action of your thyroid hormone. This is very complex, and adding in oestrogen alone at this time might not help.
8. EVENTUALLY OESTROGEN AND PROGESTERONE ARE BOTH DECLINED AND POSTMENOPAUSALLY THE FSH HORMONE RISES.

In the interim time before you become truly menopausal you may thus actually experience symptoms of **oestrogen dominance** as illustrated below.

Symptoms of decreasing
progesterone and relative
oestrogen dominance

decreased libido
mood swings
irregular or abnormal periods
bloating and water retention
breast swelling and tenderness
weight gain (tummy and hips)
cold extremities
headaches (especially premenstrual)

If breast swelling/pain is also a problem for you make sure your B vitamins are balanced in your diet, omega-3 and healthy fats are regularly eaten (see nutrition chapter), and try gradually reducing or stop caffeine (see breast chapter).

What is everyone saying about the menopause? I am terrified!
Fortunately for our younger allies the conversation is more open about this natural stage in our lives.

Symptoms you hear of that used to be kept quiet are:

- **Hot flushes or flashes – you may have sweat, dizziness, palpitations**
- **Night sweats accompanying above**
- **Sleep disturbance from above**
- **Vaginal dryness, soreness, itching**
- **Urinary symptoms (cystitis, frequency)**
- **Low libido**
- **Pain on intercourse**
- **Migraine sufferers may suffer more**
- **Mood disturbance (especially if you tended to PMS when younger), anxiety, panic, depression**
- **Sleep problems (often related to the sweats or flushes)**
- **Joint pains (oestrogen helps our joints be lubricated and calms inflammation so the decrease can elicit some stiffness and aching)**
- **Skin and hair changes**

Looking at those symptoms it is simple to predict that a vicious circle can arise. The lack of sleep will affect mood and libido and a general downhill spiral can develop. *Not all women are going to suffer all symptoms though.* One of my dear colleagues used to sit on the front desk of our practice and literally beg me to find something to cure her hot flushes. Others sail through with minimal symptoms.

Why the flushes?
Scientists still have some discussion as to the cause of hot flushes or flashes. It was thought to be due to low oestrogen but younger women can have lower oestrogen for other conditions and not always suffer flushes. It was then decided it was due to the CHANGE or DECREASE of oestrogen levels and that this may be causing the hypothalamus area (like a hormonal control centre at base of brain) that normally deals with temperature regulation to detect too much heat. Then the brain releases hormones to try to regulate temperature and effectively lower it. The blood vessels on the skin dilate or expand to dissipate heat and the increased blood flow then activates the body's cooling mechanism and sweating occurs.

Hot flushes can also be called *vasomotor flushes* and they are characterised by a feeling of heat and sweating, particularly around the head and neck. Thus, the embarrassment and discomfort can be really upsetting, especially in the workplace. It can affect up to 85% of women at some point in the menopausal time; but having said that, for many it is just a sensation of warmth and slight sweating. It can be out of the blue or linked to certain food or alcohol, e.g. wine. Night sweats can be dramatic, requiring a change of sheets.

The textbooks say that 'about half of women have slight perimenopausal symptoms that last for a year. A quarter of women usually seek help for their symptoms'.

For up to 15% it is worse – **hourly waves of intense heat and drenching sweat** so day and night are constantly interrupted. The sleep disturbance can of course in that case soon lead to feelings of depression and low mood (see sleep chapter). We can never know of course what proportion of women suffer as many may never discuss their symptoms.

So, let us say that you are suffering enough to want to seek help. Talking to your doctor is essential. You can first of all try what you can do at home if you feel you are not desperate. Let's start simple.

Avoid triggers for flushes: spicy food; limit wine if this makes you worse – try sulphite-free organic wine (anecdotal as can help with allergies as less histamine is released – may help with flushes). Reduce caffeine as it might exacerbate anxiety and flushing.

Cooler bedroom and clothing. Cool clothing not only includes cotton. Fabrics have been developed for women's comfort. Read my interview later on with the ladies from 'Cucumber Clothing' who saw a need for their sustainable and revolutionary sleepwear to wick away moisture and aid cooling at night.

Remember if you have had a night of sweats you must **recoup fluids** lost by keeping some water beside your bed. This will reduce the severity of any headaches and reduce the risk of urinary symptoms from dehydration.

Think sexy. This may be a time when you have more time for each other and, once you are properly postmenopausal (see contraception below), no longer need to worry about the risk of unwanted pregnancy. Some women **feel reborn** as they may have less day-to-day exhausting responsibility – children leave home, or their nine-to-five ends. It is important not to dismiss your sex life. Hell no! Before we get onto HRT think about lubricants and vaginal moisturisers that could help. There is no shame and we need to stop the stigma around vaginal dryness or soreness. It is debilitating and could affect not just your sex life but your day-to-day comfort, cause burning, itching and urinary symptoms. More of that later.

Yoga. May help **sleep** and in turn deal with other symptoms.

Cognitive Behavioural Therapy. May reduce impact of hot flushes by 50% – group therapy improved quality of life more, but self-help was good for symptom management. Power of the mind is strong, and stopping a cycle of panic and anxiety in its tracks may take the edge off.

Read my Meditation*, Acupuncture** and Meditation** app sections (*Happiness **A broader approach).

Acupuncture is effective but not as much as HRT of course.

Hypnotherapy. Clinical hypnosis has studies showing its efficacy on flushes.

Look at your plate. We now know that the gut and the brain are directly linked, and the gut microbiome communicates directly with the brain via chemicals or hormones that act as messengers and may influence our mood and behaviour. Give your gut plenty of plant-based nutrients and encourage healthy bacteria and you will inevitably have more chance of being happier. Feed your gut with over-processed white carbs and white sugar and the less good bacteria thrive and you could potentially be down in the dumps. Alongside that, flushes and symptoms related to menopause may be worsened if you are low in minerals such as zinc and magnesium. Making sure you have a plate enriched with all the nutrients you require before, during and after the menopause may massively help you and can do no harm.

Think of your bones. Please see the bone chapter.

Supplements. The supplements I was taught about have survived in being recommended years later but some have been considered possible to cause harm. My favourites for hormone-related mood swings or depression always included a trial of vitamin B6 50mg which may make the boat ride a little less jumpy and smooth things out. You may need to wait six weeks to three months for the benefit. Do not take excess or there may be side effects and talk to your doctor first. Evening primrose oil and starflower oil are ones to read about, and then we come to red clover and black cohosh. Some women find they help, but black cohosh can affect the liver in some ladies and cause toxicity, and they can both interact and cause problems with drugs like tamoxifen. As with any causes of depression some people turn to St John's wort, and just as this can reduce the working of the contraceptive pill in younger life it can also affect the metabolism of other drugs and cause problems because it speeds up the chemicals (enzymes) in the liver. All things natural are not always without power to cause harm; remember, many conventional powerful medicines are derived from plants. Speak to your doctor to advise you.

Contraception in the perimenopause

Some women believe that because fertility declines with age, they can just stop using contraception in their 30s or 40s. **Contraception should be continued for at least one year after your last menstrual period if this was after the age of 50, and for two years if your periods stop before 50.** This is because sometimes periods may restart even after several months without bleeding. Some hormonal contraceptive methods such as 'progestogen only' will mean you only have occasional periods or none, so discuss with your doctor what to do to evaluate if you are menopausal. Alternatively, it is thought that after 55 fertility is incredibly low, so contraception can *then* be stopped. Hormonal contraception or HRT means that blood tests are unreliable. HRT is not a method of contraception. Use barrier methods or discuss with your doctor using the Mirena as the progesterone component.

Seeing the doctor about menopause symptoms

You are suffering, and all this just isn't kicking it. You book an appointment with your doctor who knows you, or maybe the doctor in your practice who has a special interest in the menopause, or maybe you found a doctor in the **Menopause Society** who is noted for their interest and knowledge (www.menopausesociety.co.uk).

Before your appointment, just like if consulting for heavy bleeding, prepare. Write out your symptoms along a timeline. Doctors love a *prioritised* list – not your most bothersome thing at the end as you go out the door. Come with a written list and lay it on the doctor's desk. They know immediately the reason for you attending and it is easier then to prioritise what can be dealt with today and what may need a repeat visit for another day.

What might the GP do?

The GP may refer you for a blood test and a scan if they think there is another gynaecological cause (this will be an ultrasound and, depending on the view needed, will be done through the tummy – *transabdominal* – or via a sterile probe in the vagina – *transvaginal*). Many of the conditions listed in the abnormal bleeding section of this chapter and others may be checked for this way – fibroids/polyps/ovarian cysts/checking the lining of the womb for overgrowth or hyperplasia. These may all need to be dealt with alongside menopausal symptoms.

If you are over 45 and having irregular periods and symptoms of the menopause it is not likely that the doctor will need to do blood tests to diagnose the menopause. If you are younger than this they may do an FSH test (follicle-stimulating hormone), and if this is raised it may indicate you are menopausal. It can also be raised in other situations, such as polycystic ovarian syndrome or some chromosome abnormalities, and it will be important for the doctor to know of other symptoms/contraception and so on before interpreting the test when you are younger. Younger women may also be referred for a bone density scan (DEXA) – see bone chapter.

LET US TALK HORMONES AND HRT

Until menopause the primary oestrogen a woman produces is OESTRADIOL. During perimenopause the body starts making more OESTRONE, produced both in the ovaries and body fat. Testosterone is still released from the ovaries after menopause although production does decrease with age. PROGESTERONE FALLS PERIMENOPAUSALLY, OFTEN AS THE FIRST CHANGE. Oestrogen and androgens (like testosterone) maintain bones and vaginal and urethral tissue. Oestrogen and progesterone maintain a healthy layer of collagen in the skin. We naturally make all of these hormones from the precursor cholesterol molecule.

Why looking after yourself is key

Perimenopause is a natural state and our bodies are designed to produce the correct amount of hormones but *only if we are healthy physically and emotionally* as we enter this period. The ease of transition can be influenced by our lifestyle, general health and the demands we place on ourselves. The ovaries still function, they just slow (if still intact), and other tissues such as fat, skin, brain and adrenals share some of the hormone production. Synthetic or other hormonal-affecting supplements or medication may be the answer but also consider managing stress and how you look after yourself. I am not saying we should lie down and give up; to the contrary – look holistically and use this time positively as a wake-up call to order things in your life that have been neglected as well as seeking professional help.

Why stress needs to be dealt with

At the risk of too much chemistry in this book I want to explain why stress is so tough with menopause change. In our bodies we make cortisol (the stress hormone) from cholesterol and we also make oestrogen and testosterone from cholesterol. If we are stressed the body favours the cortisol path so you can see you can lower your natural oestrogen and testosterone levels if you are stressed. The extra cortisol will encourage fat around the tummy too. So meditating and relaxing actually encourages the healthier path to more oestrogen. Relaxing is paramount. This also explains why with our demanding lives menopause can be such a physical struggle both in the workplace and at home.

Previous hysterectomy

If you gave oestrogen **alone** to a woman with her womb intact, the oestrogen would stimulate the lining of the womb to build up and in some cases undergo cancerous changes.

Progesterone has a protective effect on the womb by stopping the lining building up. Progesterone causes the lining to shed or not build up in this way and thus protects from the stimulating effect of oestrogen. Thus you can see that just because your friend after a hysterectomy may only use, say, oestrogen gel, doesn't mean you can have exactly the same HRT as her if you still have a womb. **HRT should be tailored to the individual lady and her needs.**

If you have no uterus

If you have had a hysterectomy and have no womb, then you have no womb lining (endometrial lining). You can have HRT that does not include progesterone and just have oestrogen.

You have a uterus

You will need to have progesterone and oestrogen combined HRT. For the first year you will usually have it as what we call *sequential or cyclical* – for some days of the month you will take progesterone and this will allow the womb lining to shed. Once you have taken this for a year you can often change to continuous combined HRT. This combines both hormones and does not usually result in bleeds but you may bleed in the first six months due to your body acclimatising. If women are starting HRT more than one year after their last period they are often given continuous combined HRT, and this is thought to be better for the womb lining than sequential HRT by 53 years.

Risks are complex. The lower risk is oestrogen – in gel or patches – as it does not have to go through the liver to be used in the body. Transdermal preparations (through the skin as a patch or gel) are associated with lower cardiovascular risk and may often be chosen for smokers, migraine sufferers and so on. The Women's Health Study in 2000 reported some of the risks in a way that frightened doctors away from prescribing HRT. The study was done in older ladies over 60 and was not the same as giving HRT to women just going through the menopause. HRT has also evolved somewhat, and the patient will always be managed on the minimum dose possible. Most of our HRT was derived from pregnant female horses' urine that could contain up to ten different oestrogens and other metabolites we may not need as humans. Now we also have other HRT formulations to choose from. Doctors may now choose newer formulations and use the equine-related medications as second line.

What are bioidentical hormones?

These are plant-derived hormones which are structurally identical to those we make in our body. They contain a variety of different hormones (including oestrogens and progestogens) at different potencies.

These are prescribed in many independent private clinics. They **are not generally prescribed** by conventional doctors within the NHS. Often the dose is calculated after symptoms are written down in a questionnaire, or in some cases after a saliva test that measures hormone levels. Saliva tests can vary greatly in accuracy and may be affected by time of day and so on. Bioidentical hormones are usually a mixture of 'oestrogen and progesterone like hormone' *allegedly* tailormade to the individual. **The problem with them from a conventional doctor's standpoint is that they are not regulated, we need more efficacy and safety data and, if you take natural progesterone as an example, if given in an unsupervised dose this may not be enough to protect the endometrium lining and protect from the oestrogen component of the compound HRT. Speak to your specialist.**

Body identical hormones

These are licensed for prescription in the UK. They are more similar to our natural hormones and are derived from yam (root vegetable). They tend to be 17 beta-oestradiol combined with micronised progesterone. Micronised progesterone means it is made into very small drug particles that can stay active once in the body (biologically active) and work where **needed** in the womb lining and have less side effects than other progesterone HRT in terms of metabolic and vascular risks. **There is evidence of reduced risks with HRT preparations containing micronised progesterone.**

Conventional HRT

This is usually bioidentical oestrogen as above but with a synthetic progestogen. There are various preparations and the doctor will choose the best for you to maintain you on the lowest dose to relieve symptoms. There are various routes of delivery – patches, tablets and topical gels/vaginal capsules. There is a new preparation for those women with a womb and who cannot have progesterone but more studies are needed to assess long-term safety.

When you go to the consultation, a doctor who is informed will decide with you what is appropriate and whether the advantages outweigh the risks for you. The risks of HRT include blood clot, migraine, stroke, breast and ovarian cancer, and the advantages are increased libido and energy, bone and cardiovascular protection while you are on it and skin and hair changes and so on. The symptoms of the menopause will disappear, but it is important that this is managed on the *minimal possible dose* for you. There should be a chart of risks, as shown in the NICE guidelines, that the doctor discusses with you and possibly prints out so you can assess whether you are happy to go the HRT route or would rather try other approaches. The first type you try may not be the right one for you and if, say, HRT patches irritate your skin you may need to change brand – one of my patients used to find her HRT patch was sweated off at night and often found stuck to her husband!

How long to stay on HRT?

This is really a discussion to have with your doctor regularly, monitoring being essential. It is important that you realise that you *may* go through a menopausal change of sorts when coming off HRT as your hormones return to their natural postmenopausal level.

Even during the time of researching and preparing for this book new research arose looking at risks and advantages of HRT. **What is important is that each woman is different.** Our risk factors, our symptoms and our needs are all different and ever-changing. Having any risk increased is too much for some women psychologically; others will weigh up factors and choose to take medication. Our risk is altered by age and the type of HRT. Being **overweight, drinking alcohol, smoking, not exercising** may give you a raised risk of breast cancer that may be higher than that from HRT, so everything needs to be taken into account. HRT started close to the menopause may also reduce mortality and cardiac death, as shown in a recent systematic review. Oestrogen-only preparations are lower risk than combined HRT. This is a complex ever-changing field. What is important is **talking to a doctor you trust** who can guide you to the correct route for you that is regularly checked and reviewed. Many women choose to take HRT and their quality of life is improved by it, for others HRT will not be a suitable decision personally or medically. This needs to be an individual doctor–patient decision and not one to decipher from reading a book.

Read about testosterone in my chapter on motivation and muscle.

A NOTE ABOUT THE THYROID

This book can never cover everything but it is worth noting that thyroid problems (the thyroid is the gland on the front of the neck that produces thyroxine) can cause many symptoms for women and exacerbate symptoms of the menopause or even almost mimic some of the symptoms if it is say, underactive or overactive. If you have new symptoms of fatigue, unexplained weight change, anxiety, hair loss, tiredness, sensitivity to cold, memory problems than discuss with your doctor and the thyroid may be an issue.

OTHER NON-HORMONAL MEDICAL TREATMENTS FOR THE VASOMOTOR SYMPTOMS (FLUSHES AND SWEATS)

- **Clonidine**. This works by acting on certain receptors in the cardiovascular system and can be helpful for flushes – side effects can be dry mouth, insomnia, dizziness or constipation.
- **SSRI-type antidepressants** (citalopram, escitalopram, paroxetine, fluoxetine) and **SNRI-type** (venlafaxine). Side effects include dry mouth, nausea, dizziness, constipation, tiredness, sexual dysfunction. None of these non-hormonal agents are recommended by NICE as first-line treatment alone. Paroxetine and fluoxetine have to be avoided in women on tamoxifen as they reduce its ability to work in the body.

Resources
British Menopause Society www.thebms.org.uk
NICE guideline: Diagnosis and Management of the Menopause
A great resource is www.positivepause.co.uk, which aims to put colour into a grey subject – the menopause! With their colourful, cheerful website, social media platforms and innovative events for women and organisations, PositivePause share the latest evidence-based expert advice on women's health and wellbeing before, during and after menopause, helping women to make informed choices about managing the menopause based on their unique health history and values.

ABNORMAL OR DYSFUNCTIONAL UTERINE BLEEDING

THIS INCLUDES ANY BLEEDING OUTSIDE OF THE NORMAL MENSTRUAL CYCLE

This can be caused by something gynaecological, your general medical state or from medications you are taking. We call abnormal uterine bleeding anything that includes:

- Bleeding between periods if you are still menstruating
- Postmenopausal bleeding if you have actually reached the menopause (i.e. 12 months after your last period) and then bleeding has occurred after this 12-month gap. **Bleeding after a year of no bleeding should always be investigated so make sure you talk to your doctor.**

This list may not be exhaustive, and by your doctor taking a careful history and examining you and sending you off for further investigations an answer will be found and prompt treatment can be given.

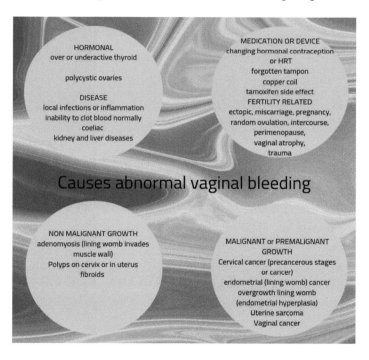

IN BRIEF, OTHER POSSIBLE CONDITIONS IN MIDLIFE

Uterine polyps

Small growths in the inner wall of the womb formed by overgrowth of the endometrium (lining). These are usually benign but some can become precancerous or cancerous. They can be from millimetres to a few centimetres in size and tend to be pedunculated on a stalk or with a broad base. They are more common postmenopausally.

Symptoms: bleeding between periods/irregular/heavy postmenopausal

Treatment: surgical removal

Cervical polyps

Small growths on the cervix that can be seen by the doctor when passing a speculum. They can sometimes be removed in outpatients by a specialist or may require surgery. They can be a cause of bleeding after sex/between periods and discomfort.

This is obviously a time to keep up with your (Pap) cervical smears until you are no longer recalled for them.

Uterine fibroids

Benign lumps in the womb wall made of muscle and fibrous tissue; they almost never develop into cancer. They can be tiny, all the way up to those that distort the whole uterus.

Symptoms: may be none or can cause heavy or prolonged periods. Larger fibroids can cause pain, frequent urination and sometimes problems opening the bladder or bowels depending on position.

Treatment: may shrink after menopause. They are sometimes injected or operated on to remove.

Adenomyosis

Tissue normally found in the womb inner lining that sheds with a period; found deep in the womb muscle wall and every month can cause intense pain and heavy or prolonged bleeding. *This can also develop at the site of previous surgery like caesarean or fibroid surgery in the scar area.* Its growth is oestrogen dependent and should reduce/shrink back after menopause. Endometriosis is similar but occurs at other sites – less common postmenopausally.

Endometrial hyperplasia

The lining of the womb (endometrium) becomes thickened and may return to normal without treatment but if left *can go on* to develop into cancer of the womb lining (**endometrial cancer**). **A biopsy or sample of the lining of the womb can be taken by a specialised GP or gynaecologist** and the cells examined under the microscope. If the cells are normal and just overgrown this is less cause for alarm than atypical (abnormal) cells requiring treatment.

VAGINAL DRYNESS

Yes, let's go there!

This can manifest as:

- itching, soreness
- pain or discomfort on intercourse

- frequency of peeing increasing
- recurrent urinary tract infections

This can affect your libido, self-esteem and any relationship. Causes of increased vaginal dryness include breastfeeding, contraceptive pills, some antidepressants, after hysterectomy, chemotherapy, radiotherapy. Occasionally dryness and atrophy as explained below can be related to diabetes or syndromes involving dryness elsewhere such as Sjogren's.

Temporary dryness can be caused by:

- not being aroused during sex/anxiety
- using perfumed douches/washes/soaps in and around the vulval and vaginal region.

Before consulting your doctor, if it is a new problem there are some simple remedies you can try:

- water-based lubricants PRIOR to sex used by either partner; plus/- vaginal moisturiser (in certain clinical situations your GP may prescribe these). Both these products are recommended by leading UK menopause specialists.

   Sylk is paraben-free and made with plant-based ingredients: www.sylk.co.uk.

   YES has a vaginal moisturiser and a personal lubricant (both water-based). They are certified organic and not made with parabens, hormones or other concerning chemicals. They are also pH matched to the vagina to help maintain vaginal health and avoid bacterial and yeast infections www.yesyesyes.org.
- only unperfumed soaps and shower washes around this area, or simply water.
- taking your time with sex so you don't feel rushed.

If this is not working, then see the GP. *See the GP sooner if there is bleeding or discharge that is not normal for you or if you have bleeding after sex.* If you are very uncomfortable in the daytime, seek help from the doctor. Be reassured that the surgery will understand if you want to request a female doctor and that doctors are quite used to looking at these problems to find a solution and are not remotely embarrassed. They will be anxious to find the cause and offer you a solution.

If **vaginal atrophy** occurs, where the tissue shrinks (so thinning and drying of the vaginal walls) in response to declining levels of oestrogen, in certain situations it can cause shortening and narrowing of the vagina and cause great discomfort on a daily basis in routine activities (and sex may become downright impossible). It is thought that half of postmenopausal women won't actually seek help as they are embarrassed and think they should put up with the symptoms, which is nonsense. This needs to be examined by the doctor who can in most cases prescribe **topical** (applied just to that area) oestrogen. As the tissue becomes resupplied with oestrogen, not only can tissue become thicker and less likely to cause discomfort, but the tissue becomes recolonised with healthier bacteria (lactobacilli) and symptoms reduce. It is important not to leave this too late as a vicious cycle of symptoms called urogenital syndrome can occur with urinary and vaginal symptoms. Oestrogen gel or cream or pessaries is used in a minimal dose; if required long term, then progesterone may be given to protect the lining of the womb building up.

Vaginismus

For various reasons in many women, sex can feel impossible or uncomfortable because the walls of the vagina squeeze down and this area cannot relax. This can be due to psychological reasons and may be related to traumatic experiences in the past, childbirth or episiotomy scarring as well as being triggered by general discomfort. It is important that women seek help with this. Physiotherapists and sex therapists often recommend objects called vaginal trainers of differing sizes to gradually encourage relaxation of the area. Relaxation techniques can help and strengthening your pelvic floor paradoxically gives you the control to relax the area when needed.

If there is discomfort or itching there, do not assume it is thrush. If there are symptoms of soreness or a spot/lesion develops it is important to discuss this with your doctor. Swabs can be taken and, if lesions seen, referrals made for investigation. Medical professionals are trying to encourage women to not be shy about examining themselves with a mirror and noticing any changes and reporting them, so they can be treated at early stages.

Jane Lewis has written a fabulous book, *Me and My Menopausal Vagina: Living with Vaginal Atrophy*, which has started an open conversation for many women.

Risk factors for vaginal atrophy

Smoking can increase the chance of vaginal atrophy as the blood and oxygen supply to the area is reduced. All causes of hormonal change and menopause can affect this area. It is important that symptoms are addressed so that opportune infections here cannot arise.

A worthy note about lichen sclerosus

This is a skin condition causing white patches on the skin and can affect the genital area. If you find a patch around the vulval or anal region, and it is likely to be itchy and may bleed or hurt if rubbed or scratched, then see your GP. The skin can become scarred and tightened over time and it is easy to see how that would then cause discomfort around this area during sex/opening bowels or weeing. The condition does carry with it a greater risk of vulval cancer. The risk is still low but worth checking regularly and seeing your GP for advice.

Vulval cancer

This is rare and can affect any of this area. It is mainly in women over 65 but can occur earlier. Any changes around here – persistent itch or soreness, changes in the skin (can be raised and thickened – red, white or dark or even wart-like or an open sore), bleeding from the area or bloodstained discharge, pain passing urine that is persistent – need to be checked by the GP.

Here is a good time to hear from Clare and her own experience and great insightful work setting up an organisation to raise awareness of these conditions.

A PERSONAL STORY FROM CLARE...

I was diagnosed at 43 with lichen sclerosus and vulval cancer stage 3. I had never heard of either condition before.

I had been diagnosed with cystitis and thrush many times, and when I looked back at the struggle to find a diagnosis, I realised there needed to be more awareness and understanding of my conditions in both the public arena and healthcare system. I had already started a closed Facebook vulval cancer support group and was in a lichen sclerosus group where I met my colleague Emma. We wanted to raise awareness of both conditions so teamed up together and launched our website, Lsvcukawareness.weebly.com, linking to our Facebook awareness pages.

By the site and running annual campaigns we aim to raise the understanding of:

- Vulval cancer
- Lichen sclerosus (LS)
- Vaginal atrophy

and we offer information and support.

I also created a UK support group for those diagnosed with vulval intraepithelial neoplasia (VIN) and for those with lymphoedema from gynaecological cancer treatment that can affect not just groin and legs but pelvis and genitals.

Getting the message across

We produce information leaflets for LS and vulval cancer, and I have presented at the RCOG world congress as a patient representative. I am also a member of their forum which aims to improve gynaecological health for women.

Future plans

To improve medical professional training in both conditions and campaign for more research so we can better understand the causes and save more women's lives.

"Our hope is that gynaecological issues, that many women face daily, will be openly discussed and women will no longer have to suffer in silence."

Thank you so much Clare.

OVARIAN CANCER – THE SILENT KILLER

Ovarian cancer is often called a silent killer but this is a little of a misnomer. It does usually have symptoms but these can be ignored or misdiagnosed. One way to improve this is to educate women and medical professionals about the signs and symptoms that could easily be mistaken for other conditions or ignored. Average women living in the UK have a 2% lifetime risk of developing ovarian cancer. Unfortunately, most are diagnosed only at the time they have advanced disease. Less than a third are diagnosed at early stages. More than half of the deaths occur in women over 65 years. Survival rates have however improved, especially in younger women. Of all the gynaecology cancers it still has the worse prognosis. Whether this is from delay in seeking help and just ignoring symptoms, or a delay in actual diagnosis, the figures show we need to identify it earlier. Some women will only be diagnosed when they present in a casualty department with severe symptoms.

Doctors learn many facts about disease and risk factors. Risk factors make your chance of getting a disease more likely but of course this is not absolute and does not apply in every individual case. What we do know is that the risk factors for ovarian cancer are:

- Obesity
- Smoking
- Risk increases with age (80% diagnosed over 50 yrs)
- Patients with a history of endometriosis
- Patients with a family history of ovarian or breast cancer
- Those with BRCA1 and 2 genes have a lifetime risk of ovarian cancer of 40%
- Genetic testing and counselling is obviously a much debated topic over recent years and has to be handled delicately and professionally by medical teams.

Having children and having taken the contraceptive pill can protect you to a certain extent from ovarian cancer as at these stages the ovaries are kept quiet (not ovulating or releasing an egg). If you took the combined contraceptive pill for more than 15 years, the protective effect on your ovaries can last 30 years! Talcum powder – using this between your legs has been suggested in some studies to increase the risk but studies are inconsistent and the risk may still be small but worth bearing in mind.

Many women have symptoms in middle age and beyond that can be difficult to pin down. Many people label themselves as having irritable bowel syndrome; there can be some overlap between bowel symptoms and what happens in ovarian disease.

Symptoms with ovarian cancer do not tend to be intermittent, but permanent and worsen over time...

- Feeling constantly bloated (not relieved by opening bowels)
- Swollen tummy

- A feeling of feeling full all the time or feeling full up with minimal food or loss of appetite
- Pain or discomfort in the tummy or pelvic area
- Needing to wee more frequently or more urgently

Other symptoms:

- Pain on intercourse
- Loss of weight unintentionally
- Back pain
- Tiredness
- Changes in bowel habit
- Bleeding that is not normal for you or postmenopausal

It is obvious that all of these symptoms can occur in other conditions, and this is where the doctor should be your first step to ask you more questions to decide whether further tests are needed. If you have been feeling bloated, particularly more than 12 times a month, it is suggested you see your doctor.

The doctor can then decide whether a blood test and ultrasound are needed and these will be interpreted carefully along with all of the symptoms.

What is worrying is that many women have had symptoms up to a year before diagnosis.

In conclusion, there is real wisdom in your femininity...

The general message of this book should be that if something does not feel right then get it checked. So many of us are frightened or reluctant to be examined – don't be. Many recent campaigns in the UK are addressing just this issue.

Further Resource
@eveappeal on Facebook, Twitter, Instagram
www.eveappeal.org.uk

The Eve Appeal is the UK's leading gynaecological cancer research charity with a unique focus on the prevention, risk prediction and early diagnosis of all five gynaecological cancers. As well as funding research, they raise awareness of the signs and symptoms of the gynae cancers, break down the culture of shame surrounding women's bodies and run a nurse-led information service, Ask Eve, to answer gynaecological questions and concerns.
nurse@eveappeal.org.uk 0808 802 0019

Women are complex.

Not just our minds! Our bodies are **extremely** complex – like men, only different. There are a large number of organs in a small space in our pelvis. The bladder, the womb, ovaries and intestines are all within this bony space sitting above the pelvic floor, which is a muscle group across the area, shaped like a bowl. In a woman's lifetime she may go through pregnancy, childbirth, heavy lifting, sports, weight gain, and the delicate pelvic organs are all supported by this muscle group. When things are stressed too much and when the muscle strength declines with age and hormonal change, there may be a shift in the anatomy and things don't end up exactly where they used to be.

The pelvic floor can be damaged by pregnancy, childbirth, chronic coughing, straining, constipation or connective tissue disorders and this causes the walls of the vagina to become weakened as they are not supported by the sling of the pelvic floor, and then either the front (near the bladder) or the back (near the rectum) descend into the vaginal space. In severe cases the uterus is not supported and the cervix area can descend downward. If this happens to you then see your doctor to discuss management.

The importance of Kegel exercises

Pelvic floor exercises are mentioned to us at different stages of our lives and most of us do not take notice until something goes wrong. A leak of urine on coughing/sneezing/laughing or a need to run to the loo quickly, problems related to opening your bowels, or a dragging sensation below as though things aren't in the right place, and one can immediately panic and feel completely desperate and lonely.

Urinary incontinence

This is the unwanted or involuntary loss of urine – out of our control. It can cause embarrassment, worry and even fear of leaving home, massively affecting self-esteem and quality of life.

This can affect women at any age and we divide it into **stress incontinence** (loss of urine when bladder is under pressure – sneezing, coughing, laughing hard, jumping) and **urge incontinence** (need to run to the loo quickly). Sometimes the scenario can be a combination of the two.

Up to half of us may experience incontinence at some time in our lives. The problems can range from mild leaking to uncontrollable wetting and needing to constantly wear a pad.

Stress incontinence

This occurs when you increase your intraabdominal pressure so much with, say, a cough or sneeze that the muscle holding the urethra closed (urethral sphincter) cannot hold back the urine that is in the bladder.

Causes of stress incontinence

Pelvic floor muscle weakness, during pregnancy, after childbirth, chronic cough, excess tummy fat increasing the pressure in the abdomen, and sometimes genetic causes of connective tissue weakness in which case there is a family history. Diabetes and multiple sclerosis, etc. can all affect the nerves associated with this area.

Getting help and helping yourself

At this stage it is a good idea to **visit your GP** who will examine you, exclude anything else going on such as infection or pathology, and give you a diagnosis. They may advise you to reduce caffeine which may be making your bladder more sensitive or look at the effects of any medication you are taking, like water tablets (diuretics). If they do not need to refer you to a specialist they may talk to you about physiotherapy or doing Kegel (pelvic floor) exercises yourself. These can be difficult to perform at first, much helped by explanation from a physio. You need to know you are doing them correctly and with adequate rest for the muscle to relax in between. Up to three-quarters of women can have symptoms resolved by doing physiotherapy. Kegel exercises involve squeezing the pubococcygeus muscle which is the same muscle we use to stop the stream of urine. It is not a good idea to practise this while passing urine though. Relaxing in between squeezing this muscle is just as important in treatment as contracting. The exercises will not work well if you are contracting other areas at the same time like the tummy, thigh or buttocks as you will be overall increasing the intraabdominal pressure and compounding the problem. If you are being taught by a physio, which is ideal to start with, they will recommend that you maybe place a hand on your tummy to start to remind you to keep that area soft and relaxed. Some women find a weighted cone that they hold in the vagina for a period of time up to five minutes helps them, increasing the weight of the cone as strength progresses. These can be helpful if there is straightforward stress incontinence. In theory if you are practised at performing Kegel exercises you can do them whenever you have a moment without anyone knowing (if you do not facially contort simultaneously which I personally have a tendency to do!). With regular exercises you may also be increasing the blood supply to this area making you generally more resistant to infections possibly. Interestingly caffeinated and decaffeinated coffee can both be a bit of a bladder irritant but make sure you replace any java you give up with water.

If you want to help yourself and you have no contraindications after checking with your doctor and physio (pelvic cancer, pacemaker, recent surgery or pregnancy) then I cannot recommend a pelvic floor machine like Kegel8 Ultra 20 highly enough. This is my personal opinion, not an advert. There are different internal probes for different uses, clearly explained on the website, and if you do not feel that using a probe is right for you, you can try the electrodes that are placed on your back – a little like a TENS machine given in the hospital during labour. Many of the probes can be used while you keep active. At first you will probably want to use it reclining peacefully on your bed, following the instructions and finding the correct frequency and programme that works for you. You may find it more comfortable and supportive to wear a large sanitary pad and pants while using the probe so you can get on with daily activities whilst secretly pelvic training.

We need to start the conversation with our daughters and each other, to encourage awareness to strengthen the pelvic floor to prevent these conditions and possibly reduce the need for future surgery. See my fantastic interview with the lovely Christien Bird at the end of this chapter for more information about our pelvic floors and everything down below from the point of view of a specialist physio.

Urge incontinence

This is another name for an overactive bladder. If bladder muscles become too active you can sense the need to go to the bathroom even with a small amount of urine in your bladder, as occurs with cystitis. Women with urge incontinence can find themselves repeatedly visiting the bathroom in the day and planning trips out around locations of toilets. If infection is not present then this is something the doctor can advise you about in terms of trying medicine to make the bladder less active (although these anticholinergic medicines can have side effects like causing a dry mouth), exercises and bladder training, or even referral to a specialist doctor. Bladder training involves trying to train your bladder to go to the bathroom at more spaced-out intervals, gradually increasing in time! A recent review study showed that behavioural therapy (exercises to strengthen bladder floor or bladder training) was more effective than drugs in treating stress or urge incontinence in women.

A urologist or gynaecologist referral may be an option in all cases. Choices for some cases include surgery but sometimes the solution might be a pessary that is a plastic or rubber device within the vagina to support any prolapse while exercising or to be worn permanently in certain cases. These are fitted to the correct size by an experienced nurse practitioner. Incontinence pessaries lift up the bladder neck and restore your control of urine flow. If the problem is only during certain activities, like dancing or exercise classes, then a Reliance Urinary Control Insert can be used, rather like a small tampon, and these can be disposable.

Postmenopausal incontinence

The outer third of the urethra is oestrogen sensitive and this can mean that after menopause this area thins, increasing the chance of urine infections and stress incontinence. The topical use of oestrogen gel can be very helpful and is done in a controlled way with a dose that gradually reduces to the minimum to control symptoms. A very small regulated amount is needed, and as it is used locally only the systemic effects are reduced.

As you can see there are many options before a lifetime of using urinary pads is the only choice. Talking to your doctor or nurse is a brave and essential first step and something they will be well used to dealing with.

A physio appointment may change your life in this scenario.

Christien Bird is an expert physio at the White Hart Clinic in London. Here she shares some wisdom with me...

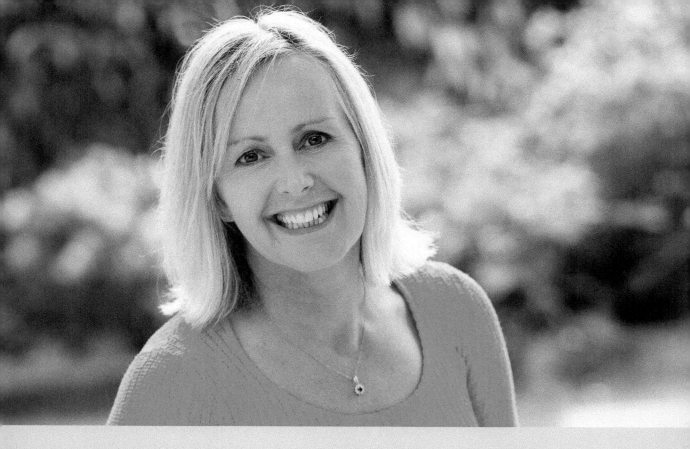

Tell me about a general pelvic floor check around the menopause

Oestrogen is like water to the garden, nearly all cells in your body have oestrogen receptors. Your vaginal & bladder tissue needs more oestrogen (the plant in the garden that needs lots of water) than other tissues. It means once oestrogen starts fluctuating you can start experiencing an increase in urinary leakage, urgency (that key in the door moment), bowel issues, prolapse symptoms, and your sexual experience can start to change. This is a key time to have a pelvic health check.

A women's health specialist is a chartered therapist that has specialised training in pelvic health. A 'normal' physio will treat movement issues related to all your joints and muscles; a women's health specialist assesses and treats problems related to your pelvis (pubic symphysis or sacro-iliac joints), abdominal wall, vulva, vagina, uterus, bladder and bowel.

We also work closely with other disciplines, including gynaecologists and osteopaths.

What can I expect at my first appointment?

We will ask you what your expectations are and ask about your general & gynaecological health, bowel, bladder & sexual history or symptoms. We will talk about current activity levels and work on an exercise plan that works for you. During the first assessment we perform a full pelvic and movement assessment, including the abdominal wall, core and internal assessment.

Do I have to have an internal examination?

Most women's health assessments involve an internal examination; however, we will make sure that you are fully comfortable with this before we do. We use medical gloves and lubrication to assess your pelvic floor muscle function as well as the position of your bladder, rectum and uterus at rest and during movement. We provide a non-judgemental and safe environment. There is no such thing as a 'normal' vagina; you can talk to us about anything that concerns you, it is all totally fine.

Which parts will you examine?

The external pelvis & vulva, internal vaginal walls and abdominal wall and anything else that is relevant to any issues you may have. If you present with bowel issues, occasionally a rectal exam may be helpful; again, we will discuss this with you first – the most important thing is that you are comfortable.

Will it hurt?

A women's health specialist internal assessment does not usually hurt (but please let us know if you have a history of pain with sex or with previous internal examinations).

Do I need to look?

You don't need to look. We do generally encourage women to look with a mirror and become familiar with their anatomy. This will help you to check yourself for any changes, similar to a breast self-examination.

What type of things do you treat?

Bladder leakage, bladder urgency, pelvic floor muscle weakness or over-activity, pelvic pain, tummy separation (diastasis), painful sex, constipation, bowel urgency, bowel incontinence and prolapses.

What will you teach me?

Depending on what we find during the assessment, we might work on the breath or teach you how to do a pelvic floor muscle activation; we will make sure you can go home confident you are doing the right thing. We may give you pelvic floor muscle strengthening or release work, teach you strategies on how to best activate your core, bladder retraining; a whole range of things depending on your expectations and our findings.

How many sessions will I need?

It all depends on what we find – we will discuss and agree on a plan with you – sometimes one session is enough, possibly four to six sessions are needed; few people need to come for a longer period of time. We always work towards helping you to be as comfortable with self-managing your condition as possible.

What type of things will you get me to do at home?

Almost certainly pelvic floor muscle exercises and/or release connected to your breath. Depending on our findings, it might range from bladder retraining, abdominal work to knowing how to do a perfect poo!

Are they all GP referrals or can a woman self-refer?

We receive self-referral, GP and consultants, doulas, women's health charities that recommend, as well as companies we have close links with.

What exercises do you commonly advise women to try when they go home?

There are great apps like 'Squeezy'. Do make sure you see a NHS or private women's health physio if you do have symptoms, as it is not as simple as just doing your exercises.

We will also look at your weekly general exercise you currently do and find ways to ensure that you include the components that are so important during the perimenopause and beyond: 300 mins a week (WHO recommendations, 150 mins activity + 150 mins of exercise). This is so important for reducing the risk of heart disease (we catch up with men quickly postmenopause!) and cancer; impact and strength training for bone health.

We will work with you to find a way that is something you love and decompresses you from stress.

Are there any simple pieces of equipment that women can be taught to use for their pelvic floor? Can you explain in terms of mechanical and also some electrical stimuli probe-type equipment?

There are lots of pieces of equipment on the market, and some of them are great devices. We recommend an internal assessment first before trying anything out.

We may use electrical stimulation if there is a very weak pelvic floor contraction to help the neural pathway connection, or help to reduce bladder urgency if you present with an unstable bladder. Electrical stimulation can also help with 'bulking' of the pelvic floor muscles which helps to support the pelvic organ and strengthen pelvic floor muscles. It never replaces your active exercises though!

Electronic pelvic toners (such as Kegel8 Ultra 20 that you have mentioned) are electronic devices which use neuromuscular electrical stimulation (NMES) to stimulate the muscles for you to strengthen them. This is particularly beneficial for weak muscles that don't respond when your body tries to contract them.

Mechanical devices like Elvie, the Kegel8 vaginal cones (considered biofeedback tools as they do not do the exercises for you but show you if you are doing them correctly manually) can be helpful for sensory feedback and additional strengthening (especially if you are aiming to return to high-intensity sports or lifting, which is much more common in midlife now).

We may also fit you for a pessary (an internal device to give some more support to the vaginal walls).

I would imagine that if a woman had a severe degree of prolapse you would refer her back to her doctor but in all but the most severe cases can you get good results with incontinence and prolapse?

NICE guidelines recommend pelvic floor muscles training guided by a healthcare professional. It is important that prolapse assessment treatment stays in primary care; surgery is rarely needed and women's health physios work closely with uro-gynaecologists if a referral is appropriate. Exercising and maybe additional support is always the first line of treatment, supported by evidence. We may combine that with fitting a silicone pessary, which will give you additional support if needed.

Women of menopausal age may need some additional vaginal oestrogen to improve bladder & vaginal tissue, and we would work with your GP to make sure your vaginal health is the best it can be.

Tell me about your magic great advice for opening our bowels in a protected manner that you explained at your recent talk.

https://www.whitehartclinic.co.uk/blog/how-have-perfect-poo

Any last golden nuggets of advice?

You will MOT your car; we so much would like you to MOT your pelvic health and general health. Continence, prolapse and sexual problems are miserable and often women feel isolated or believe there is not much you can do. There is much you can do and most of it is simple: book in with a women's health physio, the Squeezy app has a good directory https://www.squeezyapp.com/directory/, or our professional organisation https://pogp.csp.org.uk/public-patient/find-physiotherapist/physio2u will find a physio near you.

Thank you so much, Christien, what a bonus for women to have all of that information.

CYSTITIS

Most women in their lifetime have suffered with cystitis – after a time of dehydration, sexual intercourse or other triggers. Acute uncomplicated cystitis in healthy non-pregnant women affects up to 15% of women annually. True cystitis can be immensely painful and feels like you are 'peeing razor blades', or the symptoms may only be urgency (having to run to the toilet) or frequency (feeling the need to go regularly and there being a smaller amount of urine than you thought).

Over-the-counter preparations like Cystemme are mixed with a certain volume of water and work by alkalinising the urine so in theory will help to reduce symptoms but they have not been proved alone to eliminate infection. They may work in milder cases because the amount of fluid being drunk helps flush out the system. My own remedy I would tell my patients if their packet of remedies had run out was a 200ml glass of water with a small teaspoon of sodium bicarbonate and a dash of cranberry juice. We know that cranberry has a component that is supposed to stop bacteria adhering to the bladder wall but I feel honestly you may have to drink an impossible amount of cranberry to have a real beneficial effect.

Acute cystitis requiring a trip/call to the doctor and a three-day course of a simple bladder-specific antibiotic is common. There have been lots of studies regarding the development of antibiotic resistance and side effects if more broad-spectrum antibiotics are used longer term, so the message is to keep it simple with a short course. Plenty of fluids will be advised and general hygiene measures – wiping front to back – simple analgesia like paracetamol and maybe a warm hot water bottle.

Recurrent cystitis or chronic cystitis are more complex problems. Recurrent cystitis can seem relentless. There are benefits to be had from investigating preventative measures. *D-mannose* (supplement) has some good evidence that taken early it can be as effective as low-dose antibiotic prevention. Again it works similarly to the component in cranberry that reduces adherence of bacteria to the bladder wall. Chronic cystitis can be extremely debilitating. Let us look first at why this might be more of a problem around and after the menopausal time.

Postmenopausal cystitis
Recurrent lower urinary tract infections are common after the menopause and occur in more than 10% of women over the age of 60. A rise in vaginal pH (more alkaline than acid) promotes an alteration in the normal vaginal flora with a decrease of those healthy lactobacilli and more likelihood of colonisation of the area by bacteria from the bowel or faeces. As awful as this sounds, women are not designed perfectly here with the proximity of all the openings in one area.

This increases the incidence of urinary tract infections, especially in sexually active women. Oestrogen deficiency also results in urogenital atrophy, and the risk of infections is raised further.

Oestrogen therapy does promote recolonisation with the healthy bacteria as I said, and sometimes careful use of vaginal oestriol cream or vaginal oestrogen pessaries, both prescribed by a doctor, will be more effective than a placebo in reducing UTI.

Examination by the doctor will include a urine sample and, if necessary, a urologist examination of the bladder with a camera (cystoscopy) and a bladder biopsy; sometimes further studies of the urinary system are also performed.

Options are long-term preventing antibiotics if no other cause is found, or vaginal lubricant and prophylactic antibiotics before intercourse and hygiene methods of voiding after sex.

Sometimes cystitis is not bacterial, and a condition called interstitial cystitis is possible. This diagnosis really should only be made after bladder camera examination and a bladder biopsy showing specific immune inflammatory cells (mast cells). In all cases the diagnosis of bladder cancer must be excluded. There are many different treatment options and these can vary in popularity depending on where you live in the world e.g. low dose steroid or bladder nerve pain medication. There have been many trials of other preparations and it will be up to the protocol of your local urology team.

Book resources

Holding the Ball by Julia Kaye

Prolapse Exercises Inside Out by Michelle Kenway

The Calm Bladder: Freedom from Cystitis by Dr Tim Whittlestone

Great Sex Starts At 50 How to age-proof your libido by Tracey Cox

The Wisdom of Menopause by Christiane Northrup, M.D.

Va Va Voom The 10 – Day Energy Diet by Jackie Lynch

CHAPTER 9: SKIN AND SKIN PRODUCTS

Invest in your skin, it is going to represent you for a long, long time

INTRODUCTION TO SKIN, ITS FUNCTIONS AND HOW IT CHANGES WITH AGE

Skin is what we see, what we feel and what we compare. When looking for beauty or recognition we are looking at skin; were we looking at a skeleton our perception would be different.

Despite years of medical training I still NEED to be reminded that skin is an organ, indeed the largest. A **living** organ, just like the liver, kidneys, lungs and heart.

To this end we should think of it as something that requires protection in its own right. When young, we mentally *separate* this 'covering' from our internal body when often our skin is crying out for TLC. We need to be aware that skin may absorb what is placed upon it. Be mindful about what you give your skin to drink, albeit if it only reaches the skin cells in many cases. This applies strongly to our children's delicate young skin.

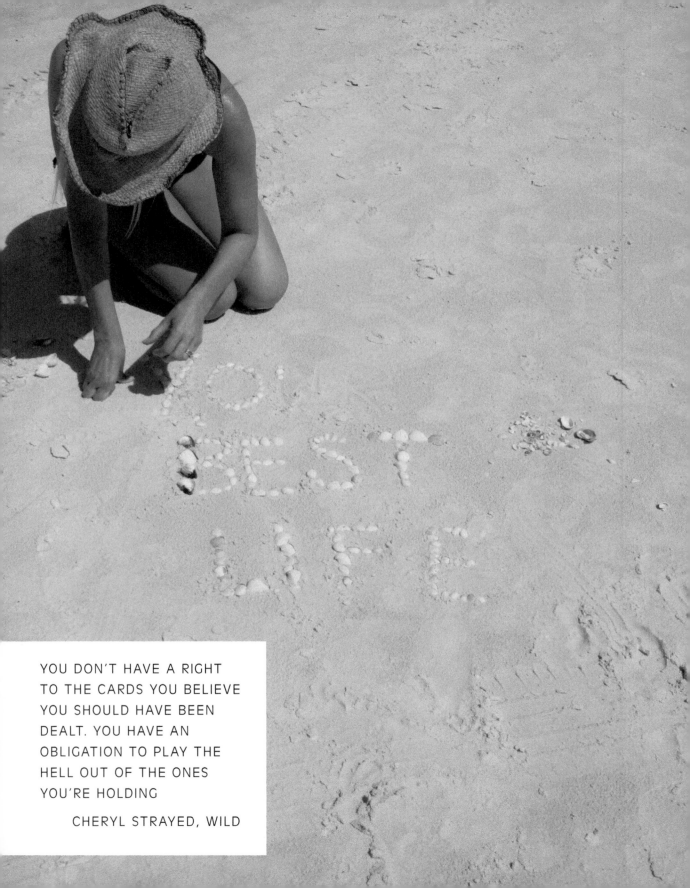

YOU DON'T HAVE A RIGHT
TO THE CARDS YOU BELIEVE
YOU SHOULD HAVE BEEN
DEALT. YOU HAVE AN
OBLIGATION TO PLAY THE
HELL OUT OF THE ONES
YOU'RE HOLDING

CHERYL STRAYED, WILD

Diseases of the skin are psychologically inescapable – they call for attention. What we might ignore were it within our body, we cannot ignore on the surface. Anyone who suffered acne can testify. It can dominate our thoughts as our skin is what we present to the world. We can become obsessive if we see something as imperfect on the outside, triggering a myriad of negative emotions within, *if we are so inclined. Add in signs of ageing and skin can become a source of negative and hopeless emotion.* **We judge a lot by skin**, we make assessments of others aesthetically with many different, often subconscious, cues. We estimate age, social stature, character – just based on someone's face.

The world would be bland were we all to appear identical. In applying makeup or changing our looks we are presenting a message of *how we want to be seen*. It may be very different to the face we wake up with or were born with. In the case of some plastic surgery or physical 'corrections' we can alter our appearance dramatically. We still remain **a person with skin judging other people with skin.**

Surgery aside, what can *you do* to present the best version of YOU? Not you trying to copy a beauty pageant idol, but the best version of you *as yourself*. You cannot live in a dark box, we are all going to be exposed to sun, smoke and pollution at different stages in our lives. I am purposefully not including in this book the wealth of amendments and procedures we can turn to these days to alter the physical appearance of our face. I am not a specialist or surgeon. I am interested in how you can change your **lifestyle and actions** to enhance or naturally maintain your 'youth'. I think we should not judge what other women have done but **women do judge women**. The only person you should compete with is the one in the mirror. So, from now on, my philosophy must be to make my own reflection the healthiest, happiest version possible. If we have done this and then choose to alter our looks in more interventional ways then so be it. I have friends and colleagues that Botox and fill (rather than Netflix and chill) and friends that would never. My opinions are largely irrelevant to them and I would not want their disparagement if I were to choose that route in the future.

What is skin?

Far from a simple sheet of tissue, skin is divided into three layers: epidermis, dermis and subcutaneous layers.

The **epidermis or top layer** consists of 'stratified epithelium' which regenerates from a base layer so successive cells are produced, and as they reach the surface they are dying. Skin cells turn over roughly every 28 days, or less when we are young. The very outer layer is called the stratum corneum and is made up of the dead skin cells that are then shed. Hence the skin is *constantly regenerating*.

The **dermis (deeper) layer** contains blood vessels, nerves, sweat glands, hair follicles, muscles, lymphatics (to drain waste) and connective tissue fibres. These connective tissue fibres consist mainly of **collagen** which forms a scaffolding in both skin and bone. Cells called **fibroblasts** lie between the collagen bundles. Fibres made of **elastin** run parallel and enclose the bundles. Fibroblast cells make new collagen. This layer is what gives the skin its **elasticity**. We know how young skin stretches and springs back and older skin may just not be so 'elastic'.

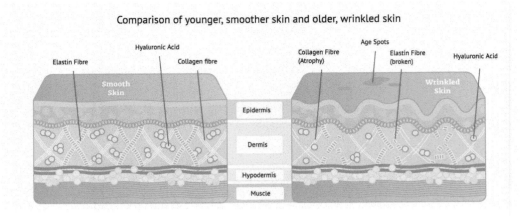

Comparison of younger, smoother skin and older, wrinkled skin

Within cartilage, joints and also skin are compounds called glycosaminoglycans (or GAGS as we amusingly called them as med students). These can form large molecules that attract water, forming a 'hydrated gel'. We find them as the ground substance in many areas of the body, and in skin and cartilage they provide a framework. One of these is **hyaluronic acid**. This, along with holding up to 1,000 times its weight in water, also has protective effects in the skin-fighting free radicals, wound healing and anti-inflammatory. Sadly, our production of hyaluronic acid reduces with age. In youth we have about 15g in our bodies.

It is important to have a vague idea of the layers to understand where your creams can reach and where they work.

Phew. Enough anatomy. You just want to look younger. But you get the idea – the skin is regenerating and renewing naturally. But what does skin do for us?

- physical barrier to infection
- semi-waterproofs us (prevents fluid loss by keratin cells in epidermis)
- pigmentation (melanocyte cells in epidermis) prevents injury from UV light
- touch sensation, pain and temperature provided by nerve cells
- immune response to threats dealt with by immune system cells in the skin.

Part of the function of the skin is protection. Free radicals are protective when produced in the skin to help fight any virus or bacteria, but if produced in excess (as with radiation, pollution, smoking) the free radicals can damage our own tissue and lead to sun spots, ageing and inflammation. We call this *oxidative stress*, and if we counteract this with antioxidants we can reduce ageing sun damage. Antioxidants *may* also repair and brighten our skin and reduce the risk of skin cancer.

Why all the interest in skin ageing and why all the science NOW?
We are living longer. This has inevitably promoted a demand for people to *look younger for longer*. In response to this demand, products have been designed that *may help* hold back the

arms of the 'clock' of your face. Or at least make us *look like* we have longer to go. You will have recognised words that are incorporated into beauty speak – elasticity, hyaluronic acid, collagen.

Skin ageing really has two distinct, different components. The first is **intrinsic** ageing – changes within you that *you can prove under a microscope* possibly from the moment you emerge as a baby. This ageing process can be accelerated in the latter decades of life. This is genetic in origin and largely pre-programmed. Or at least we think it is. Whatever I tell you in this book, you will have intrinsically aged by the time you reach the last page. Turn to the genetics section as de-ageing your chromosomes may have implications for your skin.

The second component of ageing is **extrinsic** ageing attributed to ultraviolet radiation causing photo-aged skin and other external factors, thus this is somewhat induced by **lifestyle**. Studies of twins and how they age are proving that this is very multifactorial and the two types of ageing cross over.

Why wrinkles?

Breakdown of the elastic fibrils or loss of their function in the skin naturally occurs with ageing – from early adulthood but more noticeable from the 60s. Wrinkling results and irregular pigmentation becomes more noticeable on areas of exposed skin. Skin can gradually appear more irregular in colour and slightly 'yellow tinged'. Such subtle nuances we pick up visually when we meet someone and try to guestimate their age. Our minds are trained to pick up the visual clues.

Also altering the skin appearance is the degree of exposure to ultraviolet light, hormones and nutrition. Studies of pairs of genetically similar or identical twins with different lifestyles are revealing. In a 2009 study in Ohio, Dr Guyuron et al. studied the factors contributing to the facial ageing of identical twins who had different lifestyles but the same genetics. In some cases, both of a pair of twins may have a genetic predisposition to a disease or ageing but an *environmental trigger* like smoking is needed for it to be active. We call this **epigenetics**.

- Lifestyle stresses like divorce added 1.7 years to the perceived age of the face.
- Women who did not drink alcohol at all looked younger than their drinking twins.
- Being slightly overweight under the age of 40 made the face plumper and look older but over 55 it could result in a younger appearance.

Catherine Deneuve famously stated that beyond 40 a woman needed to choose between her derriere and her face, as too drastic a weight loss could cause the face to look gaunt and aged. Just what is a girl to do when the jeans don't fit? I suggest everything in moderation!

Just as our priorities change with age so does our skin and its needs. Your skin care now may need reassessment if you have not changed it for five years. Products now have *ingredients clearly labelled* so we can see whether they have relevance to us. Looking at the 'decades of ageing' is an oversimplification but as a doctor I like to break things down into bite-size chunks – I'm a simple gal like that. You can read what is relevant to YOU NOW.

You cannot, and why would you, erase all ageing naturally. You can lessen the effects and keep skin healthy if you choose.

THE DIVINE DECADES OF SKIN

20s

Skin may be affected by the contraceptive pill here. There is naturally increased oil from sebaceous gland activity but eventually the hormones stabilise. Acne should improve but may be worsened with some progesterone-only pills. Later in the 20s, skin can become drier. Women should moisturise if they have dry skin. Use a sunscreen. Dry skin may mean fine lines start around the eyes and mouth. Targeted skin care in terms of moisturisation can prevent premature signs of ageing. Cleansing should be routine. The skin becomes less able to deal with oxidative stress. STOP SMOKING NOW. Many dermatologists recommend using a light eye-specific product.

30s

Skin may still be affected by the contraceptive pill, some acne may flare as women come off the combined pill. Pregnancy may affect skin. Collagen production slows. Skin can appear thinner and less full. Skin may become drier and the undereye area is more delicate. Now is a good time to start thinking of being proactive in skin care – a light hyaluronic acid preparation and other night-time moisturisers to nourish the skin. 'Dynamic' wrinkles from smiling and frowning develop (NOBODY MOVE!) – 'static' wrinkles from sun damage if skin has not been protected. Niacinamide (vitamin B3 containing products) may help reduce signs of ageing as will moisturisers such as glycerine. Use a sunscreen. Careful cleansing should be routine. Skin may be affected by stress as responsibilities increase. Consider ways of counteracting this – relaxation, exercise, meditation, mindfulness, yoga...

40s

Oestrogen declines and as it is involved in collagen production so elasticity and thickness of the skin may decrease. The lifecycle of skin cells changes from the 28 days to around 40 days. Skin will overall be drier with fine lines and wrinkles. Deeper lines around the eyes, mouth and forehead develop and age spots may occur. Neck skin may start to sag.

Moisturiser and sunblock are essential. Look for SPF in day creams to combine products. Hyaluronic acid is still a good ingredient for moisture. Wear a hat in the sunshine. Remember, sun damage and skin cancers can also occur around the forehead and tops of the ears, and legs in women. This is when basal cell carcinomas (vascular (blood vessel appearance) type, raised, almost pearlescent lesions that if removed early do not spread) may appear and moles may change.

Long-term medication may age and dull the skin. Look for **retinol-containing products** and **peptides** to help lessen the signs of ageing.

50s

Unless you are on HRT, oestrogen will decline and skin will be less elastic and firm. Women may feel their skin has lost some 'glow'. Skin will be drier with fine lines and wrinkles and the effect of gravity will be more apparent. Reduction in oestrogen also reduces melanin production so skin becomes more susceptible to UV light. Wrinkles deepen and pigmentation and age spots appear. These may be very apparent on the hands. Moisturiser and sunblock are essential. Hyaluronic acid is still a good ingredient for moisture. Night-time heavier duty moisturisers will be well tolerated. Wear a hat in the sunshine. Regularly check skin for new spots or lesions. Report any changes to your doctor. Make sure your diet includes lots of healthy wholegrains, essential fatty acids and omega-3 to help balance hormones and skin from within. Exercise will stimulate blood flow to the skin.

60s, 70s and 80s

Continue skincare as above.

Hormones are more stable. Skin is thinner, wrinkles are heavier. Purpura or bruising may appear under thinner skin, more visible in patches. Aspirin and blood thinner medication may make this more likely. Continue advice as above and continue to make time, and self-exam for skin lesions or ask a dermatologist for an annual review. Seborrheic keratoses or warty lesions are more likely at this time. These and skin tags can easily be removed by cryotherapy or curettage – may have to have this done privately if it is entirely cosmetic. Exercise will stimulate blood flow to the skin.

YOUR LIFESTYLE, YOUR SKIN

Food and skin

'You are what you eat' and there is now much information in the stratosphere regarding nutrition. **'This month's food is next month's body'** is a great motivator for eating well but what about the effect on your face? To do the best for our skin and our bodies we may need to make changes to the decisions we make about food. Long term we will start seeing the results not just in our waistlines but in our faces.

What you ingest through your mouth can have a serious benefit that is felt within and seen outside. A diet rich in overly processed food full of saturated fat and sugars and low in nutrients is going to leave your skin *sagging and dull*, with breakouts of inflammation, and your hair limp and lifeless. Actually if you retrain your body to eat whole foods and nourishment your taste buds will learn to crave the healthy ingredients.

YOU WILL GLOW!

Water and skin

We are two-thirds composed of water (see food is life chapter) but you will notice a change in your skin if you replace a large proportion of any caffeinated beverages, fizzy or sugary drinks with pure water.

Even though no one seems to have studied whether water intake at the correct level will increase the smoothness of skin, it stands to reason that water will give skin more turgor or bounce. Doctors look for signs of dehydration in extreme cases as lack of elasticity showing within the skin to the touch. Our skin itself is about 30% water. Flushing our system with a healthy amount (not excessive as beware that excessive water intake can be harmful in extreme cases) will help remove toxins from the body, keep our liver and kidneys healthy and reduce accumulation of waste. In turn a healthy fluid intake will reduce constipation and reduce transit time for waste in our gut and this can be reflected in our faces. However, as Ruby Hammer recounted to me in her interview: 'We all know where the tap is but how many of us get our eight glasses a day?!'

Alcohol and skin

Dehydrated skin, broken capillaries, blood vessels more noticeable giving a reddish appearance – alcohol does not love your skin. The dehydration will only worsen the appearance of wrinkles. You will simply look tired if you drink very regularly and excessively. The possibility of a heavy reliance on alcohol may mean healthy food intake is compromised. Of course, we would all recognise the bloodshot eyes and yellow complexion of a jaundiced alcoholic, but subtle changes are apparent with alcohol on a more 'socially acceptable' level. Effects will show ON YOUR FACE whatever your vice if taken in excess. The sugar content of alcohol also has a direct effect. If you think you are gluten sensitive, some gin, vodka and whiskey contain gluten. Wine can be sugary, and 'clean' drinkers will indeed advocate grain-free vodka with soda. What you mix the spirit with will have a big impact. Committed wine drinkers may try organic sulphite-free wines with less allergy reactions potentially in the skin.

There is the option of rarely drinking or not at all. There are massive benefits for general health and your skin will thank you. I am not however a preacher or teetotal and you will have to read this whole book then make your decision.

Smoking and skin

On a pure vanity level, stop. Smoking reduces the very life, the blood supply, of the skin. You will look older if you smoke and simply more unwell. The effects are cumulative. The sneaky fags in your 20s aren't just sneaky now, they are the death toll for your skin. The longer a woman smokes, the older she looks, with more, deeper wrinkles and more uneven skin tone. You are literally starving your skin of oxygen. Every ten years of smoking allegedly adds a subjective 2.5 years to guessed age. I suggest this increases rapidly if you add in sun damage and a life spent burning the candle...

Stress and skin

Stress is a major player in disease but also in our appearance. Aside from the frown lines (consider meditation/facial acupuncture/yoga), stressful life events can show on our faces.

Turn to the happiness chapter ;-)

Sugar and skin

Three years ago I made a conscious effort to cut out processed sugar. Apart from a drop in dress size, there was an added bonus! My skin LOOKED different. Brighter and more evenly toned. We are becoming increasingly aware of the inflammatory effect of sugar on our bodies. This could explain increased spots with a higher intake of processed foods. Sugar promotes **glycation** in the body, and in skin it causes 'crosslinking' of collagen rendering the collagen fibres less able to repair. Glucose and fructose link the amino acids present in the collagen and elastin that support the dermis. In time this can cause it to stiffen and **wrinkles worsen**. *Try a healthy morning smoothie with avocado (good fat), cashew butter (protein boost) and greens as a beauty elixir instead of a sugary breakfast.*

There is also evidence from diabetic studies and studies with introducing a sugar load in the form of sweetened sugary drinks, that sugar can affect the circulation in our skin. In fact, it is of course a well-known complication of diabetes affecting circulation elsewhere.

Sleep and skin (see sleep chapter)

During sleep many restorative and repairing mechanisms occur driven by the rise of the biological marker melatonin. We also release growth hormone which has a restorative effect. Deprive ourselves of sleep and we know our skin looks lacklustre and our eyes puffy.

Great food for great skin

This month's snacks/meals could be next month's face. Make them good...

```
                    SKIN FOOD
Omega 3* e.g. salmon, mackerel, herring, linseed, chia
seeds, walnuts, cold pressed extra virgin olive oil
ANTI-INFLAMMATORY, SMOOTHER SKIN

Selenium e.g. brazil nuts (2-4 gives RDA*), fish,
shellfish, eggs, tomatoes, broccoli, mushrooms
POWERFUL ANTI-OXIDANT, ANTI-INFLAMMATORY,
ELASTICITY

Zinc e.g. fish, wholegrains, poultry, nuts, liver, eggs,
chia seeds, chickpeas, quinoa
GOOD SEBACEOUS GLAND FUNCTION, WOUND HEALING, ANTI-
INFLAMMATORY, UV PROTECTION, HAIR BENEFITS

Silica e.g. raw organic fruit and vegetables
COLLAGEN FORMATION, ELASTICITY, WOUND HEALING, HAIR
AND NAIL BENEFITS

*we need both essential acids omega 3 and 6 but we need the
right ratio of 3 (anti-inflammatory) to 6 (inflammatory)
*Recommended daily allowance adult
```

Alongside this, having plenty of good carbs like beans, pulses and porridge will give a steady supply of energy without reaching for the wrinkle-causing refined sugar.

```
                    SKIN FOOD
Betacarotene e.g. oranges, carrots, sweet potatoes,
spinach
ANTIOXIDANT, NATURAL SUNBLOCK

Niacin e.g. fortified cereals, legumes, milk, poultry,
fish, tuna
Role in preventing dermatitis

Vitamin A e.g. egg yolks, carrots, kale, spinach, liver
ANTIOXIDANT, REPAIR, CLEAR ELASTIC SKIN

Vitamin C e.g. oranges, tomatoes, sweet potatoes,
berries, broccoli
ANTIOXIDANT, REPAIR, STRENGTHEN COLLAGEN AND
CAPILLARIES OF SKIN

Vitamin E e.g. avocadoes, hazelnuts, pine nuts,
olives, olive oil, egg yolks, spinach, fatty fish,
sunflower seeds
ANTIOXIDANT, ANTI-INFLAMMATORY, REDUCE EFFECTS OF
AGEING AND SOME SKIN PROTECTION FROM CANCER
```

Ideally then: five portions of colourful fruit and veg a day, 'supersnacks' like walnuts/almonds/ seeds at the ready when you are on the go, plenty of water and fresh food all round. Make sure you have plenty of protein and great fats as a woman needs them! It might take 6 to 12 weeks to see the difference in the skin but you are going to feel better before that. You might prefer to just take the supplement vitamins and minerals and forget the healthy diet. This is obviously *never as good* and in some cases there can be risks of excess (n.b. beware excess vitamin A in pregnancy). Speak to a professional, always be aware that your body can't get rid of fat soluble vitamins A, D, E and K by weeing them out so take care with supplements.

Sunshine and skin

As a teenager I loved the sun. The book I treasured though was a Cosmopolitan 'guide to beauty'. On the cover was a girl with the sun on her face, wearing a hat, with the breeze blowing through her sun-bleached hair. As a teenager, I would grab any opportunity for a suntan. In my 20s, with more days on hot beaches while studying abroad, 'melasma' or 'chloasma' hit me (pigmentation). This is a pattern of pigmentation that gives you a kind of butterfly shaped tan pattern on your face and in my case a horrendous pattern looking like a heavy brown moustache.

I suddenly became obsessed with blocking the sunlight's path to my face. A complete reversal from my younger years of loving the feel of the sun on my skin. I had to block the sun, and without the current sunscreens it was not so easy.

I even wore a tea towel on my head on a Mauritian beach, much to the squeals of hilarity from my friends. It was only because *I could see the pigmentation*, **but what if I had not been able to see it** – would I have bothered protecting my skin at all? Do you bother?

Let's think about the damage we cannot see and what we can do to preserve this valuable asset wrapping our bodies.

Be skin cancer aware

Check your skin regularly and if you have a friend or partner who can cast a second pair of eyes even better. WATCH FOR ANY LESIONS THAT: change shape, colour (darker, lighter, variegated) and/or start itching/bleeding.

Brand new lesions (other than normal injury/spots) need to be reported to your GP. Women tend to develop seborrheic keratoses or warty growths (skin tags) around the neck and bra line where clothes rub as they pass middle age. These are benign but unsightly to some.

Any lesion that is not healing similarly needs to be checked by a doctor – do not assume it is an ongoing infection.

Skin cancer nearly always develops on areas exposed to sunlight, but not always. Common areas are scalp, face, lips, ears, neck, chest, arms, hands and legs. Less commonly it can even develop on palms, beneath nails or around the genital area.

Non-malignant melanoma type skin cancer

Basal cell carcinomas are waxy or pearlised bumps that appear almost 'under the skin' with a blood vessel rich surface. They can be flesh or brown coloured and can bleed or scab and re-heal repeatedly. These lesions are less likely to spread than other cancers and are usually successfully entirely removed.

Squamous cell carcinomas are usually firm red nodules or can be flat with a scaly crusted surface. They can present as painful which may help the doctor in diagnosing. Picking up squamous cell carcinomas early is essential for a good prognosis.

Malignant melanoma type skin cancer

Malignant melanoma can occur in existing moles that change or appear as new. There are various appearances so any change or *anything new* should be looked at. They can occur on our external skin but also mucous membranes such as mouth, nose, vagina or anus. Picking up these lesions early is essential to give the best chance of successful treatment and survival.

There are further types of cancer affecting skin and even the trained eye cannot always diagnose accurately without a biopsy and histology. This is why great dermatologists insist on a **full body exam** at any consultation as often diagnoses are made when a patient is attending for something else.

With all skin cancers, I repeat, early detection is key.

Protecting skin from the sun

There are two types of ultraviolet radiation which we are exposed to every day:

- **UVA** radiation is associated with accelerated skin ageing (A for Ageing!)
- **UVB** exposure is associated with skin burns (B for Burning!).

Sufficient exposure to both types of radiation puts us at major risk of skin cancer. The risks of sun exposure are raised even more if the exposure is from a young age. The pattern of two weeks' intense sun exposure from a holiday 'abroad' annually after a year cooped up is often a risk factor for malignant melanoma, especially when we look at exposure in childhood.

By using sunscreen to protect against the harmful effects of the sun we also look younger longer. It is well documented that those of us with fair skin that burns easily, many moles or freckles, red or fair hair and light-coloured eyes are most at risk. Ethnically darker skin is at risk of skin ageing and has a lower *but not absent* risk of skin cancer, and of course lesions may be less obvious and diagnosed later. It is also well publicised that the risk of sunbeds is just as high or worse, and there is additional concern here as sunscreen is often not used.

What about vitamin D though? I hear you! For this reason, the British Photo-dermatology Group states on its information sheets that absolute sun avoidance is not advocated. This is because casual brief sun exposure, well below that leading to burning, helps maintain bodily vitamin D. If for medical reasons it is completely contraindicated for you to be exposed to the sun,

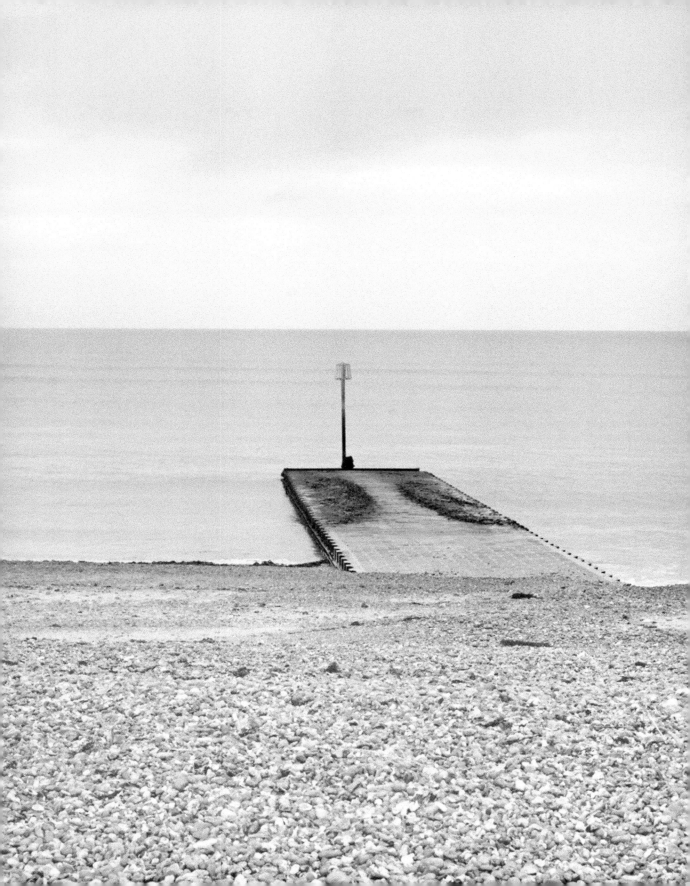

then oral supplementation with vitamin D3 (the form most similar to UV-induced vitamin D) is advised – read more in my nutrition chapter. There is a recent study, brought to my attention by Dr Hextall (see specialist interview at the end of this chapter), that suggests that sun cream does not reduce our manufacture of vitamin D. It is also important to note that darker skins may need more exposure to the sun to produce adequate levels of vitamin D.

You are, of course, advised to limit exposure between the hours of 11am and 3pm to short periods during warm weather from April to September in the UK, and all year round in tropical areas to limit the chance of burning. Ultraviolet radiation is significantly increased at high altitude and by reflection from light sand or concrete. Water can also reflect 30% of ultraviolet back up at us, and ultraviolet can also penetrate to 50 cm water depth. Sailors and swimmers must take care. Cloud cover is actually poorly protective so we cannot assume a cloudy day will not age us or damage our skin. Clothing may only block a percentage of strong sun.

All sunscreens have instructions on them about application, e.g. applying chemical sunscreen 15 mins prior to exposure (not the same with mineral type) and applying adequate amounts and reapplying frequently. Some medications and medical conditions can increase sensitivity to light so such photosensitivity means extra added precautions need to be taken.

The sun protection factor (SPF) on sunscreen ONLY refers to the UVB blocking. What you need is both UVA and B so it is recommended to have a **high SPF, e.g. 30 or more,** plus a UVA star rating of around 4 to 5. The news is the same in the USA; the US Food and Drug Administration announced new regulations for sunscreen labels to emphasise the importance of both UVA and UVB protection now known as **BROAD SPECTRUM PROTECTION**.

We need to be aware of sun protection on cloudy days and behind glass. You sadly cannot obtain vitamin D when behind glass. Normally, UVB rays hit the skin and lovely vitamin D (7-dehydrocholesterol) is formed. But normal glass blocks this wavelength so active vitamin D is not formed. In northern/mid-European climates I would suggest a spray or liquid-drop vitamin D3 preparation with the recommended dose as in my chapter on bone. As vitamin D is a fat-soluble vitamin it cannot be eliminated from your body in your urine. You cannot simply pee the excess out. I was very deficient a few years ago and took a higher dose under consultant supervision only to find on a re-check blood test that I had gone to high toxic levels! You should not be taking anything other than the Public Health recommended dose of vitamin D during the winter unless you have had blood tests and are being supervised by your doctor. Vitamin D is involved in many delicate systems in the body and a toxic high level can be very dangerous. If you have symptoms of deficiency this is something to discuss with your doctor – tiredness, bone aches, stomach aches, feeling down, hair loss, but of course all of these symptoms can be related to other problems within the body so it is a case of getting a proper diagnosis.

Dosage can be described in international units or micrograms (mcg):

- 2.5 **mcg (micrograms)** = 100 **IU**
- 5 **mcg** = 200 **IU**

- **10 mcg** = 400 **IU**
- 15 **mcg** = 600 **IU**
- 20 **mcg** = 800 **IU**

The Public Health recommended UK dose in winter *for adults* is 10mcg or 400iu but many argue amounts should be around 25mcg or 1000iu. Look at your lifestyle and discuss with your doctor to decide. Check Public Health England's current advice on the NHS website regularly regarding vitamin D.

UVA rays are not stopped by glass so we must protect against the sun and ageing behind glass, e.g. driving. So you don't end up a hot mess you want to find a non-greasy everyday sunblock for your face that can sit under make-up if needed. You want to find a well-scoring sunscreen with non-comedogenic (not pore blocking) and maybe slightly 'mattifying' properties if you want your make-up to survive the day and not slide off your face. You need a sunscreen with safe, non-irritating ingredients and adequate UVA/UVB protection – a dermatology recommended type is, for example, Heliocare 360, La Roche Posay Anthelios.

A small habit of using sunscreen daily can give huge benefits.

A study in the USA in 2016 wanted to look at whether a facial sun protection factor (SPF) 30 formulation could improve previous photodamage with a year's use.

The subjects applied a broad-spectrum (UVA and UVB) sunscreen to the entire face for 52 weeks. They looked at skin texture, clarity and mottled and discrete pigmentation. THE RESULTS: there was a 40% to 52% improvement from baseline in 100% of subjects. So, although this was a small study it almost is a **no-brainer**. You could not only prevent additional sun damage to your skin if you start today, you may very well VISIBLY reverse the signs of existing photodamage. What is not to love?

There have been popular valuable studies showing that the use of moisturiser per se also is a great preventer and reducer of signs of skin ageing, so don't underestimate it.

Important differences of note between sunscreens

Because a thick coat of sunscreen is required to work effectively and it is applied often to the entire body as well as the face, it is of no surprise that the chemicals are then found in our bloodstream, urine, sweat and even breast milk isolates. If you use a spray formulation the ingredients can also in theory reach the lungs and bloodstream this way. There is concern that chemicals in sunscreen such as oxybenzone may work as hormone disruptors and have negative consequences in the body. There is still ongoing research and it is not always clear, for example if reactions are due to allergy to sun or to ingredients in formulations. Some people veer towards choosing **mineral sunscreens** that, instead of penetrating and working via chemicals, sit on the skin surface and act as a mirror reflecting the light. These generally consist of zinc and titanium oxides. A layer of zinc oxide around the eyes/nose/ears/vulnerable areas as a second layer of protection can also be great. Mineral sunscreens used to be well known for leaving a white hue on the skin but new formulations can be worn invisibly with or without make-up. Mineral formulations can also be more successful at preventing melasma as they form a physical barrier.

It seems not everyone can agree regarding mineral vs chemical so it must be your choice.

Blue light

Dr Hextall explained that sweating my make-up off whilst typing this book in front of a large screen was likely due to the infrared radiation coming off it. Also, we know that screen blue light can cause changes in the skin, and we can counteract this with some antioxidants to scavenge the free radicals produced in our skin. Heliocare 360, Anthelios 50+ and Ladival all have formulations with antioxidants that mitigate this effect (see sleep chapter re blue light).

Unwanted skin pigmentation

'Melasma', 'chloasma' and 'mask of pregnancy' are names for **hyperpigmented** (so, excessively pigmented) areas mostly on the skin of the face due to increased production of melanin, the skin pigment that gives us our colour. It tends to occur on the forehead, cheeks, nose, above the upper lip and the chin and can actually affect anyone. It can also occur on the forearms and neck. It is more common in women.

Causes of melasma

1. HORMONES AND SUN EXPOSURE: Oral contraceptives, pregnancy, HRT and (recently proven by clinical trial) stress are all contributing factors. It is still *not entirely clear* what causes melasma. Because the cells that produce the pigment melanin (melanocytes) are making too much colour then the darker the skin pigment naturally, the more likely you are to suffer.
2. COSMETICS: Cosmetics that irritate/sting/burn the skin can worsen melasma. As with spots/inflammation, the result can be a pigmented area – this is **post-inflammatory hyperpigmentation** and can cause the same significant stress as melasma. Waxing as a form of hair removal may irritate and in turn worsen the melasma.
3. MEDICAL CONDITIONS PREDISPOSING TO MELASMA: For example, ovarian dysfunction, thyroid autoimmune disease, liver disease. Melasma usually worsens in the summer and lightens in the winter in Europe. Sunlight is of course a major factor.

How is it diagnosed?

Often a GP will diagnose melasma from talking to you and examining the affected areas and will give you simple advice as I have here. You may be referred to a dermatologist. To see how deep the melasma goes the dermatologist may use a device called a dermatoscope or Wood's light. This can see whether it is epidermal only (top layer), dermal (deeper layer) or both. In some cases, if the diagnosis is not clear, a skin biopsy may be taken safely by the dermatologist.

Treatments for melasma

As time goes by melasma may fade, as mine did. As hormones of pregnancy/the pill subside the degree of melasma often reduces. If not, the dermatologist can discuss the following with you before prescribing them.

Hydroquinone cream

A preparation applied to the skin to lighten it. It can actually come in the form of a cream, gel or liquid. A dermatologist would prescribe these in higher concentration than would be available over the counter. I personally feel that unregulated use of very much higher doses of hydroquinone (say more than 4%) can be dangerous when performed by unregulated products bought over the internet with no physician supervision, and there are reports of women trying to drastically lighten their skin with horrific unwanted long-term damaging consequences. This really is one to use under the guidance and review of a doctor.

Corticosteroids and tretinoin

These may be prescribed by a dermatologist to enhance skin lightening. There are preparations that are a combination of hydroquinone and these substances in a kind of 'triple cream'. As stated in the anti-ageing section, the tretinoin can have side effects and should be avoided in pregnancy and breastfeeding.

Azelaic or Kojic acid

Can lighten melasma.

Tranexamic acid (as a cream and oral)

Is being studied as a potential treatment for melasma.

More interventional treatments for irregular pigmentation

Dermatologist-performed **peels**, **microdermabrasion** and **dermabrasion** have been used. These should always be performed by a proper **dermatologist** only. In more recent years with the use of **certain laser therapies** there are potential options for melasma – this is really something to be discussed with a skin doctor with a special interest as some therapies can potentially worsen pigmentation.

Sunblock for melasma

In my time I tinkered with hydroquinone but then settled on stronger SPF sunblock for my face. I had to be patient. The psychological effects and the potential damage to your self-esteem cannot be underestimated. Whatever treatment you opt for long term, sunblock is key to maintaining any improvements and preventing recurrence after treatment.

Photosensitivity over 40

Some medicines can cause a reaction in the sun similar to sunburn, called photosensitivity. The medicine plus the light have to be present for this.

These reactions are of two types:

1. PHOTOTOXIC: The drug is activated by the sunlight and causes skin damage – this happens fast and the skin looks like it has been sunburned. UVA causes this more than UVB. If the burn comes up as a rash, it will be in the area exposed to the sun. This reaction tends to clear up once the medicine is stopped and has been cleared from the body.
2. PHOTOALLERGIC: Light acts to change the chemical structure of the drug so the body's immune system sees it as an *invader*. The body then initiates an immune response to it like you would have with a food allergy and this causes skin inflammation in sun-exposed areas. This looks more like eczema and is more long-lasting than phototoxicity. This can linger in the body after the drug is stopped and can recur.

If you develop a rash after sun exposure, look at medications and discuss with your doctor. Many medicines have warnings on the information leaflet and your doctor will let you know at the time of prescribing. If you are a committed sun worshipper now may be the time to change your lifestyle or discuss the use of a different drug. It is thought that if photosensitivity were allowed to persist it MAY have the potential to increase the incidence of skin cancer, so this should be taken seriously but in context. There are thoughts now that good antioxidant levels in the diet may reduce sensitivity.

It is important to remember that we may all use medication and we have a responsibility to ourselves to be aware of the benefits and the side effects in making a decision WITH our doctors regarding what to take.

Midlife acne

When you are a young child if you are lucky you have perfect skin. As a teenager hormones change skin. It secretes more lubrication (sebum) and eruptions can occur. These can be mild/severe/painless/painful. If you suffered painful spots you will be able to remember what they felt like. You will also remember the dread on wakening when you ran to check the mirror. In my time, magazines would run articles on spots – should you pick them, put toothpaste on them, go out with a paper bag on your head?

A doctor's stance on the issue will now be more informed but it is likely that anyone consulting about their acne is *desperate* enough for a solution to have plucked up the courage to walk into the surgery, especially as an adult.

Acne can be a socially isolating condition, and feeling confident in your own skin is a massive predictor for our wellbeing and health.

'Mature acne' is said to be from the age of 24 years. It is increasing in incidence and the age distribution is widening – 12% of 40- to 50-year-olds. In all patterns of acne there may well be a genetic predisposition but our hormones and bodies can be changing.

Pregnancy, breastfeeding, contraceptive change and the stress of our lives can all have an effect.

What is acne?

Acne is a chronic inflammatory disease of the skin. It is more commonly diagnosed in women in midlife possibly due to hormones but maybe because men are less likely to visit the doctor.

Basically, skin produces more sebum, the hair follicle becomes 'keratinised' or thickened resulting in a whitehead or blackhead, a bug now called Cutibacterium acnes (not cute) arrives and the area becomes inflamed.

- Whitehead = closed comedone
- Blackhead = open comedone

A beauty product labelled 'non-comedogenic' should give you neither!

Spots or acne?

Whatever the distinction, a chronic recurrent problem needs a doctor appointment. Scarring is thought to mainly occur in the first few years of suffering, and even mild to moderate cases of acne account for about 60% of scarring. Patience is needed throughout treatment, and you thought you would just be contending with gradual ageing and middle-aged spread so this may totally knock you for six. You need to seek out a sympathetic medic to see you. Your doctor or nurse may also be able to reassure you that further time may be needed to see the results you are praying for. Similarly, if the medication is put onto a repeat prescription it should not be taken endlessly as, especially in the case of antibiotics, your body may develop resistance to it and gut changes can occur, etc.

There is a vast quantity of helpful information on the web but nothing should really replace your nurse or doctor consulting you in a way tailored to you alone.

A shocking factor is the often unrealistic expectation of skin quality that we may now have, even as adult women, with the liberal use of camera filters, skin smoothing apps and so on. Real skin is rarely perfect unless it is airbrushed.

Lifestyle advice for acne

Smoking cessation
Most studies have shown that smoking worsens acne so it goes without saying – stop.

Nutrition

There were lots of old wives' tales – 'she has spots because she has a bad diet'. This was both refuted then discussed in the medical profession – see the gut health section (gut–skin axis) – and it seems that some of us are more genetically susceptible to what we eat affecting our skin, and this is not true of all individuals. Not all acne should be blamed on sugar.

Medical reviews of research prior to 2007 concluded that diet played no important role in actual **acne** and that it was mainly down to hormones and genetics. Family studies have shown that there is a major heritable factor influencing sebum production but that the development of acne is mediated by environmental factors. Recently, well-designed trials have shown there are associations between specific dietary factors and acne. This was reviewed in 2009 by Spencer et al. in 'Diet and acne: a review of the evidence'. These found low fat, high fibre diets may be beneficial, and so reducing saturated fat is all for the better. Increasing the ratio of omega-3 to omega-6 fatty acids, as previous – this is naturally higher in Japanese diets and reduces the level of inflammation in the body. These are in fact important principles for general health.

My conclusion from a check through research in 2020 is that it is emerging that processed foods worsen acne, probably because insulin and something called insulin-like growth factor 1 (IGF1) are raised with a high-sugar or calorific diet. Also dairy is thought to be an issue for some but make sure if you eliminate dairy you have other sources of calcium and iodine in healthy foods. Vitamin D deficiency may also exacerbate acne potentially, as vitamin D confers some protection from inflammation.

Dr Hextall has found great benefit from addressing gut health with the use of probiotics such as Symprove, a good intake of prebiotics from vegetables and fruit, a diet rich in antioxidants and a high SPF. Don't underestimate the power of improving gut health on any inflammatory process in the body (see interview with Dr Jenna Macciochi).

Wearing make-up with acne

One of the fears embedded in us when we were teenagers was not to do anything to worsen the spots. I really believe that choice either way is key and to cover up with concealer an essential option for a teen or a grown woman.

An informed woman with an arsenal of information and a makeup bag with some worthy concealers is more in control of her life. Studies have shown that skincare advice and make-up had beneficial effects on quality of life and no worsening symptoms. A study showed that cleansing with a weakly acidic foaming facial cleanser plus correct moisturiser and calming preparations can greatly help acne. Dr Hextall often advises patients to try such cleansers as Cetaphil and CeraVe as they have less of a drying effect and do not upset the acid mantle of the skin.

Makeup has become an artform in the public forum now and I think this is a positive step. You are not obliged to wear it but if you want to improve your skills you are able to open a Pandora's box of information on techniques and products.

Concealers for scars, pigmentation and acne

- Dermacover – prescription or buy over the counter
- Vichy Dermablend
- Dermacolor – prescription or buy online from Kryolan.

Treatment of adult acne

- *Avoid over-cleansing – use mild cleanser but be reassured acne is not a hygiene issue*
- *Use non-comedogenic make-up and preparations only*
- *Avoid picking/fiddling, to reduce scarring*
- *Look at improving nutrition if applicable (see previous)*
- *Your GP may prescribe a topical retinoid (not in pregnancy or breastfeeding) which may be added into benzoyl peroxide (beware bleaches fabrics)*
- *OR they may prescribe an antibiotic cream with benzoyl peroxide (the latter stops bacteria becoming resistant)*
- *OR they may prescribe azelaic acid (care with darker skins as can cause depigmentation)*
- *Any preparation can irritate (you may need special moisturiser) and you may have to start cautiously using trial and error. There are further treatments such as antibiotics for resistant cases either from the GP or a consultant.*

The dermatologist may discuss the use of retinoids as oral medication (serious side effects exist – skin dryness, redness, sun sensitivity, mood changes which can be severe and special counselling and blood tests will be needed concerning this and also ensure pregnancy must be prevented as retinoids can affect the baby in utero) and further treatments beyond the scope of this book. See interview with Dr Hextall in this chapter. If you have a single bad spot in an emergency, try cleansing gently, then with a cotton bud apply tea tree oil or crushed aspirin (if not allergic) or sudocrem or benzoyl peroxide spot preparations carefully to that area.

Acne rosacea
The blight of many women and a very important condition to receive professional help for. It causes redness and visible blood vessels in your face and may also produce small, red, pus-filled bumps, which mimic acne in a way, and sometimes skin can be thickened or the eye area be more affected. It may be brought on by hormonal changes in middle age and often women are wrongly embarrassed to seek help, or simply think it is natural with age and must be put up with. It can be socially debilitating, worsening with the stress or heat of anxiety of social interaction.

Triggers for a flare can be:

- temperature extremes
- cold wind
- sunlight
- sunburn
- stress
- anxiety
- alcohol
- caffeine
- spicy food
- strenuous exercise
- treatments such as chemical peels
- microdermabrasion
- local irritants such as menthol.

Treatment of rosacea
Getting a diagnosis, recognising your trigger and maybe even counselling can be essential.

- **Moisturising** – flushing and redness also increase water loss from the skin and a vicious cycle of redness and dryness and hence irritation can develop.
- **Sunscreens** can actually block some of the chemicals that trigger rosacea.
- **Antibiotic gel** can be prescribed but the gel components can actually be irritative and sting, so cream is often preferred. Ivermectin is a popular choice and can be very helpful, and also a chemical called **azelaic acid**. Retinoids are used ahead of oral antibiotics these days.

See Dr Hextall's interview for more detail on this.

Chemicals and skin

I love the word organic. I trust it and often spend extra pennies and pounds on it. However, as I have reiterated throughout this book, be wary of 'organic' labelling and do your research. Do not assume that for you all organic substances are not harmful – you may still react to natural compounds/develop allergies, and some materials are mixed with less natural chemicals in a product for stability. Get to know your brands. If, like me, you like a lot of chemical-free products (but I am not exclusively so personally), discuss with those selling the product about ingredients.

A strong word about smoking, pollution and ageing

The link between smoking and wrinkles has been known for many years. Women seem to be more susceptible to this than their male counterparts. Fine lines around the eyes (crow's feet) and mouth (smoker's lines) appear at an earlier age than non-smokers. Smoking women also seem to suffer with more facial redness, thinner skin and more obvious bony contours to the face. Smoking increases chemicals called enzymes to literally break down collagen and elastin in our skin, free radicals are increased and these generally have a detrimental effect on skin. Smoke literally constricts our blood vessels in our skin just like the rest of our body. Supply of goodies and removal of waste is thus reduced.

Longer-wave UVA radiation added to pollution can also worsen pigmentation in those susceptible.

Combining smoke or environmental pollutants with UVA light can have a synergistic effect and is more likely to cause ageing and other skin changes. All the more reason to say no to the fag on the beach and put your SPF on...

Now I have the honour of handing over to a wonderful Dermatologist and friend...

SPECIALIST INTERVIEW DR JUSTINE HEXTALL FRCP

Consultant Dermatologist,
Medical Director Tarrant Street Clinic
website www.Justinehextall.co.uk
Special interests: skin cancer surgical and non-surgical treatments, acne and rosacea, connective tissue dermatology and skin rejuvenation

Tell me about your approach to treating acne in midlife?

I will look immediately at triggers, hormonal changes, stress and dietary issues with an interest in gut health. I look carefully at skin products being used and any in-clinic or at-home skin procedures. I will look to make changes to diet considering the gut microbiome, balance any hormonal issues, look at exercise, stress management and sleep. I will make sure the skin regime is gentle, respecting the skin's barrier. Once this is all in place I will look at active treatments. I will try to avoid antibiotics, especially long courses, and will mostly start with a combination of a retinoid and benzyl peroxide. I will be very aware that retinoids can irritate skin at first and will introduce slowly, alongside emollients to soothe the skin after application. I sometimes combine with physical therapies, e.g. mandelic peels in combination with LED light. Less commonly I may use intense pulsed light. In most patients this approach works very well. Rarely I may need to step up to an oral retinoid.

Rosacea?

I take a very holistic approach to rosacea. Firstly, I will look for triggers such as UV exposure, stress, foods, alcohol. All patients with rosacea have a sensitive skin barrier. I introduce a specific gentle and hydrating skin regime to repair the skin barrier. I discuss probiotics if there seems to be a link between the skin and gut (which there often is) and I introduce a high-factor sun cream with protection against UVA/B and longer wavelengths to give broadest possible cover. This should be worn all the year round. I may suggest antioxidants, and then I prescribe a combination of topical metronidazole cream (not gel) and Ivermectin 1% to reduce the Demodex mite count. It is not certain the role Demodex mites play in rosacea, but topical Ivermectin has been shown to be very effective. If there is a telangiectatic (thread vein) element, once I have calmed the rosacea I will treat the erythema with intense pulsed light (IPL). I now try to avoid antibiotics in rosacea patients, even though in the short term they are effective, as I am concerned about their effects on the gut microbiome.

What is your personal view on supplements for the skin – collagen, antioxidants, vitamins and minerals?

I am interested in supplements, but firstly I would stress that no supplement is a substitute for a healthy balanced diet. I think marine proteins for example are good for nail and hair health. There are interesting but small studies looking at the effect of resveratrol in skin rejuvenation. There is some evidence that hydrolysed collagen may be effective, but definitely more studies are needed. Topical vitamin C is very effective for skin brightening and I always recommend vitamin D3 from October to April in the UK.

In terms of anti-ageing if we consider good skincare a done deal, what are the next steps of treatments you consider?

There are some very good long-term studies with large numbers showing the benefits of IPL in skin rejuvenation. There is no doubt that micro-needling is good for improving skin tone and texture and giving the skin a lift. I have found in my practice that combining micro-needling with PRP is particularly effective. As we lose hyaluronic acid from the age of 26 years, with a steep drop around menopause, injecting it into the skin in the form of a skin booster really helps to improve skin texture and hydration. In my view skin treatments should leave the skin looking fresher and brighter with improved texture and preferably lifted. Most importantly the face shouldn't look 'changed'. In my view if a procedure is obvious, it is a failed procedure.

What is your personal ethos for patients/clients in terms of more interventional procedures – Botox, fillers?

I think when Botox is done well it works brilliantly. In order to be successful a knowledge of anatomy is crucial. With good Botox, lines that age the face soften and may disappear, e.g. the angry furrowed brow, heavy forehead lines. The face looks lifted and fresher but moves normally. The heavy, flat, shiny forehead – the Botox giveaway – can and should be avoided.

What do you see in the future of skincare?

I think some of the current in-clinic procedures will definitely be available to do at home. I think skin treatments will become more bespoke, creating skin repair products specific to that individual. Products will become much more effective at protecting us from environmental stressors.

Any take-home message for the reader wanting to keep their skin optimal for their age?

Always wear a high-factor broad-spectrum sun cream, make sure your skincare regime respects the skin barrier, balance active ingredients such as retinoids with gentle cleansers and hydrating moisturisers. Consider topical antioxidants such as vitamin C and resveratrol to protect against environmental aggressors such as UV and pollutants to brighten skin. Always cleanse the skin at night to remove pollutants that will, if left, damage skin. Apply any active serums as night time, a great time for skin repair. Finally, sleep is vital for general health and especially for skin – hence the term 'beauty sleep'.

Thank you so much, Justine – all so helpful for many women who do not realise what help there is out there for their skin.

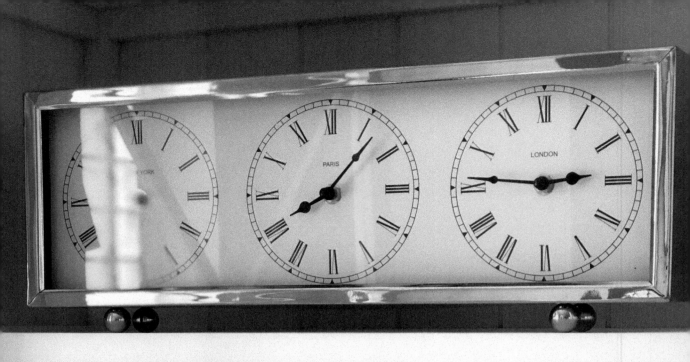
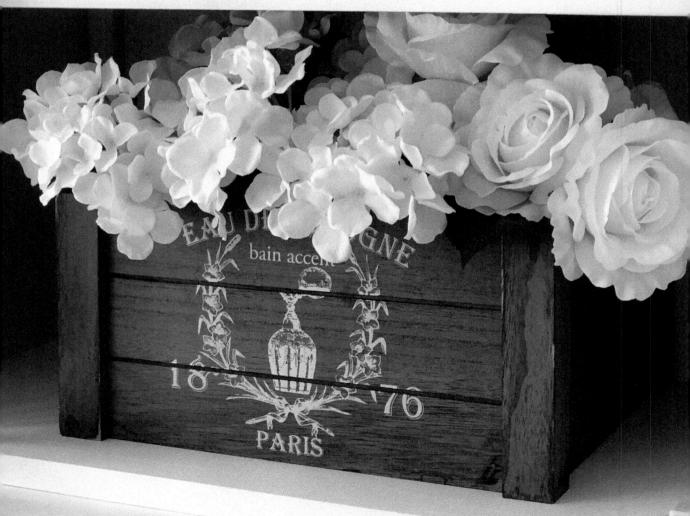

SKIN PRODUCTS

Okay... so possibly one of the most important parts of the book for many of you. Possibly the one important question my friends ask me over dinner. Information is everywhere. They are all products 'guaranteed' to make you look 'younger'. We want them now. I want them now.

I have spoken to many who are in the serious business of making others look younger. They know what they like in their beauty cupboards and they know what works for them. You can read it in 'The Women' section of this book and see what *you* think. I hear what they tell me and if they recommend something I want it!

I am a doctor writing this though, not just a woman reader, and I guess you want some scientific backing? I have an arsenal of serums that slide in and out of favour with me. I want scientific proof so I went through the papers in Dermatology and Plastic Surgery both sides of the Atlantic. Having spent a good portion of my time in the last five years living in the USA I can see how shared the market is. This is a level playing field. I can sit here in England and watch 'Annie from Minnesota' (name and place changed) show me on YouTube what retinol has done to her face over the last eight years. I can read the comments made by other women around the world about the 'good and bad' parts of this lady's face. Never before has beauty been quite so UNIVERSAL. We think we are unique but everywhere, right now, women are looking in the mirror and looking for answers. The only thing accurate to write here would be the ingredients backed by scientific research. A 'medication-like' substance can be introduced into a cream, branded a cosmeceutical, be on the market and thousands will apply it to their precious skin. Thus it is an unregulated business!

Beware, this information is subject to change. In 2021 something else may be discovered or side effects be revealed. The only way is to read around this and make your own informed choice. Always bear in mind my first words of this chapter – *your skin is an organ. It might absorb what you put on it.* Tattoo ink has been isolated as deposits in liver. That's evidence. Your body is a collection of systems that all communicate so be mindful. I could have written this book from the frame of mind of being all natural; I am all for that ethos and *many* of the products I choose to use on *myself* are naturally derived, certified not animal tested and won't allegedly give me cancer in ten years, but not all of them and where is the guarantee? Research your own brands. It is beyond the scope of this book to do this for you.

CLEANSING

Cleansing must remove grease, pollution and make-up but protect the skin's natural defence mechanisms. It should be **gentle** and effective. Not too harsh or drying. If it is too stringent then the skin reacts with rebound greasiness and inflammation. Creams, oils and balms are often less drying than *some* lathering foams or soaps. Remember, it is a delicate equilibrium. Alcohol-containing toners may temporarily remove excess grease but potentially over-dry skin. Work out what is best for you. Micellar waters are great if you don't have time to cleanse properly but not as good as a proper primary cleanser with water. Oils can be good at dissolving dirt and grime but these may be too oily for some. My good old favourite face wipes in my 30s just don't cut it as a cleanser unless I'm on an aeroplane.

Work out what is best for you. Our skin thins as we age, especially over 50, and the waterproof, fatty barrier may not be as resilient so cleansing should be gentle, not drying or harsh.

Ruby Hammer introduced me to the concept of double cleansing – so, using two different cleansers in the same routine. A face caked in make-up may require one clean to remove make-up and another to remove what is left from the day. Whatever you choose, single or double or even triple, do it carefully and thoroughly. Never use water too hot as broken capillaries and rosacea will be inflamed and the heat may dry your skin – use 'tepid' water to help dissolve grease away.

Mindful cleansing

What you cannot read on a product label is a concept I learned from Lee Pycroft. Be mindful of our cleansing routine and our mental associations with it. Use it as an opportunity to calm your breath and indulge yourself. Embrace this moment of stillness. Your face will relax and the process itself becomes therapeutic. Hocus pocus? Try it and no harm will be done. You may learn to love and relish those few quiet moments.

MOISTURISERS

The models and make-up artists I have spoken to all shared the same approach – cleanse, maybe tone and *always moisturise*. There are countless 'anti-ageing' creams on the market and all make exciting claims about reducing wrinkles, fine lines and sun damage. When you look at the actual ingredients many of them are remarkably similar. The most important component of is often moisturiser, making up about 80%.

I spoke about skin being a waterproof layer. This was essential in evolution for us to survive on land. It protects us from infection, desiccation (we are not coconuts), chemicals and mechanical stress. The stratum corneum layer cells (corneocytes) are tightly packed next to each other. The stratum corneum provides a barrier against water loss but some water does move out into the atmosphere through it. This is called *transepidermal water loss* (TEWL). Healthy skin has low levels of this loss but if you have eczema or psoriasis it can be excessive. Doctors love this measure because you can measure a moisturiser's ability to stop the TEWL, and we love some numbers.

Moisturisers temporarily smooth and enhance the protective barrier of the skin, temporary being the key word, and many a doctor will have tried to emphasise to a patient with eczema the necessity of **frequent reapplication** of moisturiser.

Moisturisers work in different ways...

1. Occlusives form a water-repelling layer over skin, even better applied to damp skin, e.g. petrolatum (Vaseline), cocoa butter, beeswax, shea butter. They are greasy but very effective. You might not want this over your face though and there are reports of the flammability of such moisturisers and sad, horrific stories. Dimethicone is occlusive but doesn't block pores or cause acne. It is a type of silicone and is found in oil-free moisturisers. Petrolatum actually works better on fine lines and dimethicone does not prevent water loss quite as much as petrolatum. However, if you think about sunscreen when you are sweating, this is a good feature as sweat can pass and also pore blockage spots don't develop. Smothering Vaseline on your face may flare up your acne.

2. Humectants enhance the water content of the skin by helping water move from the dermis deep up into the epidermis nearer the surface. They attract and hold water molecules. However, you can lose too much water from the dermis to the outside. These are things like hydroxyl acids, propylene glycol and urea. Sugars such as honey work in the same way. The one that is seen the most and has been discussed recently in the popular press is glycerol or glycerine. It also has the ability to reduce scaling by its work on that stratum corneum layer and can also produce moisturising effects in the skin long after it has been present. If you add an occlusive moisturiser to glycerine you have a bit of a powerful combination on a moisturising level as you stop that water escape.

3. Emollients improve the texture and appearance by filling in crevices between those corneocytes. Emollients include essential fatty acids and these are found in natural oils. Feeding your skin with a lovely body oil after a skin-stripping shower is a good habit.

4. Rejuvenators are supposed to replenish essential proteins in the skin. Proteins or peptides such as collagen, keratin and elastin are skin proteins found in these rejuvenators. They are large molecules and cannot get through that stratum corneum so they may not reach the dermis but can improve your skin appearance by creating a film over the skin. Aesthetically this smooths the skin, stretches it out and fills in fine lines. A bit like a filler in a cream on a small scale.

Many moisturisers are in more than one group. The best moisturisers have a combination of emollients and humectants.

A non-moisturising chemical group called **ceramides** are similar to fatty components of skin and these are often added to face creams and are oil soluble and so mix in easily with moisturisers. They are expensive but have been shown to improve the barrier function of damaged skin so are quite exciting. Recently, more research has shown some cheaper versions are effective.

So, the words are now familiar and you may find that some better value products have good ingredients. To be informed is power – right, ladies?

So, onto more exciting goodies.

ANTI-INFLAMMATORY AGENTS

Inflammation is caused by everyday life – pollutants, alcohol, sugar, poor oral hygiene, gum disease and infection. Change in lifestyle and diet will massively reduce the impact and so can skincare (see anti-inflammatory food for skin earlier).

Caffeine and alcohol have an inflammatory effect – they increase the levels of cortisol and this can exacerbate inflammation and wrinkles. Abstention may not be necessary but moderation may help (see alcohol section). Aloe vera gel has an anti-inflammatory effect on our skin.

Antioxidants in skin products

Antioxidants are formed naturally by the body to counteract the oxidative stress that occurs through pollution/stress/radiation and so on. We can help with natural antioxidants in our diet but also topically on our skin.

Topical vitamin C

This has been found to have a brightening, tightening and exfoliating action on the skin and seems to help collagen synthesis, confer some ultraviolet protection, lighten hyperpigmentation and reduce inflammation. Vitamin C is a strong antioxidant. It can also lighten dark spots on the skin and revive dull skins. I have talked about chronological ageing from birth that you cannot avoid – without the sun you have just skin thinning and a few wrinkles – have a look at your lovely bare behind. In sun-exposed areas damage is from photo-ageing and this is added onto what the ravishes of time have done. Vitamin C is thought to reduce ultraviolet-induced photo-injury – so, what the sun has done to your skin – by being such a powerful antioxidant. It also partly restructures your collagen. Powerful stuff. We think it also helps maintain the fatty waterproof layer of the skin by its action on some fatty cells. In summary, it has a brightening, tightening and exfoliating action on the skin and seems to help collagen synthesis, confer some ultraviolet protection, lighten hyperpigmentation and reduce inflammation. The formulation though has to deliver enough of the active ingredient so it is usually stored in darkened bottles. As storing is tricky, a good diet is still important and some studies are looking at supplements.

Green tea (catechins are active antioxidants but can be harmful in excess in some oral supplements) **and resveratrol** (more than you get from a glass of red vino) are making their way into topical skin products.

Vitamin E

This moisturises and heals and, when combined with vitamin C, can be more active as the vitamin C regenerates oxidised vitamin E!

Vitamin B3 (niacinamide)

This seems to have a broad range of action in skin when used on the skin and is well tolerated. Reduces hyperpigmentation, red blotchiness, reduces fine lines and wrinkles, improves elasticity and reduces skin sallowness (yellowing).

Vitamin D

This has important antioxidant roles in the body. See bone and nutrition chapters.

Vitamin A

Beta-carotene and the other carotenoids are the pre-active forms of vitamin A we get from food. Its active forms are retinal, retinol and retinoic acid and these are linked with many beauty products.

Retinol

I have talked in 'skin food' about the importance of vitamin A in the health of skin and in reducing ageing signs. I want to be clear about the difference between retinoids (prescribed by a doctor for acne or ageing – one name is tretinoin) and retinol. They are all vitamin A related but not the exact same thing. **Retinoids** work by initiating the skin to rapidly turn over cells, killing old cells to boost new cell growth. They also excitingly stimulate collagen production and thicken deeper layers of the skin which are the source of wrinkles. They can correct brown spots and curb melanin development. **Retinol** will do similar things but on a *more gentle* scale as it needs to be converted to the active form of a retinoid before it can work.

However, retinoids can have effects we just do not want. Tretinoin (Retin-A/trans-retinoic acid/retinoic acid) is a prescription drug launched by dermatologists over 40 years ago to treat acne. Doctors and patients noticed that it boosted collagen, reduced wrinkles and smoothed the skin. Retin-A is 100 times stronger than retinol and is already in the active form – retinoic acid is powerful on the skin and in your body. Your body does not need to convert it so it has quick effects, maybe within four to eight weeks. Sometimes the irritative effects are so high it is prescribed for ten-minute application then washed off so as to limit the skin's exposure. Because the tretinoin is strong and active when applied, the side effects of, say, irritation and peeling can be severe if too high a concentration is used, so the dermatologist titrates it up slowly. It is not advised to take in pregnancy or breastfeeding.

All fine if you are under the care of a doctor you trust but what can you do at home?

Retinol is a form of vitamin A that naturally occurs in the skin. Retinol in creams is artificially produced but works like vitamin A. Just using retinol often gives the results we are after. The body can almost self-regulate it as it has to convert retinol into the active retinoic acid form so it cannot 'overdose'. It may take three to six months to see the difference. Retinol can still irritate but this is unlikely in the dose found in most formulations as, remember, your body has to activate it first. Recently, manufacturers are concentrating retinol into higher concentrations in creams, and irritation may be more likely. Thus it is advised if changing to a stronger formulation to maybe use it once or twice a week initially and see if your skin tolerates it. If you are using a standard formulation ideally you can use it at night every day after cleansing.

It is absolutely imperative that with retinoids and retinol you properly adequately sunblock your face every day when using it and for a week or so after discontinuing. The skin is far more susceptible to damage from UVA and UVB rays while using it. A good plan of action is to use retinol more in the winter months and still sunblock.

Because retinol can destabilise it should be in darkened or opaque containers to maintain its potency. A good starter would be 0.2% retinol, then 0.3% retinol, then progress to 0.5% then 1%. Consider 2% but keep reading. If you get redness and dryness, reduce the number of nights you apply it weekly and wait for tolerance. Avoid the eye area unless the cream is specifically for that or you know you can tolerate it. There is a theory that high-concentration retinol may actually thin the skin and I have seen evidence of this on videos on YouTube of enthusiastic retinol users. If you want it combined with vitamin C there are formulas that do that; if you prefer an oil-based formula for extra moisturising then there are many for that. The fabulous thing these days is choice. My instinct is to start with basic creams that have just the ingredients I want.

There is an entirely natural compound called **Bakuchiol** which is a plant-based alternative to retinol, used in Ayurvedic medicine (from the BABCHI plant) with promising results. Watch this space.

Other antioxidants include **alpha-lipoic acid.**

Hyaluronic acid (HA)

This is a wondrous compound. It is naturally occurring in our bodies (you can see how beauty companies try to recreate the young functioning physiology of the skin) and is involved with manufacturing cells in the top layers of the skin and their reactions with the environment. It is also in our joints, eyes, internal fluids and is important for lubrication of connective tissue. One gram can hold six litres of water. That kind of doesn't sound right, does it?! As we age the amount of HA reduces, so why not add some back in to your daily routine? It is too large a molecule to penetrate so it sits on the skin's surface and grabs and holds moisture there. Babies have loads of HA in their skin hence their lovely soft skin. HA also helps the skin's healing and repairing ability. In studies they looked at that important stratum corneum layer of cells, and a statistically significant moisturising effect was found whether you used a serum, cream or lotion. There are also new smaller molecules being studied that can penetrate deeper. Because hyaluronic acid is naturally occurring in our bodies, the serums (albeit manufactured versions) present very low risk for allergy or irritation. It is also something you can use all year round. You might see formulas with sodium hyaluronate in the ingredients – this is the salt of hyaluronic acid and some say it goes deeper in the skin, but essentially it does the same job. Hyaluronic acid can draw water from the dermis deeper in our skin and thus from below so we can trap it in the stratum corneum by putting a lotion on top.

Hydroxy acids (alpha and beta) and peels

Peels offer instant exfoliation and can clear pores and in theory make them 'look' smaller.

Hydroxy acids which have this effect have been used in many cosmetic formulations. There is still some doubt as to how they work, although we are well informed of how they benefit the skin. Examples are glycolic acid, lactic acid and salicylic acid. They are used in a variety of concentrations and pHs to treat warts, photo-aged skin, psoriasis, sunspots and so on, often under the careful control of a specialised doctor. In the last 30 years alpha hydroxy acids (AHA) have been incorporated into cosmetic products for daily at-home use. It is thought they reduce roughness, discolouration and pigmentation and increase density of collagen and elastic fibres in the skin. Some formulas containing them act as exfoliants and moisturisers. In very high concentrations they are used as chemical peels.

Alpha hydroxy acids do include lactic acid so maybe Cleopatra bathing in milk was not such a bad idea! However, glycolic acid for example can increase the sensitivity of the skin to solar-type radiation and studies have tried to evaluate this, with differing results. It would seem that after stopping use the skin reverts to normal sensitivity after a week or so. This becomes important though if it is in a large number of products and being used daily, even if in small amounts, by a large number of the population. In the USA the Cosmetic Ingredient Review panel decided in 1998 that the acids were safe and did not cause cancer but that to reduce sensitivity the concentration should not be above 10% and that users should be advised to use sun protection separately or use acids in formulas incorporating sun protection. The sun risks have to be considered along with the benefits on reducing pigmentation and, interestingly, post-inflammatory pigmentation. It still seems there is some caution with using and *maybe occasional use or in low concentration* might be preferable. They do seem however to have antibacterial and anti-inflammatory effects and can be brilliant for acne. Glycolic acid can be good for scarring and can help skin regenerate.

Collagen

As this is such a large molecule, placing it into creams and onto the skin may not actually reach the places it needs to – smaller molecules may work better in delivery. Some collagen to be taken orally is thought to be from cow or chicken parts, which many people will not ethically consider or tolerate. Certain preparations that are acceptable have some successful trials. The main component is hydrolysed collagen, and although my first thought as a doctor would be that the digestive acids would destroy the proteins and break them down to amino acids (so you might as well have a good amount of lean protein in your diet) actually it seems bizarrely that the presence of the collagen fragments in the supplements encourages the body to use these for repair and also signals to the body that there may be damaged collagen and encourages it to make more, allegedly.

Maxine Laceby, founder of www.absolutecollagen.com, created a collagen supplement after she experienced amazing results from drinking homemade bone broth. She believed after research that the collagen in the bone was having an effect on her skin and wellbeing. Researching further, she developed her liquid product of 8000mg high-grade marine collagen and only deals directly with consumers via her website: www.absolutecollagen.com. The company has an increasing number of users reporting a reduction in the appearance of fine lines and wrinkles and thicker and faster growing hair.

A recent review in the Academic Dermatology press (January 2019) concluded that 'preliminary results are promising for the short and long-term use of oral collagen supplements for wound healing and skin aging. Oral collagen supplements also increase skin elasticity, hydration, and dermal collagen density. Collagen supplementation is generally safe with no reported adverse events'.

I really do think along with some of my dermatology colleagues that this is an area to be watched carefully. Do your own research and see (taking into account tolerance of ingredients) whether collagen supplementation is something for you.

Peptides
These are amino acids (building blocks of proteins) in small chains or chunks called peptides, and by being present on the skin they signal to cells that collagen has been lost and this encourages the cells to produce more collagen.

THE POWER OF LIGHT

Aside from the ageing effect of UV light, blue and red light has been found to be anti-inflammatory and antibacterial. They stimulate collagen so are becoming popular as face mask beauty treatments in salons and now at home. The *British Journal of Dermatology* stated that blue/red is better than blue and better than placebo. Machines for home use are likely to be weaker than in salon but watch this space.

A WORD ABOUT LIPS

As we age we know that our lips lose volume, definition and moisture. The effect will be dependent upon your genetic starting point. Fine lines develop around the lips naturally – not always related to smoking. Exfoliation of the lips with a gentle product and use of a lip cream can really help. Look for lipsticks with a moisturising not drying action.

HANDS, NECK AND DÉCOLLETAGE

These areas get a hard time with exposure to light and the elements and often a second-rate skincare regime. The chest can be more sensitive to ingredients so try with care. Start protecting and replenishing the area with moisturisers and active agents. We often look to hands to betray chronological age; protect these areas from skin cancer as well. Many side sleepers find their upper chest area folds and creates passive wrinkles during sleep. Back sleeping would of course relieve this but a lot of us cannot manage to adhere to this. I have tried gel-like patches that adhere to the skin here but find they end up somewhere else on my body by the morning!

SLEEPING WRINKLES

This is my name for the passive wrinkles we acquire through our faces being squished overnight. They have been studied in clinical trials by plastic surgeons. We tend to often favour one side and the wrinkles may be more pronounced here. You can try various pillows – wedge pillows, U-shaped beauty pillows, silk pillowcases (we know they snag and catch hair and skin less), pillows that have a structure that moves with your face... It really is a case of trial and error. I am a great advocate of silk eye masks as you will read in the sleep chapter but make sure yours is not so tight as to leave railroad markings across your face!

EYES

The cells around here produce the least oil and are the thinnest in the body and get thinner with age. Eye preparations can be soothing and depuffing (caffeine extract, a cold spoon(!), eye cream, cucumber slice) and they can also help if they contain peptides that stimulate collagen synthesis so skin is less thin and maybe less of the blood is seen beneath that gives rise to dark circles. Retinol can be used here but with great caution as the area can be so sensitive. Remember, non-caking make-up will be the least ageing here.

Eye serums contain more active ingredient and less additives like emollients and they are water based. In theory they are used before emollients. Many of the items mentioned, such as vitamin C, come in serum form.

It is imperative that you carefully use sun protection around the eye area; studies have shown that most of us miss this area and put it at risk of wrinkles and cancers. Sunglasses also confer protection, dependent upon their style.

CONSIDER 'LUXING UP' YOUR ROUTINE

Massage with serum, oil or balm is thought to be a great aspect of self-care if you are not receiving it in facials. Massaging upwards and towards the lymph node areas can help stimulate blood flow, and reduce tension in muscles, increase their tone and literally relax you. Use this as part of your mindful routine. A set of a jade and rose quartz roller was inexpensive and a great addition to my routine. The coolness of the roller is so refreshing. The smaller ends of a double-ended roller will reach areas on your face not touched normally in this way (such as around the nose). A Tokyo study proved all the beneficial effects mentioned in just ten minutes of use. Add a little each day and it will all add up, but keep your tools scrupulously clean!

WHAT DO I USE

Lou's Favourite Current Skincare Products in her 40s– opinion not advertisement

(sunblock has to be a priority obviously, especially alongside retinol and any resurfacing products)
Estee Lauder Advanced Night Repair
Estee Lauder Night Repair Eye Supercharged Complex
(these were game changers for me; balancing moisture, stopping any spots, reducing wrinkles and 'tired face')
Boots No. 7 Protect and Perfect range
(I used the serum from my 30s)
Aldi Lacura range
La Roche Posay (sun protection products – tinted and untinted, eye preparations and retinol formulations)
Tropic (face masks, fruit peel resurfacing serum, bamboo face cloth, body creams and oils, perfecting leg serum)
The Ordinary (need a product – buy exactly what you need by ingredient)
Elemis (soothing apricot toner, daily defence shield sunblock, procollagen range)
Liz Earle Cleanse and Polish Hot Cloth Cleanser (must have for me – effortlessly removes eye makeup and gently cleanses and balances skin)
Pra Ageless Throat and Decolletage Cream and **Mio Skincare Boob Tube** for the chest and throat area.

I nearly omitted this – who wants to know about me – but my friends ask me product advice and then seem to report great improvements after trying my favourite products. I make things last and some of the more expensive items I have had as samples and only invested after trying. I have not been paid to promote any of these, this is purely opinion and your skin is not the same as mine. Research product ingredients before you buy and read reviews.

THE PRACTICAL SIDE OF SKINCARE – WHAT AND WHEN

Look at your product stash. Make sure you take time to cosy up to the labels, discard what is out of date, work out the main active ingredients in what *you have*. Fill the gaps with what you need and get into a routine. What we do now should show in our faces in five years so if you are in it for the long haul get streamlining with me. Talk to your friends about what works for them – it may not work for you but recommendations are often valid.

Keep everything clean and ordered. You will enjoy using it more than chaotic bottles caked in last year's foundation that leaked. Make sure you don't run out of disposable cotton wool/buds, and better still get a stash of muslin or bamboo gentle cloths on daily wash rotation where you can easily grab a new one so you are not ladling last night's bacteria back onto your face.

Create night and day routines. Go that extra mile. Daytime is all about protection and night-time about restoration, repair and treatments. Leave time for layers of products to sink in by working them into your morning regime.

Remember the mantra 'thinnest to thickest'. Skin is designed to keep things out! We want the active ingredients that need to penetrate the skin to actually get in, so they are best first after cleansing. The products that we want to just sit on the surface can go last – like emollients and humectants – and then they keep the moisture and our serum in.

It makes total sense as water will not penetrate oil.

Chemical sunscreen will need to be absorbed to be effective and this would have to be applied before a moisturiser if you are not using a combined moisturiser/sunblock. Physical sunscreen does not need to penetrate so can be placed last.

Some combos are just not meant to be. Retinol and benzoyl peroxide can cancel each other out. Hydroxy acids can reduce the potency of vitamin C and increase irritation from it as they change its pH.

Dermatologists are divided but maybe keep retinol for night and vitamin C for day.

IF YOU ARE USING TOO MANY PRODUCTS YOUR SKIN MAY START FLAKING OR THE PRODUCT MIGHT RUB OFF OVER YOUR FACE. NOT ALL STAGES ARE ALWAYS APPROPRIATE EVERY DAY. DERMATOLOGISTS OFTEN ADVISE LISTENING TO WHAT YOUR SKIN IS TELLING YOU FOR THAT DAY OR NIGHT AND BEING SELECTIVE OR HAVING PRODUCTS IN ROTATION.

Korean concepts are filtering into mainstream skincare. Beauty essences are one. An essence is more 'creamy' than a toner and primes the skin for the next product as the skin will accept moisture better if it is already slightly 'damp'. Essences are lightweight hydrating liquids and have a higher number of active ingredients than a toner. Choose one designed for your needs – moisture or brightening.

Active products like retinol and acids may need time to absorb so try to leave 20 minutes after them in your evening routine. Ruby Hammer taught me to pause between serum and moisturiser to let the layers seep in with less residue.

DAYTIME DELIGHTS ROUTINE

CLEANSE
Lightly clean with warm water +/- your cleanser

TONE IF YOU ARE A TONER GIRL

ESSENCES IF YOU ARE AN ESSENCE GIRL

EYE CREAM
Apply this carefully with clean hands. This way you won't be contaminating this delicate area with irritative ingredients from your other products.

SERUM
Your antioxidant dose of goodies.

SPOT TREATMENT
If there are areas that need topical treatment try to apply *just the treatment* to the area and nothing else.

MOISTURISE
You may choose a combo product with SPF, if not...

MINERAL SUNSCREEN
Choose a product that doesn't leave a white pasty layer on your skin. If you are in front of a computer all day consider those with claims to protect against blue light as well.

MAKEUP

STARRY NIGHTS WIND-DOWN

CLEANSE
Oil or gentle balm cleanser of your choice.
Double cleanse if you feel it is necessary.

SERUM OR ESSENCE FOR HYDRATION
A good chance to ladle on some hyaluronic acid content.

EYE CREAM
Again with cleansed hands.

RESTORE AND REPAIR AND TREAT
If using acne or rosacea treatment incorporate this at this stage.
Retinol (heeding advice above).
Peptides and growth factors often in the form of 'anti-ageing' serums. Use this
stage for a roller treat if you are not using a facial oil.
Hydroxy acids – carefully heed warnings above.

FACE OILS
For skins that tolerate this, add in a few minutes with a jade roller if you
have the time, or treatment masks can be used that can be left overnight.

NIGHT MOISTURISER
These tend to be thicker than daytime preparations and
sit on the skin, stopping water loss overnight.

There is no doubt, despite this plethora of goodies at our fingertips, that it is tempting to only rely on the creams. Just like you can't out-train a bad diet by exercise, you can't expect a cream to give you youth and beauty if you are puffing on cigarettes and drinking wine and spirits nightly. You should discuss with a dermatologist or doctor if you have specific concerns and take advantage of a beautician's knowledge, bearing in mind she may be gaining commission on certain brands. Saying that, these days ingredients are clearly displayed and you can go home and have a think about what you want to buy and how, with no pressure. Beauty care providers are a fabulous source of information and if you find someone you can trust it's a great coup.

Another thought is the decluttering or 'going without' scenario. Overloaded heavily moisturised skin could in theory lose its ability to maintain moisture naturally – is it worth intermittently detoxing your skincare regime every so often and giving your skin a chance to find its own equilibrium? I am sure this will become a topic for discussion more as we think eco wise and revisit and reuse products we already have, maybe in different ways just like we revisit our wardrobes.

One proviso: don't think just because I have written about creams to reduce the visible signs of ageing that I am against ageing naturally. Completely the reverse. A woman is her true beautiful self with the wrinkles of her experience on display in her laugh and around her eyes. The age you appear is defined more by your attitude and the way you carry yourself than the number of lines around your mouth – I bet they came from laughing too.

CHAPTER 10:
HAIR LOSS

Hair loss is a hugely emotional subject. Hair is our crowning glory and part of our identity. When it doesn't look the same because there is less of it, it is not just a bad hair day – it hurts. As it cascades down the plughole or clumps of it lie at your feet in the shower, the pain is of losing something precious, like a bereavement. As you look under bright lights and see more of your scalp showing at your parting or your hairdresser notices patches of, dare I say it, baldness, it cuts like a knife.

Most women would not welcome hair loss and, although half of women by 65 have suffered it in some way, we do not talk about it much. It is a final taboo. Men go bald and they can still look sexy, but women – they might not feel the same. Doing a combover is not what you expect as a woman. Hair loss can trigger depression and anxiety symptoms and massively affect self-esteem, resulting in social isolation.

HAIR FACTS

We are born with about five million scalp follicles. All of the hairs that grow are at *different* stages of the growth cycle. There are three cycles:

- ANAGEN – this is the growing phase.
- CATAGEN – this is the transition phase where new growth stops but the hair is held in the follicle.

- TELOGEN – this is the resting phase where hair is shed, and then the cycle normally starts again. This phase usually lasts 100 days before re-entering the growth phase so the hair is *naturally lost* before another grows. This is fine when not many are lost at once.

We can all go through periods of increased shedding and it does not make much perceivable difference to our hair appearance. The recovery and regrowth naturally happen on their own with no treatment. We naturally shed around 50 to 100 hairs a day. When it goes beyond this we may notice our parting and our hair feeling thinner.

GETTING A DIAGNOSIS

It is important to establish the *cause of the hair loss* – it may be multifactorial – and the *type* to work out how to treat it. This is where it becomes more complex and, depending on the severity, an appointment with your GP may lead to referral to a dermatology consultant. They will take a careful medical history and blood tests and a possible scalp biopsy to reach their diagnosis. For any appointment about hair loss it helps to focus if you write a timeline first of symptoms and when they occurred and any triggers you can think of (illness, stress) to help the doctor understand easily.

FOOD AND HAIR

Food types that are great for hair alongside protein include:

- **Iron** (chicken, fish, lentils, spinach, leafy greens like kale and broccoli, and salad greens)
- **Vitamin C** is needed for collagen production so strengthens blood vessels supplying the hair root (fruit, sweet potatoes)
- **Omega-3** is involved with the production of oils in scalp (oily fish, avocado, pumpkin seeds, walnuts)
- **Vitamin A** helps us make sebum and provides a natural conditioner for hair. Hair can be dry and the scalp itchy without it; get this from food not supplements as an excess can be toxic. Found in orange and yellow veg (the beta-carotene that makes vitamin A gives it the colour), so carrots, sweet potatoes, pumpkins
- **Zinc and selenium** A lack of zinc makes the scalp dry and flaky. Get this from fortified cereals, wholegrains, oysters, beef and eggs.
- **Vitamin E** helps protect skin and hair from the sun. Nuts are great as they contain zinc, selenium and vitamin E.

LOUISE'S 'FOR HAIR' SALAD

There are many ways to incorporate these elements into your diet. Chuck salad greens, chopped up peeled orange, walnuts, grated carrots, pumpkin seeds, chicken or salmon together and make a salad with some or most of these ingredients, and if you vary it through the week you are covering the bases for your hair.

It goes without saying that having a healthy Mediterranean diet and a diet rich in protein from eggs, fish, chickpeas, etc. will benefit the hair but sometimes these things happen without your control and women can feel they have 'done something wrong' and are losing hair because of it. There is wrongly so much shame associated with hair loss and it can have causes beyond our control.

TYPES OF HAIR LOSS

1. Telogen effluvium (TE)

This is when there is a **diffuse shed of hair** – more in the resting (telogen) phase is shed than normal so we notice the difference. Hair is non-essential to our bodies, the last thing to receive nutrients and so is shed when nutrition, etc. is under par.

TE can occur:

- in cases of under or active **thyroid**
- naturally **postpartum** when hormone levels subside (but remember, postpartum can also be a trigger for alopecia areata)
- with some **contraceptive pills** (or stopping them)
- with some **medication** (*some* antidepressants/anti-epileptic medication/anti-ulcer drugs/betablockers)
- after shock, trauma, bereavement
- **postmenopausally** – as oestrogen reduces it cannot oppose the effects of testosterone
- after **weight loss** surgery or simply after drastic weight loss
- with low **iron STORES** (we know now you do not actually have to be anaemic to get hair loss from this – it may occur with just low iron stores but otherwise normal blood tests). A large French study of 5,000 women confirmed that low iron stores caused hair loss with a ferritin below a certain point – to regain hair, try to get levels well above 60ng/l.
- **joggers** can suffer hair loss due to possible haemolysis (breaking down of blood cells with trauma) and possibly low iron stores if a new regime is started without a supportive diet. Any sudden change in diet and exercise needs to be supported by care and nutrition – don't let this stop you running!
- **zinc and copper** and other mineral deficiencies

- **vitamin D deficiency**
- you have a higher amount of free **testosterone** in your blood (this means testosterone not carried by a protein called sex hormone binding globulin but *free active hormone*). This active testosterone called DHT can cause the hair follicles to shrink and hair to become finer with successive cycles.
- complete shedding at time of **chemotherapy** (sometimes reduced by wearing a cool cap – frozen gel in cap constricts blood vessels during chemo so less meds to scalp – not always effective); or after **radiotherapy that may cause scarring alopecia to hair-bearing areas**. Hair generally recovers well from chemotherapy and may come back curlier or different due to hair shaft changes, as I have seen in one of my close friends who says she is now Shirley Temple!

Diagnosis and history of telogen effluvium

The **history** of your symptoms is important. Shocks and physiological events usually take about three months to show in your hair due to the timing of the hair cycle, so that is why the history is vital. **Examination** by the doctor will show that generally the hair is diffusely thinner and 30% or more of the hair is lost. Blood tests help to make the diagnosis and may not all be done by a GP – you may need specialist referral for:

- thyroid function
- routine blood tests and ferritin (iron stores)
- zinc (this may not be done by your GP, only a specialist, as the results can be thought inaccurate)
- vitamin D and testosterone levels (free and bound).

Treatment for TE

There may be spontaneous resolution, such as postpartum when hormones balance out again. If the underlying cause is treated the hair may recover. Zinc, copper and iron all compete for absorption in the gut so if you end up needing iron and zinc replacement then take the supplements at different times. Copper is not always recommended as a supplement per se as its absorption profile is extremely complex, so you will simply be encouraged to have a mineral-rich diet. Remember, patience is required with any treatment as the hair cycle means it can take six months for improvement to show.

Vitamin D3 is very effective as a supplement in the form of a spray or liquid drops dissolved in oil. Take the recommended dose or that stated by your doctor after the blood test. **Viviscal** hair supplement may be recommended as there is strong evidence that this helps although may take six months for you to see a difference, as with all these things. Shedding should decrease with treatments before changes are actually seen. **Nothing better than an excellent diet though**.

HRT may help in postmenopausal cases (if it is deemed right for you by the doctor) when taking into account general health and any contraindications. It would not be a sole reason for taking HRT but would be a very motivating reason for many women.

Vitamin B12, biotin and selenium are far better obtained from a healthy diet than a tablet – we do not have enough evidence really for biotin as a supplement helping hair.

2. Female pattern hair loss (FPHL), also called androgenetic alopecia

This is the women's equivalent of male pattern baldness. This is partly genetic and can also be related to hormone imbalance, part of **polycystic ovary syndrome (PCOS)** or related to the menopause.

Diagnosis and history of FPHL

Examining the scalp, the hair loss is around the top and sides, especially temple regions. The issue is that many women will have a combination of TE and FPHL so it may not be just one cause.

Treatment of FPHL

The mainstay of treatment is **minoxidil** as a topical solution – **the women's preparation** – a solution applied to the scalp once or twice a day. It extends the growth phase of the hair so that there are more strands on the head. IF YOU STOP using it YOU LOSE THE HAIR YOU REGAINED. This is a commitment. A study at King's College London showed significant results.

3. Hair loss associated with lupus

Lupus can cause inflammation that involves the scalp and can cause general thinning of scalp hair, or sometimes round discoid lesions on the scalp which may scar hair follicles causing permanent hair loss in these areas. In the hairline region hairs can become brittle.

4. Alopecia areata (AA)

This is an autoimmune condition which usually starts with one or two isolated patches of complete hair loss on the scalp. It may be associated with other autoimmune conditions such as vitiligo. The body is basically reacting against itself to work against the hair. There can be a family history of autoimmune disease. Not just head hair but also underarm, arm and even eyelashes and eyebrows may be completely lost. In the event all hair is lost we call this **alopecia totalis**. There is the possibility that the hair may grow back but there is always the chance of the condition recurring at a later point.

Diagnosis of AA

This will usually warrant referral to a dermatologist, and scalp biopsy, blood tests and examination after taking a thorough family and medical history is appropriate.

Treatment of AA

Patches of AA can be injected with a steroid by a dermatologist – the earlier caught the better. Steroid creams, dithronal, UV light and immune therapy are all further options to be discussed with a specialist. There is emerging evidence for some disease-modifying drugs.

5. Frontal fibrosing alopecia

This is a form of lichen planopilaris that causes gradually progressive alopecia and scarring on the scalp at the front near the forehead. In some cases, eyelashes, eyebrows and other areas are affected. It is not really known what causes it and may be genetic or an autoimmune response. Some medication prescribed by a dermatologist may help but there is really no known cure. It can be associated with FPHL in some cases.

6. Eczema, dandruff, ringworm or psoriasis related alopecia

These can all cause hair loss and can be fairly easily treated. They will worsen with stress and also if you leave hair damp and not ventilated after washing, or covered as you tie it up, as the moisture will encourage yeast growth on the scalp.

Treatment of scalp irritation

An antidandruff shampoo containing zinc pyrithione (as in Head & Shoulders) can help if used two or three times a week, or Vosene or a tea tree oil based shampoo. This all has an antimicrobial and anti-inflammatory effect on the scalp so may stimulate hair growth. Stronger topical treatments or shampoos may be prescribed for psoriasis, along with managing stress and potential UV therapy. Ringworm will require a specific treatment or shampoo from the doctor. You can read a lot more about scalp conditions, ringworm and dandruff in my articles at www.netdoctor.co.uk.

7. Traction alopecia and trichotillomania

Pulling your hair too tight with clips and bands can have a permanent damaging effect. The compulsion to pull out hair and it acting as a kind of release in trichotillomania is a complex issue that needs to be handled delicately and with psychological-based treatments. In many cases the hair will return but in recalcitrant cases it may be permanently lost as the follicles are damaged.

General advice

Have a diet rich in protein – especially important postmenopausally – and some specialists recommend complex carbs too. Many other remedies for improving hair have been tried. Vera Peiffer in her book advises using jojoba oil on the scalp to keep the pores clear but massaging the scalp with the oil and maybe covering with a turban at night. She also believes nettle tea stimulates hair growth and advises washing with the cooled-down liquid. Olive oil may be an alternate massage oil or aloe vera gel. Any massage should increase blood supply and encourage hair growth. This is often part of facial acupuncture as well.

Try to think holistically and, in terms of hair and skin, really try to avoid strong detergents that tend to strip our skin and can *in theory* cause hair loss, eczema and so on...

CHEMICALS IN OUR PRODUCTS

The Environmental Working Group (www.ewg.org) exists to empower people to live healthier lives in a healthier environment. It is a non-profit, non-partisan organisation dedicated to protecting human health and the environment. Based in the USA it looks scientifically at many aspects of life – from cleansers, water quality and the environment to what is found in food. Because this is USA based not all data can be extrapolated back to the UK and we have different guidelines for contents of products and so on.

The Cosmetic, Toiletry and Perfumery Association (ctpa.org.uk) has a role in trying to make sense of risk versus hazard. It aims to promote best practice, ensuring cosmetics are made to the highest possible safety standards. This works as a voice to the UK government, the EC authorities and the media. We are very demanding upon the cosmetic industry and in many cases chemicals are safe or are used in concentrations that deem them safe.

It is beyond my scope to examine all of this in detail. I think you have to find the margin you are happy with: no chemicals, limited chemicals, organic, partially organic? This will all be a personal choice based on your own research. Read labels on products. Not all skins tolerate products the same. Invest in what you feel strongly about. You may dismiss this research or you may choose to never use chemicals again. On the matter of animal testing of products this is for you to investigate yourself. *Be mindful* when making decisions related to products used on scalp and skin: some things may be absorbed, some may not.

Here are a few chemical facts...

Sodium lauryl sulphate (SLS) – found in soaps, shampoos, shower gels, toothpaste. Works as a surfactant, trapping oil-based dirt so it can be rinsed away. It can irritate skin, eyes or lungs. It is used in certain cosmetics for which it has been deemed safe because of the low concentration. It is thought to disrupt the natural oils that maintain the skin's integrity, so less protection from allergens as it has a drying effect. Palm oil is used in the production of SLS and has a well-known destructive effect upon tropical forests and livelihoods. By reducing the amount of SLS in products we are heading in the right direction. The trouble is, it creates the rich foams we are used to.

Sodium laureth sulphate (SLES)

Diethanolamine irritative, linked to many health problems and potentially carcinogenic

Propylene glycol irritative, allergy

Isopropyl alcohol irritative, may have other harmful effects

Parabens (methyl, propyl, ethyl, butyl, isobutyl) are thought to cause hormone disruption, irritative, allergy.

Remember, many products contain these chemicals at allegedly safe levels. Many of the effects may only be seen in research at **high dosage**.

Organic is produced without pesticides, synthetic fertilisers, genetically modified organisms (GMOs), sewage, ionising radiation, antibiotics or growth hormones. Natural just means derived from nature.

Natural *or* organic (you will have to research each further) skin and hair care brands include:

- www.tropic.co.uk
- www.myroo.co.uk
- www.100percentpure.com
- www.truebotanicals.com
- www.juicebeauty.com
- www.honestbeauty.com
- www.honestskincare.co.uk

Natural hair brands include:

- www.thinknatural.co.uk (Avalon, Jason)
- www.aubreyorganicsuk.co.uk (Aubrey Organics)
- www.soorganic.com (Barefoot Botanicals)

Natural hair dyes include:

- Aubrey Organics
- www.suvarna.co.uk (Logona)

BACK TO HAIR AS YOU AGE

Generally, after menopause look for a milder shampoo and lighter conditioner. Try not to apply conditioner to the roots; and if your hair is thinning, colour techniques can thicken the hair shaft as colour swells the hair cuticle. Some colouring techniques thicken the appearance of the hair but others can cause it to break off and become brittle. Darker hair colours have been hypothesised to increase the risk of cancer in some studies. It seems dark dyes before 1980 were potentially more harmful, but evidence is both ways for later dyes. There is an increased risk of bladder cancer in hairdressers and this is thought to be related to the use of chemicals. Whatever you choose, use the advice of a hairdresser you trust. Colours can be more naturally produced now.

Shampoos containing caffeine are on the market. There is good evidence for them helping hair growth in lab conditions and we need more clinical trials. There is some emerging evidence of this helping women with hair loss, but we need more long-term studies. They may help hair appearance by improving the health of hair by helping blood flow to the scalp. The beneficial effects may be more in leave in products or when combining with other hair loss treatments.

Condition-improving products like 'Olaplex' have revolutionised the colouring market but should be used under the guidance of a professional hairdresser as they work on the bonds within the hair. 'Philip Kingsley Elasticizer' is a great product for helping soften brittle or damaged hair. 'Thicker Fuller Hair Revitalizing shampoo and conditioner' can help cosmetically improve the appearance of thinning hair. Always be aware of product build-up and of not overloading your hair with conditioner. Protection of hair from ultraviolet light with a hat or UV protective spray should be as important as your sunblock in sunny hot weather. When buying products that may be more expensive than your typical supermarket shampoo, make sure you are purchasing from a recognised retailer and receiving the genuine article.

Hair – to wear or not to wear

Life being the way it is, sometimes, despite extensive investigation and treatment, hair loss becomes a chronic condition and you may choose to *lose the stress* and start wearing hair. If you are undergoing chemotherapy or radiotherapy you may have a temporary window when you will want to wear hair.

This can be in the form of **extensions** (be careful to discuss with the technician the state of your own hair as wrongly fitted these can cause long-term traction if the extensions are too heavy). These can be attached by bonds, rings and other methods. Research carefully and look at the quality of hair.

There are **'hair integration systems'** where your own hair is integrated with a hair piece, and these should ideally be discussed with your dermatologist and the company you are going to – do your own research and find out if this is the right route for you.

Synthetic wigs and hairpieces ('toppers' not designed to cover the entire scalp, only the top part) are available from the NHS in the UK and privately. There are strict criteria depending upon where you live in the UK for obtaining a free wig. If you want a *real hair* wig or topper you will need to seek this on a private basis as they are not given on the NHS (except in exceptional cases such as allergy to synthetic hair or having an incurable condition and so on – all criteria decided by the dermatologist). Synthetic hair is easier to look after but the wig may only have a longevity of six to twelve months (which might be appropriate for chemo patients, say). There are care points with a synthetic wig – do not allow it to be exposed to intense heat (e.g. opening oven door) as it may melt! Cleaning is relatively simple. The NHS tends to supply a new wig every six months *to those who are entitled to it*. The criteria are helpfully laid out with a great wealth of information on the Cancer Research website: https://www.cancerresearchuk.org/about-cancer/coping/physically/changes-appearance/hair-loss/wigs-other-ways.

An NHS synthetic wig costs between £50 and £200 upwards, depending on the type. Speak to your clinical nurse specialist if you are not sure what you are entitled to.

Real hair wigs are something you must research. Thanks to a particular American family, 'wearing hair' no longer bears the same stigma it used to. Most good wigs have a lace front and a silk top – designed to look like scalp so only the wearer will know. You can stick to your old style or even go for the hair you always wanted. Styling natural hair is easier than synthetic. The price of initial outlay is quite high and you have to work out if this is the right route for you.

https://www.nhs.uk/using-the-nhs/help-with-health-costs/wigs-and-fabric-supports-on-the-nhs/
www.glamorousbutterfly.co.uk

Head coverings

It may be your choice to go glam or simple with head coverings. Buffs are an alternative to scarves and bandanas and are stretchy tubes of fabric offering some UV protection: www.lusciouslids. com, www.annabandana.co.uk, www.bohemiaheadwear.co.uk.

Future and specialist treatments

PRP, laser light therapy, can be discussed with your dermatologist.

Whatever the problem, you may feel very alone if you do not experience improvement and, remember, this may take months or a year or more. Hair loss clinics run by dermatologists may give you stronger topical lotions and medications to help but be careful you are being treated by a well-researched doctor. In some cases, hair transplantation is appropriate, albeit an expensive and permanent potential solution.

For women going through hair loss with no one to talk to, then https://www. womenshairlossproject.com/category/womens-hair-loss-network/ is an international organisation online that can be logged into in confidence, protecting your identity, and you can read stories from women suffering and share solutions. This appears to be a secure network at the time of writing but it is your responsibility to check this for yourself.

There is no shame in admitting hair is important. If you are suffering hair loss that does not seem to be resolving, seek the advice of a doctor you trust and explore all your options.

Embracing the grey?

Going grey heralds many different responses. By 30, most people have a few grey hairs; by 50 normally half of the hair will have greyed. Pernicious anaemia, diabetes and thyroid changes can cause premature greying. Grey hair will be more noticeable the darker your natural hair colour. Grey hair is actually white hairs interspersed with normally pigmented hairs. Grey hair has less protection from UV as it is lacking melanin.

Food and hormones can influence greying but a lot may be inherited patterns. Some studies have shown that some B vitamins help reverse some greying but this is really *animal studies* and would probably involve excessive dosage. Emerging results suggest stress does influence greying.

As we age, hair gets finer and drier and thus it may appear coarse but is not actually thicker. If you perm grey hair it can turn slightly yellow, and the same with smoking. The on-trend purple shampoos can cancel out this yellowness in the same way they reduce brassiness in bleached blondes, however do not use too frequently *as product build-up will turn your hair lilac*. Unless you want lilac, which can look fabulous!

Reading resources
Regrowing Hair Naturally by Vera Peiffer
The Hair Bible Philip Kingsley
The Modern Rapunzel by Jeanne Powers
What's up With My Hair? by Mary Corrigan

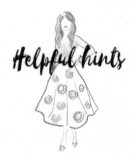

Helpful hints

- Hair loss is complex
- If things are worsening consult your GP
- Write a timeline of symptoms and events that may have triggered change
- Ask your hairdresser to check for progress on loss you can't see
- Look at what you can improve in your diet
- Look at supplements with a doctor
- Remember, hair loss is often multifactorial and patience is key. Any changes take at least three months to show and loss similarly may occur three months after a triggering event.
- Seek out a consultant with a special interest if you are not getting anywhere, PRP and other new treatments may help

CHAPTER 11: A BROADER APPROACH TO FEMALE HEALTH

Engaging the link between mental and physical health and opening up to our own version of spirituality

Western medicine is what I know. Conventional teaching for a medical degree and clinical experience of 15 years in the NHS shaped my knowledge, along with the subsequent specialised training and examinations. However, conventional medicine is only one part of the story. It is the only part that I can tell as a medical doctor. I can quote you evidence for what I have written, as it is how I operate.

There are many features of our world that cannot be explained, that have an enigma or a mystery about them. Some of these we will never comprehend. Spirituality and belief are an important, valued aspect of life for many of us and I could not encapsulate them with simple words on a page. We all have different views and that is the wonder of this world.

However, the **formal study** of other recognised fields within healthcare and outside it, which could complement my own **with their own basis of evidence**, fascinates me. As a woman studying the effects of ageing and lifestyle on health and disease, I am open to the superior knowledge of specialists whose work would be complementary, and possibly synergistic, used alongside conventional medicine.

ACUPUNCTURE

My own experience of acupuncture before 2017 was brief. I had been concisely taught some techniques to use for chronic pain sufferers when I was a young anaesthetist working in the hospital pain clinic. At this time the clinicians teaching me were quite clear that it would be greatly beneficial for some but not help all.

I understood that, in that context, acupuncture in the pain clinic was working by the 'gate theory' of pain control. Basically this theory explains how stimulating the pressure receptors around an area of pain blocks the sensation of pain travelling to the brain and thus the perception you have of it.

THERE ARE SO MANY PATHS TO CHOOSE IN LIFE, YOU WILL NEVER KNOW IF EACH ONE WAS RIGHT OR WRONG. SURELY THAT IS THE PURE FUN OF IT.

Hence why your parent may have said 'rub it better' when you hurt yourself; and TENS (transcutaneous electrical nerve stimulation) machines work on labouring mothers' lower backs. This is all working through the 'gate control theory of pain'.

Hence, me placing carefully chosen acupuncture needles in specific areas of patients, e.g. neck muscle areas, seemed to help with their pain. The needles would be left for 20 minutes or so, and often repeated sessions would see some patients improve.

My first general acupuncture as a client

I did not really know what to expect as I walked in to see the lovely acupuncturist Shelley. She had studied for a four-year BSc and more and was extremely knowledgeable about Chinese medicine and many different healing methods, dependent upon the client's needs. This was a whole new world to me!

On a very basic level I understood that it respects that the mind and the body are very much connected. The mind has a definite effect on the body – think of something tragic or frightening that you have experienced. Feel your heart rate quicken and the feeling of anxiety rise. My visit to an acupuncturist was part of my cathartic mission to improve my health and wellbeing. My ailments were upper back tension from the hours at my desk, very occasional migraines and just being a worrier. What could be done for me?

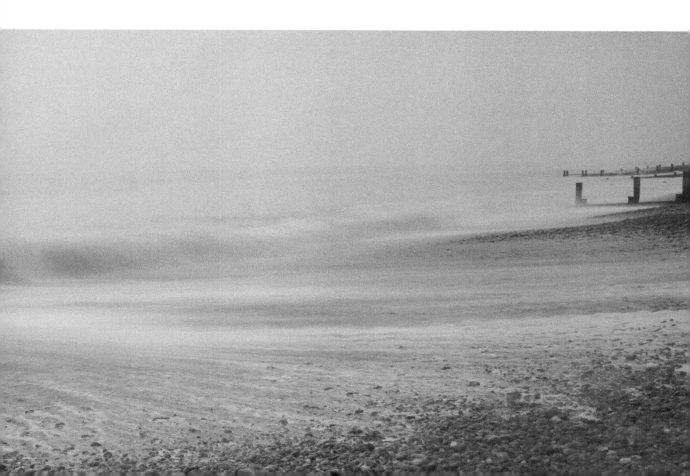

My first session was to look at my current state of health and see what could be helped in terms of illness prevention. It is common to visit a practitioner at the **change of the seasons** to prevent stress on the body and thus disease. My pulses were felt, but not in the way I would have palpated pulses. Shelley assessed different systems in the body from the pulses at varying points and depth on my wrists.

I was holding a lot of emotional tension at the time and this was described as being around the liver and kidney systems – an oversimplification really. It did not mean in the sense of disease in those organs. The kidneys reflected my increasing age and the impact that two traumatic episodes of childbirth and blood loss had impacted. The adrenal glands sitting above the kidneys were likely under strain with everyday stresses.

Needles were then placed fairly painlessly in various places in my body and left for 20 minutes or more. It was immensely calming – a perfect time of mindfulness – and my day was able to continue after as usual, ensuring I kept myself hydrated as advised. A great night's sleep followed. By my next appointment I realised my upper back tension was greatly improved – could have been exercise or the acupuncture or both.

My first facial acupuncture

We talked about what my thoughts were on my needs for my face. I laughed at this as I came up with a fairly long list! I had started to notice some fairly minor furrow lines, and my general exclaiming personality ('oh really') when people tell me gossip had started to create some wiggly lines above my eyebrows. Shelley reassured me she would work on the 'looser' facial areas.

Shelley explained all she would do. There would be some additional 'intradermal' needles to problem areas, reaching the slightly deeper dermal layer. I was warned there could be a slight chance of bruising, which I happily accepted.

My face was gently cleansed with a tea tree oil preparation and I was ready for the treatment.

The needles were placed in my ears, lower and upper body and finally the face. I have read that insertion in the ear may even have an anaesthetising effect on the face as it releases endorphins. The whole experience was relatively painless. You are conscious of the needles going in but really just the pressure sensation as they are so tiny.

Once all the needles were in situ I was left to relax for 25 to 30 minutes with eyes closed, and calm descended.

After the treatment the needles were gently removed and I was to have a head, face and neck massage to work on specific points to help the face.

My face was gently massaged with specific oils. The massage was immensely relaxing and worked gently but firmly on the areas of my scalp and neck *that felt as though they had needed this for the last ten years*. The facial massage was exceedingly soothing. Finally, my face was gently cooled with a jade roller to close the pores.

At the end I had a reaction that surprised and shocked me. I burst into tears. I could only describe the feeling as though the massage was 'something I really needed' and that the tension was now running out of my body. From my introductory chapter I wrote about my pneumonia and my escape from a shortened life at that time. In the years that followed I had completely focussed on my children and family. Maybe I was just not dealing with the emotion of the risk to my health that the illness had posed. I really felt that being ill had just made me appreciate every moment of life and want to squeeze the last drop out of it. Somehow this head massage was releasing those pent-up emotions. Whilst sobbing and laughing we tried to piece the information together. My most cynical colleagues would be hysterical now – Louise has 'gone to the other side' with that hocus pocus. All I say is, you don't know until you try it. The massage may have been the trigger for the emotional release, or the time in the consultation for one-on-one discussion of 'self'. How often does someone ask you how you are, really? Just having a good stretch or moment of yoga can energise your body, so it was no surprise really that such focussed treatment would have a beneficial effect. Whatever it was, I felt a release and more energised for the future.

My skin looked so good when I got home.

What changes did I see?

A week later I could see that I looked brighter and the darkness under my eyes was markedly reduced. I had also developed a feeling of calm. I felt more in control of my responses to stress and very invigorated to get things sorted.

The cynic would say that this could be due to now giving myself a little 'me time'. There was, however, no disputing the lightened effect on my face.

Doing things back to front and not reading instructions and jumping straight in is a little forte of mine. This is all well and good with an Ikea flatpack. I did the research into what I had experienced *after the event* this time and can hopefully enlighten you a little on the methods and beliefs of acupuncture from an Eastern medicine perspective.

The science of facial acupuncture

In Chinese medicine it is thought that many meridians (pathways in the body along which energy flows) start or finish in the face and hence the relation of health and appearance.

Changes and deterioration in muscle tone may therefore reflect imbalance in the body.

In a time when we hear of celebrities trialling natural and not so natural ways to look young, there can be phases of interest in a procedure spread by word of mouth or the internet. Facial acupuncture seems to be one of them, with mentions in the popular press as far back as 2007. However, it was of course developed many years before that.

It is known in Chinese-documented history that the Empress and Imperial concubines enjoyed the luxury of acupuncture for 'cosmetic enhancement' as far back as 475 BC.

More recently, when patients were treated for conditions like Bell's Palsy with needling, it was found that the surrounding skin improved in terms of colour, texture, elasticity and size of wrinkles!

The use of acupuncture for cosmetic purposes has gained momentum worldwide. There was little research documented in conventional medical literature about its safety and efficacy. One study in 2013 by Yun et al. first looked at this. They wanted to see if it had an effect on facial elasticity. The theory was that it must affect elasticity by restoring resting mimetic muscle tone through the insertion of needles in the face and neck.

It is thought to be more effective when combined with facial massage, therapeutic-grade essential oils and aromatherapy blends. As with all the methods I am investigating in pursuit of 'your best life', this approach combined with lifestyle management and healthy nutrition should only amplify any effects.

In a study performed in Gangdong, Korea, the female participants received five treatment sessions over a period of three weeks. The outcomes or effectiveness were measured by the patient's own assessment and also a 'topography criteria' – contour lines were generated on a photograph of the face, and the cheek and mouth regions were assessed independently for improvement.

A significant improvement was seen by the topography measure after treatment. An improvement was measured by the women themselves, although this difference was not statistically significant.

So it seemed this was a big step in assessing facial acupuncture. More large-scale trials are thought to be needed as most people have up to 8-12 recommended sessions or more. It then seems to be beneficial to have maintenance treatments to follow seasonally or monthly.

As this is an area of medicine I have not studied I was prepared to try it myself if it were to at least do no harm. I was warned that due to the high blood supply to the face there can be a risk of bruises or haematomas (collections of blood under the skin), and I found one anecdotal report on the internet of a patient suffering a skin infection. If you find a practitioner be sure they are practising in a sterile environment with sterile packed disposable needles.

Different theories as to how facial acupuncture works include:

- the acupuncture may reverse the shortening and straightening of facial muscles that occurs with age, increasing our resting muscle tone – in other words it may increase elasticity
- increasing blood flow at certain points
- stimulating collagen regeneration by stimulating the dermal layers of the skin directly
- possible evoked inflammatory response at site of needle insertion provokes wound healing response and localised inflammation that will provoke changes for the better.

Moisture in the skin
A study in 2012 by Donoyama et al. looked at acupuncture in the value of oil and water content of the skin. In this small study acupuncture increased the water and oil content of the facial skin in a female participant whose water and oil content were lower beforehand than average women of her age.

My conclusion

My personal experience:

- immensely relaxing
- luxurious moment of mindfulness
- I was approaching ageing from within with no harmful chemicals

Just talking about the natural ageing process with a practitioner starts you on a road of self-care and may secondarily improve your general health by the treatment and your subsequent approach to lifestyle. I felt the needles had stimulated more than just something in my face and felt keen to complete a full course for evaluation later.

This is a subjective personal opinion.

For general health I now see Shelley regularly for acupuncture. She has become a friend and an integral part of my life. I personally find great benefit from regular appointments; the whole experience is always enlightening. Shelley has told me things about my health from examining me that I had forgotten to tell her with words or then go on to discover. For this writing 'gal' acupuncture is now part of my health arsenal, to reset my stress levels and achieve some balance. Here's over to Shelley herself...

SHELLEY OSBORNE-SHAW BSc (Hons) MBAc.C

My passion for acupuncture sparked in my teens when I received treatment for the first time. I remember seeing diagrams on the clinic walls of the human body covered with lines and dots. I soon came to learn these lines marked the meridians, energetic pathways that circulate qi through the body, and all the tiny dots represented the 361 acupuncture points. I found the treatment to be very effective and the whole experience was fascinating, from having my pulse and tongue read to experiencing a deep feeling of peace and calm. This sparked my interest in holistic healthcare at a young age. I became interested in the connection between mind, body and spirit and this grew even more 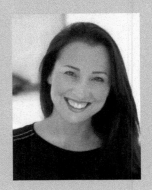 when I began meditating and practising yoga. I came to realise there is more to consider than the physical alone when it comes to treating our health.

I went on to study holistic therapies, qualifying in Reflexology, Aromatherapy and Energy Healing. I practised for some time, gaining experience, before undertaking my four-year bachelor of science degree in Acupuncture and Chinese Medicine. This really set my professional trajectory in motion and for the last 11 years I have been solely practicing acupuncture.

My special areas of interest

One of my areas of interest is the use of acupuncture for emotional wellbeing and mind health. This has led me to work in areas such as stress management, addiction, depression and anxiety. Acupuncture is a wonderful therapy to support our emotional body.

Depending on how sensitive we are to stress some of us can struggle more than others when the going gets tough – our body can go into overdrive and experience what is known as a 'fight or flight' response to normal day-to-day stresses. This response is activated by our sympathetic nervous system and is actually part of our inbuilt survival mechanism primarily used for when we perceive great danger, however in the modern world it can be triggered by events and experiences which are far from life-threatening such as sustained worry, a confrontation or a pending work presentation. When we experience this kind of stress our body is flooded with adrenaline and cortisol. If it is short-lived, we recover but when these high levels of stress hormones are sustained they deplete us of our vital resources and can impact our physical and mental health. Studies now show that acupuncture affects these systems and encourages the body to move into a parasympathetic state – 'rest and digest' – lowering stress hormones and heart rate, allowing our energy to naturally conserve and bodily functions to regulate.

I have found acupuncture to be a great support for patients working through challenging times, minimising symptoms of stress physically and emotionally, and it is now a large part of my practice.

The concept of Qi

Acupuncture has been around for over 4,000 years. The concept of qi is rooted in Eastern philosophy. One of the first medical texts on Chinese medicine dates back to 300 BC and is known as the *Neijing Suwen (The Yellow Emperor's Classic of Internal Medicine)*; this text discusses in depth the concept of qi alongside the theory of yin and yang and the channel system that provides the foundations for acupuncture today.

In simple terms qi is seen as the life force in all living things: plants, animals and humans. In Chinese medicine it is thought that the state of our health is dependent on the state of our qi. It plays a vital role in the health of our immune function, circulatory system, organ functions, emotional state and overall vitality.

The intricate network of channels known as the meridian system is thought to circulate qi at all levels of the body. The pathways are a means of communication, and when working efficiently they allow the body to function as a coherent whole. I often explain to patients that the pathways closely resemble lines of fascia (connective tissue) that similarly connect all areas of the body, superficially at the level of the dermis and more deeply wrapping around muscles, bones, nerves and viscera. There is a growing base of evidence that now explains some of the mechanisms involved in the physiological effects of acupuncture, and connective tissue planes is one of these areas explored alongside nerve transmission and blood flow.

We now know that when an acupuncture point is needled there is a release of adenosine and ATP at the site of needling; these substances are often referred to as the energy currency of our cells. Additionally, blood vessels dilate and there is an increase in nutrients and immune cells. The healing effects are localised but also systemic in that signals are fed back to our central nervous system where our autonomic functions are controlled and pain modulated.

"ATP and adenosine start a cascade of biochemical events that affect all tissues and body systems. This explanation removes doubt about biological plausibility and explains how acupuncture can be clinically helpful for such a diverse range of clinical areas" *Dr Mel Hopper Koppelman, Lecture on The Biochemistry of Acupuncture, 2019*

For information on scientific research and evidence about the physiological and biochemical effects of acupuncture visit https://www.evidencebasedacupuncture.org/.

Techniques I use in treatment other than acupuncture

Other techniques I use in treatments are moxibustion, meditation and massage.

- If I am working with someone that is highly stressed or anxious I often do a guided meditation and some breath work whilst the acupuncture points are retained (which is between 20-30 minutes). This slows down what is often referred to as the monkey mind, where we feel overwhelmed by the activity of our minds. In my opinion meditation is hugely complementary when used alongside acupuncture therapy.

- I often use mugwort (artemisia vulgaris), otherwise known as moxa, which is a dried herb either applied to the ends of needles, or used via a stick or little cones. The warming properties of the herb when burnt are thought to warm the channels and increase blood flow. It can be applied for a variety of symptoms.
- There is also a point at the end of the little toe – UB-67/ Zhi Yin (reaching yin) – that is very effective at turning breech babies; this point can be treated with acupuncture but more often moxa is applied and can be very successful. This is also offered within the NHS by some midwives. http://www.boltonft.nhs.uk/services/maternity/information/complementary-therapies/moxibustion/
- I often use massage as an adjunct to treatment, particularly when there are musculoskeletal issues; the two work well together helping to soften tissues and increase blood flow.

Symptoms I regularly see in women aged 40 and over

A fundamental principle of Chinese medicine relates to our body's ability to process change, including the natural transitions we experience through life. When we provide the right conditions for our body and mind we thrive. However, we often neglect ourselves through the constant demands of life and lose touch with what we need to feel well.

When we move into our 40s we may be juggling a completely different set of balls to what we were in our earlier years; we have also entered a phase of life where our hormonal norm begins to shift and change. Therefore, it is not unusual for me to see women in their 40s and 50s presenting with symptoms such as:

Anxiety, depression, low mood, migraine, joint pain, poor quality of sleep, back pain, weight gain, hot flushes, PMT, digestive issues, painful periods, heavy menstrual bleeding, low libido.

Referring patients back to their GP

If any areas of concern flag up on questioning or during treatment, then referral to their GP is necessary.

How often do I see patients for acupuncture to be effective?

This very much depends on the patient and the condition. Generally, for wellbeing and maintenance it can be anywhere from 4 to 12 weeks. Frequency of treatment for pain management also varies and patients tend to determine what works best for them. When dealing with more severe conditions, chronic or acute, often weekly or biweekly appointments are required until symptoms settle.

Examples of symptoms or illness where I have seen great results

I have had many cases of lower back pain, sciatica, carpal tunnel and tendonitis that have successfully cleared after a course of treatment, but the cases that really blow me away are patients that have been battling chronic illness for many years and are at a point where their medications are no longer enough. I have had transformational results with **rheumatoid arthritis** where the disease has gone into remission after many years of being active and controlled by steroid medication. I have also had cases of **colitis** where patients have been battling it for some time and then similarly the symptoms completely settle, or they suffer much less severe flare-ups that can be managed by herbs and acupuncture alone, avoiding the use of strong medications. **Polycystic ovarian syndrome** is another area where I have witnessed patients defy the odds, and after trying to conceive for some time, often years, with no joy, have fallen pregnant whilst receiving regular acupuncture treatment.

Other areas I have had great success treating are **depression, chronic stress** and **chronic fatigue syndrome**. Cases where patients have been unable to work, their entire quality of life tarnished by their condition. I have seen real transformation when working in these areas where patients have committed to regular consistent treatment and have eventually been able to reduce or completely come off medications (under the guidance of their GP), return to work, regain a social life and most importantly rediscover their joy. In cases of chronic stress patients may present with all kinds of symptoms, from insomnia, digestive issues, high blood pressure and headaches to anger and low mood; I have found acupuncture very helpful at addressing the stress therefore allowing the body to regulate.

What have I found acupuncture helpful for?

My summary of what I have found acupuncture helpful for is solely based on my experience with the patients and conditions I have seen in clinic; of course this may vary between practitioners depending on the setting they work in or their area of expertise.

I have found that acupuncture helps in different ways; I often call this RMR: reducing, managing and resolving. Sometimes it may be that a condition completely resolves during a course of treatment, other times symptoms are reduced, and in other cases acupuncture is effective at managing more chronic diseases. So, in my experience there is a vast scope for its application and it will usually help in some way. Below are some of the areas I have found it to be effective in either resolving, managing or reducing.

Gastrointestinal disorders, endocrine disorders and hormonal imbalance, mental health and emotional wellbeing, chronic fatigue syndrome (CFS/ME), pain, autoimmune disease, respiratory conditions, pregnancy induced symptoms, musculoskeletal conditions.

What should women look for when trying to find an acupuncturist? Is there an organisation they can consult?

The British Acupuncture Council is the largest governing body in the UK for acupuncturists. It adheres to a strict code of ethics, insuring the highest standards of health and safety are met and that each professional has carried out appropriate training meeting the correct standards of practice in the UK. It has a database of qualified practitioners that can be accessed by the public, enabling people to look up practitioners in their local area.

When enquiring about treatment I would also advise women to ask the practitioner if there are any areas they specialise in or any post-graduate training they have done within the field of women's health. It is also worth asking what experience they have had in relation to the problem/condition that needs treating.

What symptoms of the menopause are helped with acupuncture?

I've seen quite varying symptoms presented with menopause, from depression to panic attacks – not always what a patient is expecting to experience when entering this stage of life. What I have observed when treating menopausal and premenopausal women is that often what state their body and mind are in when entering this life phase may heavily influence how they transition through it. Therefore, lifestyle/diet and stress-reducing methods are often discussed during treatment.

In my opinion acupuncture is useful during menopause for two reasons. Firstly, its ability to bring us into a restful state, lowering our stress hormones. This is incredibly valuable because for some women the body can translate menopause as a type of stress. Secondly, by utilising acupuncture pathways that are thought to specifically influence the endocrine system (our hormonal network). Treatment doesn't focus on a singular aspect of this system such as the ovaries alone, it works holistically through the trajectories and functions of the channels that are thought to influence other team players such as the hypothalamus, pituitary, thyroid and adrenals, all hugely important in menopausal health.

I have listed below symptoms I have found respond well to regular acupuncture sessions; often weekly or biweekly treatment is needed until symptoms have minimised:

- Anxiety
- Panic attacks
- Low mood
- Joint pain
- Hot flushes
- Feeling overwhelmed
- Quality of sleep
- Muzzy head
- Poor memory

The potential benefits of facial acupuncture

Facial acupuncture uses the insertion of tiny hair-like needles to stimulate selected acupuncture points on the face depending on the needs of the patient. For example these points will vary depending on whether the patient is concerned with skin tone, fine lines, puffiness or sagging jowls.

The state of someone's complexion, location of lines and puffiness can tell an acupuncturist a lot about what may be happening at a deeper level; combining this information with a case history, pulse and tongue reading will therefore determine where the practitioner applies body and ear points to help balance the internal systems. Most of us know that depending on our state of health and how we feel it will often show in our skin, therefore you could say this treatment focusses on beauty from the inside out. It doesn't mask the signs of tiredness, dehydration, poor circulation or hormonal imbalance, it attempts to address them from within so we can once again feel comfortable in our skin.

For best results a course of treatment will usually involve 12 sessions, weekly or every two weeks, however many ladies I treat use them as they would a facial with larger time gaps in between to give the skin a natural boost and maintain wellbeing.

Many of the improvements patients see with facial acupuncture result as a combination of three different things: increased blood flow to the face, the healing response of the skin caused by the micro trauma of the needles, and the balancing effects of the acupuncture treatment. How one person responds may be different to another due to different skin types, genetics, state of health and medications but if following a course of treatment these are the kinds of benefits you may see:

- Improvement in muscle tone
- Increased collagen and elasticity
- Reduction in puffiness
- Improved complexion and radiance of the skin
- Overall feeling of health and wellbeing
- Reduction of fine lines

Thank you so much Shelley, that is so helpful to us all.

HYPNOTHERAPY

The area of hypnotherapy was something as a GP I did not know much detail of. We had a local respected hypnotherapist who was recommended to patients if it was thought to be helpful (for smoking cessation and so on). What about for the woman in midlife – could hypnotherapy be a useful adjunct to her self-care? What about in the menopausal time specifically? I was honoured to be at a speaking event with Louise Coyle and saw how her informative talk about the value of hypnotherapy in coping with menopausal symptoms captivated the female audience. Here we can find out more about Louise's practice and her vast experience.

LOUISE COYLE

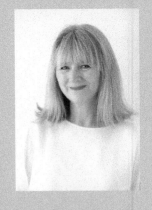

www.changingtimeshypnotherapy.com
Instagram: @changingtimeshypnotherapy
Facebook: https://www.facebook.com/changingtimeshypnotherapy/
LinkedIn: Louise (Bromley) Coyle

"I have always been fascinated by medicine and how the body works. I spent the first part of my career learning about advances in medicine as a medical journalist writing about new developments in medicine for GPs and hospital doctors and then as a medical PR specialist. On returning to work when my children were older, I wanted to do something to help people more directly, and I have found that working as a cognitive behavioural hypnotherapist offers me a rewarding and fascinating combination of helping people while continuing to learn about how the mind and body work together."

My practice

In my practice I help people with issues such as menopausal symptoms, stress and anxiety, panic, fears and phobias, confidence and self-esteem and weight problems. As well as seeing clients individually, I also run workshops for small groups of people to introduce them to hypnosis. Subjects I cover include learning relaxation skills, tackling exam stress, improving sleep and dealing with menopause symptoms.

Tell me what my readers should look for in qualifications when looking for a hypnotherapist? Is there a recognised governing body?

There are many different qualifications in hypnotherapy but some of them are of questionable quality. Hypnotherapists are self-regulating, so it is important to look for a therapist who belongs to an organisation that oversees qualifications and ethical standards of practice. For example, I belong to the General Hypnotherapy Register (GHR). This entitles me to take out full insurance and to be a member of the Complementary and Natural Healthcare Council (CNHC) which oversees a range of different types of therapy. Seeing a therapist who belongs to CNHC can give you confidence that your therapist has been appropriately trained.

Tell me about the reasons women over 40 might consult with you for hypnotherapy overall? What sort of problems can you help with?

Women over 40 consult me for a variety of issues. Generalised anxiety is one of the main issues, which may focus on issues at work, family or self. The 40s is often the time when we women face life changes, returning to work or changing careers, children getting older and leaving home, parents getting older, for example. Being the sandwich generation can be overwhelming and stressful and, often, unresolved anxiety issues become no longer manageable. So, I help women learn how to cope with stress, to build their resilience, how to sleep better, to have more self-esteem and confidence and to overcome specific fears.

Is hypnotherapy useful for anxiety that may occur with women with busy stressful lives in midlife and beyond?

There is good evidence to show that hypnotherapy can be very good in helping people overcome symptoms of anxiety and, combined with other types of therapy such as cognitive behaviour therapy, it becomes even more effective. A new study just published (meta-analysis cited below) has highlighted how effective this combination can be. Hypnosis can reduce symptoms of anxiety for as many as 84% of people who try it.

In fact, simply learning effective relaxation skills can help tremendously. People often struggle with all kinds of issues and anxieties throughout their lives, as they don't prioritise their own mental wellbeing. *They think they need to be at breaking point, not managing at all, at the end of their tether before they seek help.* But learning better stress management techniques and figuring out what changes you could make to your thinking patterns can help you stop repeating mistakes from the past and move forward with positivity. It may only need a few sessions with a hypnotherapist, rather than being a long, time-consuming and expensive process.

By the time we finish our sessions together, I want my clients to feel that they have the skills to manage whatever life can throw at them – they have become their own therapist and I am no longer needed!

Hypnotherapy and cognitive behavioural therapy were both cited in a British Medical Journal review as helping with hot flushes. Can you tell me a little about how you use hypnotherapy for this and the process?

When a woman attends one of my menopause group workshops, she will learn what hypnosis is and how it can help with menopause symptoms. I include three hypnosis exercises during the workshop: a guided relaxation, hypnosis focussed on reducing hot flushes, and hypnosis for getting better sleep. These exercises are recorded, and the women are sent these so they can continue to practise after the workshop. This workshop is enough to give a woman a very good idea of how hypnosis feels and whether it is right for her. The workshop format – usually for between 5 and 10 women – also gives the participants a chance to share their experiences.

If a woman prefers to see me for individual sessions, for example because she has other issues with anxiety that she would like help with, we usually have around six, hour-long sessions.

Often people are unsure about what hypnosis involves and how it might feel. I usually explain that it feels as though you are very relaxed, yet aware of where you are. What is important in hypnosis is to use your imagination – everyone can do this – and to focus on the suggestions for change that you are listening to. For example, for hot flushes, we focus on the idea that you are in control of your bodily thermostat and that you can practise how to turn this thermostat down whenever you need to. The more that you can practise this (by listening to the recording at home), the more effective it will be.

I also teach women simple, calming breathing techniques that can be very helpful in stopping a hot flush in its tracks.

How many sessions and how often does a woman need to see you to learn/appreciate the techniques? How long is each session?

With my individual clients, at the first session we have a detailed discussion about what the issue is, and I may begin to teach her guided relaxation skills. Learning to relax is beneficial for everybody as people often don't take the time to focus on this, yet it is very helpful for managing stress and anxiety. The second session is usually around a week later, and approximately half of the hour-long appointment will involve the actual hypnosis. As one of the key things is for the client to practise the techniques in between sessions, by listening to the recordings, subsequent sessions are more widely spaced and depend very much on each individual and what is best for them. Usually around six sessions are enough to make lasting changes.

(Louise's recommended research papers are listed in the reference section)

Do you think more doctors need to be aware of the value of hypnotherapy in menopause?

Absolutely, YES!

The more that doctors understand about the benefits of non-hormonal options for the menopause and the evidence of their effectiveness, the more options there are for women to find the right kind of help, that suits them and that will help them feel in control once more.

Thank you so much, Louise, that is so helpful for so many.

AN APP FOR MENOPAUSE

I have met Becks at two speaking events. She is so inspiring with her common sense approach to creating time for mindfulness and meditation and she has used her broad experience to create an app specifically for women.

BECKS ARMSTRONG, CEO OF THE CLARITY APP

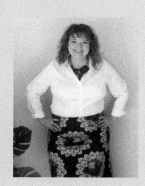

https://clarity.app

"After leaving school I did a diploma of business in hospitality where I learned all about customer service. While doing that course my father passed away from something that could have been prevented and I realised that I wanted to go into some form of medicine. Acupuncture really worked for me in many different ways so I went on to do a Bachelor of Health Science in Acupuncture and a postgrad in Traditional Chinese Medicine.

I specialised in women's health and along the way also became a doula and attended many women through their labour. I spent six years working in clinic then moved to the UK where I had to figure out a new career as the UK health system works differently and I couldn't get referrals from OB/GYNs like I did in Australia. I ended up re-training and becoming an interim COO in fast growth tech start-ups and from there decided to create my own start-up – an app called Clarity *which combines my love of women's health and technology. It's a mindfulness, relaxation and sleep app to help with the symptoms and issues that arise for menopausal women."*

What inspired you to create an app designed specifically for women and mindfulness?

All of the mindfulness apps I had seen were very generic, or they had packs that were for pregnancy but no other targeted women's health conditions. They also have thousands of sessions that are either hard to find or difficult to figure out which one to choose.

Having a good understanding of the sorts of issues women going through menopause face – like being overwhelmed and anxious – I decided to create something that was calm, easy to navigate and specific to their needs.

What do you know women can achieve mentally from following your daily introduction and subsequent sessions on the app?

The main thing I wanted to do with the introduction was to demystify what mindfulness is, what you do in a session and how it can help.

Apart from that we know by research that mindfulness can lower cortisol levels, it can help you to focus, sleep better and will also calm emotional turmoil.

This means a regular mindfulness practice can help you lower some of the symptoms of menopause (anxiety, overwhelm, brain fog) and also do unexpected things like improve your libido and help with hot flushes.

If you can create a regular daily practice of mindfulness that is around 30 minutes a day you can actually change the structure of your brain!

The value of the app seems to be not only that it handholds you through what can be a challenging concept of fitting mindfulness into the busy day, but also that is starts as bite-size chunks so is completely doable. What feedback have you had from ladies who have used the app?

I have had some great feedback from women who have used the app regularly. It has really helped with their hot flushes and anxiety, and many women have let me know that it's helped them with their sleep. One lady left a review saying that it has repeatedly been her pocket-sized superhero, which I'm so delighted to hear!

Summarise for me what the app can help with in both pre- and postmenopausal and much younger and older women? Do you encourage the younger generation who are already more aware of mindfulness to use the app?

The aim of the app is to help with life's ups and downs with curiosity and without judgement. By learning and practising these breathing techniques you can help regulate the emotional rollercoaster that can happen when your hormones fluctuate.

Due to there being younger women who have premature ovarian insufficiency or cancer, etc., I've made sure that we are open to all ages.

We all seem busy these days and for many women (regardless of age) their anxiety seems to be fairly high and they struggle with sleep. I think we can all do with a little **Clarity** in our day!

What do you see in the future for your app? Do you have any plans to create other apps or to expand Clarity?

We have a lot of plans for the future of Clarity. We are going to continue to create new sessions and open up new functionality to make the app easier to use. By the time your readers read this we will have released a Clarity Tracker app for the symptoms of perimenopause, menopause and beyond.

A lot of the feedback received when creating the app is that women do not have time to sit for half an hour every day. Where possible I have tried to show the scientific evidence around mindfulness and have created the sessions from an evidence base. You can make a difference to how you feel in only two minutes. The longer you can sit in practice regularly the better, but my aim is to get you to just do something daily – we all have two minutes in a day, it's about giving yourself permission to look after yourself.

Thank you so much, Becks, this is such an exciting and useful field.

SPIRITUALITY AND LIFE

Shelley von Strunckel

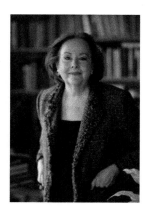

I personally knew of Shelley's work very well from reading her astrology columns weekly in the British *Sunday Times* throughout my life. I always felt I could apply her words about the Leo star sign to me but never understood why. Here Shelley enlightens us with her 'unique view' of looking at the world.

Although most known for her internationally published astrology columns, Shelley was trained as a spiritual teacher, and combines that knowledge with her merchandising background to address the often bizarre mix of unsettling events currently reshaping our world and our lives, personally and politically, financially, socially – and spiritually.

She speaks extensively, in a range of settings, from Family Office conferences to Daylesford Haybarn and WOMAD (World of Music, Arts and Dance), and recently took the stage at the legendary Wilton's Music Hall.

Her work with individual clients is strictly private and involves guiding them in personal and business matters.

Based in London, she speaks and travels extensively.

Her astrology columns are published worldwide, notably in the *London Evening Standard*, *The Sunday Times Style*, and *French and China Vogue*.

For more information, visit her website: www.shelleyvonstrunckel.com.

To apply for a private consultation, go to: pa@shelleyvonstrunckel.com.

Here I hand over to Shelley to write in her own words...

"Before I address these questions, as a writer I'd like to take a dip into vocabulary, mostly because the use of a couple of words implies one 'take' on reality and the workings of life, when mine is somewhat different. Also, for your scientific side, my responses are evidence-based, that is, what I've actually lived, not merely read or heard from a teacher or guru.

The first, crucially, is the use of the word 'believe' – in question 2, you ask if I believe benefits arise from meditation, etc. No, I KNOW it, based on my own experience, and backed by some fair science.

Also, the context of growing up not merely in Los Angeles but being born in Hollywood, where almost everybody came from somewhere else (so were already rewriting their 'life scripts'), means there's virtually none of the 'programming' so evident in life here or, really, in Europe.

So, with those two caveats, I'll proceed – with a few parenthetical phrases, here and there..."

How important do you think spirituality and feeling connected with the world is linked with our health?

Important as living a physically healthy life is; the immune system is powerfully linked to the mind and our individual consciousness, and these are deeply influenced by what's often described as 'mood'. These, in turn, are elevated by techniques such a meditation and yoga. Each gender has very different reasons for looking after themselves – men being 'strong', women 'attractive', but the actual profoundly uplifting influence of spiritual practices is the same.

What benefits do you believe arise from making time for meditation and self-care?

As above, I KNOW versions of self-care and meditation/stillness are superb tools for wellbeing. I've done a range of physical practices ranging from yoga to chi gong. And meditation is part of my everyday life – I even do it on the Underground. I can speak for myself, and others who use these methods; doing them increases wellbeing, while ceasing to practise them means those good feelings diminish.

Do you work every single day of the year monitoring charts and changes? Do you think there is anyone like you with your skills?

I write daily, weekly and monthly columns, as well as producing a lengthy voiced message about the week for each sign; it's a lot. So, usually, each day I'll do some writing or recording. Because some deadlines are for a couple of weeks ahead but others months ahead (especially magazines), I'm always juggling the planetary setup, on paper and in my mind.

As someone who read your stars since my young years, I have always found I can apply them to what is happening in my life. They are always positive in nature, never foreboding and always seem relevant. To those who are cynical can you explain a little of the mystery and why they might well resonate with my real life?

This is in two parts. First, the planets' movements portray cycles of nature, from the swiftly moving Moon to the slower Saturn. Still, each reflects (note, not 'causes'...) events, trends, changes here on earth. Part two is: each star sign views life in its own way, so responds to those cycles uniquely from others; I explain that. The positivism? Lots of psychological and philosophical study, and lots of meditation.

Is there anything about being a Leo that I might not already know, and how is it relevant to writing a book as a first-time writer, long-time doctor?

This is tough to answer because I'm unclear how much you know about your nature as a Leo...

It's the leap from the valid, but necessary, generalities of star signs to the individual chart. I would observe that being a fire sign, Leos thrive on new projects, so tackling something that requires a new skillset would suit you – such as writing a book like this.

You seem, very much, a champion of women and a great supporter of many causes, such as the Red Cross, opera and the arts. Do you have a very supportive female network? How are those friends important to you in your everyday life?

Yes, well-observed. I speak a lot on the shifting gender roles. And for this reason, I'm aware the bonds between women and men remain very different, although I have several very close male friends. My charity/cause activism combines my marketing background and joy working with those who are in some way benefitting the world. Recently that includes Montessori education, and Microloan, working to create self-supporting businesses for the poorest women in Africa.

Do you think one can train oneself to engage with spirituality more at midlife?

Each individual has their own path. Some are determinedly worldly, and for them spiritualty may not be of interest. With others – such as me – it was there from my earliest days – actually age six. If it becomes appealing to some later in life, it is because our focus is rapidly shifting from 'stuff', acquisitions of various kinds, to more subtle values. And that's where our 'inner world' comes in. It may be relating to nature, discovering the power of music, the joy of giving – none of these would necessarily be described as 'spiritual'. Now, however, many are developing an awareness of the power of their mind – their consciousness, not just for personal improvement but to contribute to the healing of our planet. Individually and collectively, we have far more power for good than we realise. However, we must use it – that begins with the simplest steps: loving oneself, and nature, and knowing healing is possible.

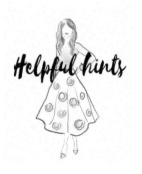

Helpful hints

Focus on Shelley's words: "our focus is rapidly shifting from 'stuff', acquisitions of various kinds, to more subtle values"
Do you engage with spirituality regardless of your religious beliefs?
Do you take time to wonder at the world?
Is there a place for meditation, mindfulness and reflection in your busy schedule?
How might you prioritise this if you currently don't engage with the peace inside you?

CHAPTER 12:
A GUIDE TO
FEMALE BONE
HEALTH

 As she danced, the music fed her mind, her soul and her swaying bones

We love our skin and spend hours comparing it with others', nurturing it with treatments. When we look for recognition, beauty or health, we are looking at skin, neglecting the bones beneath.

As women, the natural decline in oestrogen after menopause means we are at higher risk of developing osteoporosis, a condition where bones are thinned and can fracture with minimal trauma. What does this mean for you? If you have younger bones why is it important to make changes now? If you are postmenopausal what can be done to keep your bones strong so you can stay active and give the others a run for their money on the dance floor?

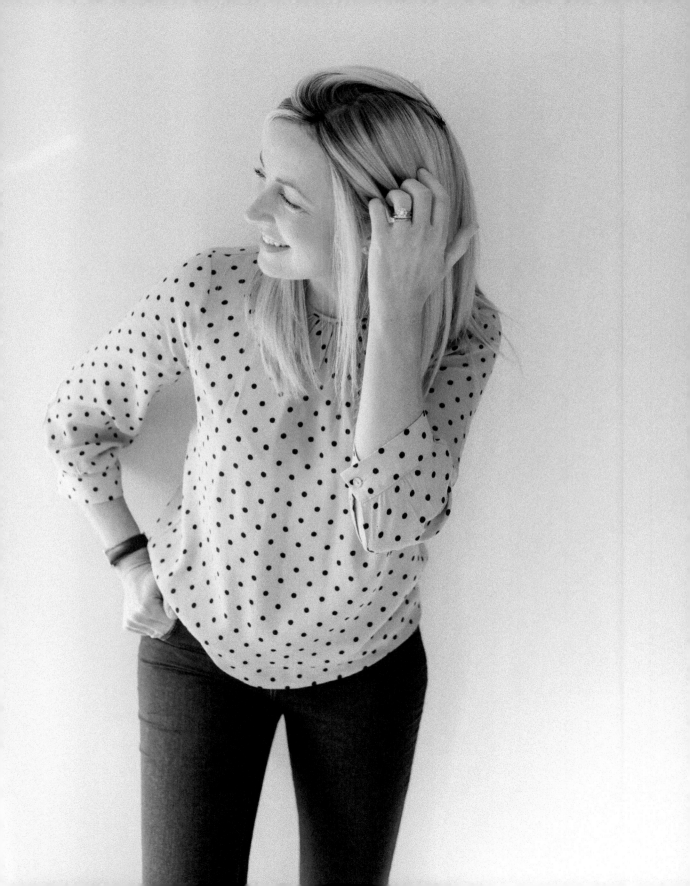

There is no point in keeping your head in the sand and hoping your bones stay strong. Bones are dynamic powerhouses with a complex system of cells regenerating and remodelling themselves. They literally *thrive* on our movement that jolts them into action. Astronaut studies have shown us what inactivity and lack of gravity can do to bone, so dancing is far from frivolous to our skeletal frame.

Turn the dial back to your teens. There is a surge of mineralisation (where bone is laid down and strengthened) from age 12 in girls, 14 in boys. During this time the body needs **more calcium and activity** to jolt the cells against gravity so that they grow bone as strong as possible. If you have teens in your life they need to be urged to **get off screens and be active** for *at least an hour* a day or their bones will never reach their full potential in strength and density. We are obsessed with how much exercise we do but scientists are concerned over our 'boxset-loving' sedentary lifestyle *between* the bouts of exercise.

Once we are in our **30s** bone remodelling slows down. There is no further mineralisation after about 35, so we must protect our bones to maintain them, especially as once we are **postmenopausal** the hormonal change will cause a further loss of mineral from bone. Osteoporosis prevalence is only 2% at 50 years but up to 25% of women at 80 years. We are living longer so need to wise up.

What are your bones like now?

What you do every day can literally **drain or replenish** your 206 bones. Osteoporosis can be due to both genetic and lifestyle factors. Whilst you cannot change your genetics, you *can* modify your lifestyle to improve your overall health. You eat well, keep fit and think your bones are in good shape? How about we get them even better?

This is a massive topic, and during a Bachelor of Science year at medical school I performed bone density scans on women (postmenopausal) who had been exercising in an aerobics class for a few years and I proved that the bone mineral density at their hip was higher than in non-exercising women of the same age. In the 25 years since, further evidence for activity reducing the incidence of bone thinning has been added to the pile.

Bone facts

Let's call it *bone drainers and bone replenishers*. Think of your bone density as an 'open-topped' egg timer with the top lid removed, slowly draining sand out of the bottom half. You can top it up, but after the age of 35 it is likely that there are always some grains of sand draining out slowly.

Bone drainers

Smoking slows down the bone-building cells (osteoblasts), almost doubling the risk of osteoporosis! Time recovering from fractures is slower because smoking constricts the blood vessels supplying bone. Smoking can also mean your menopause is earlier, and this will affect bones by the earlier decline in oestrogen.

Excessive alcohol reduces the ability of the bone to remodel and you may absorb less calcium (plus you might fall over but that's another story).

Drinking more than three or four cups of caffeinated **coffee,** so 330mg a day (effects not seen in tea), and **caffeinated fizzy drinks** *may* reduce calcium absorption. The milk taken with coffee will help balance this and we know there are many benefits to a cup of java, so everything in moderation.

Underweight women are at risk. Very worryingly if you suffered anorexia before or around puberty and in the younger years thereafter, peak bone mass will have never been reached. After the menopause a large source of our oestrogen is from fat so being underweight does not do bones any favours. Being very **overweight** increases the power of falls and stresses our joints.

Premenopausal women who **excessively exercise and reduce nutrient intake** may find their periods halt and oestrogen falls prematurely and bones can thin.

Mental stress. New studies are emerging that look at the effect of mental stress on bone density. This is a complex subject and it is thought to be mediated by cortisol and other stress hormones. Whatever the reason, this is another argument for prioritising self-care and considering the proven benefits of mindfulness and relaxation.

Lack of exercise. A screen-driven lifestyle means we are moving less. Even after 30 minutes of sitting down, our bones, circulation, immunity and metabolism may suffer. There is a lot of emerging research about the effects of inactivity on our cardiovascular system and heart health. Now the focus is also on bone health. This effect on bones and heart health does not occur while sleeping before you ask! Future medicine will tell us more – for now, move your bones at least hourly. 'Standing desks' in offices will be invaluable as we anchor ourselves electronically to this virtual world.

Medicines. Long-term corticosteroids, hormonal breast cancer treatments and certain antiepileptic medicines can put you more at risk. Some diuretics may increase urination enough to cause you to lose more calcium. Some proton pump inhibitors (used to treat excess gastric acid in reflux and ulcer prevention and so on) may at high doses in theory reduce calcium absorption from the stomach. This is **NOT** however a reason to stop any of these meds! Discuss with your doctor methods of bone protection, remembering it is all about balance and the overall benefit to your health.

Thyroid and parathyroid conditions may *sometimes* affect bone and calcium metabolism.

Early menopause. It is important to discuss bone protection with your doctor and whether HRT or other methods are appropriate for you in protecting your bone against the early decline in oestrogen. We know that HRT can help maintain bone mass by supplying oestrogen. Once the HRT is stopped, the bone density will decline as it would without oestrogen, but in many women, especially those with early menopause, it is starting them off from a better baseline bone density. This is something to discuss in detail with your own doctor.

Bone replenishers

Nutrition – calcium. Dairy is a great source of calcium. Skimmed, semi-skimmed, full-fat all give you calcium. Yoghurt and cheese are also a source although you have to be aware of the high salt content of some cheeses. If you have chosen to avoid dairy for various reasons look at the side panel of your milk replacement carton for full information on the choice you are making. We have a vast choice – almond, cashew, oat, rice, coconut. Choose responsibly and research your milk carefully, not in line with trends or fads. **Check any non-dairy milks are fortified with calcium.** (Non-dairy milks *do not have the iodine content of cow's milk.* Low iodine can be detrimental to the developing foetal brain, and iodine is essential for thyroid health in all of us. So, if exclusive non-dairy is your thing ensure you have iodine in your food, e.g. white fish, eggs, nuts, meats and fortified breads). Oat milk can be made with a large proportion of rapeseed oil which some people consider 'inflammatory' in the body. I personally love a combination of dairy and unsweetened almond milk. Check for **added sugars** in milks and their salt content. Excess salt can reduce calcium absorption.

Try adding garlic, spices and herbs to food instead of salt when cooking. Green leafy veg (such as broccoli and spring greens), fish including tinned (sardines and salmon with bones), almonds, sesame seeds, tahini, chickpeas, other pulses and fortified breads all pack a healthy calcium punch. Beware excess spinach, dried fruit, beans, seeds and nuts which have oxalates or phytates – chemicals that reduce how much calcium your body can absorb. Don't avoid these great foods, just ensure you have plenty of other calcium-rich foods alongside these beauties. There is a great summary of information available at the website www.bda.uk.com, the website of the British Dietetic Association. This also breaks down calcium needs for different ages and gives the calcium content of food points thus making it easy to work out how to meet the varying needs of your family. If you have coeliac or inflammatory bowel disease your requirements may be greater.

Vitamin D. We all know vitamin D is needed to help the absorption of calcium from our food. Most of this is obtained from the action of sunlight on our skin. In the warmer months in the UK, 15 mins outside three times a week between 11am and 3pm without sunscreen would, in theory, give us enough vitamin D but in the winter months this is not always so easy. We cannot get all of our vitamin D from our diet alone but still need a good supply of vitamin D rich foods. These include oily fish, eggs, fortified cereals/spreads. If you don't get enough sun exposure as an adult or are at high risk of becoming deficient (pregnant or breastfeeding women, those over 65, those with darker skin, those avoiding the sun, immobile in nursing homes and so on), a supplement of 10 micrograms a day all year round is recommended, or only in the winter months – you *must discuss with your doctor.* Some supplements have the dose displayed as international units (IU), and 10 micrograms is equivalent to 400 IU. Remember that vitamin D is a fat-soluble vitamin so take care not to take excess, as over time, if too much is taken, this can accumulate to toxic levels as you cannot simply pee it out. Stick to the guidelines recommended by your healthcare professional for your demographic group.

Vitamin C and protein. These are needed to build collagen (acts like scaffolding within bones and joints). Vitamin C is obtained from vegetables and fruit, protein from meat, fish, beans, pulses and so on. Always try to thoroughly chew your protein to aid digestion.

Magnesium is a major component of bones and helps the body use calcium, but its role is not entirely clear. We know it is needed but are not entirely sure why. A large proportion of the magnesium in our bodies is found within our bone. Sensible advice would be that wholegrains, fruits, veggies, nuts, dairy and seafood should all give you the essential minerals needed for your bones. In summary, a Mediterranean-style diet will be good for your cardiovascular, mental and bone health.

Exercise. If you were my best friend this is what I would tell you. (Hey, we surely are friends now you have got this far in the book?!) **Your activity NOW has a huge effect on your bone health**. You will thank me for it. You will never regret optimising your exercise schedule before or after menopause. Seek advice from an exercise professional if you feel lost in making a choice, or join a gentle class for confidence but *start somewhere*; don't underestimate the simple power of walking – read on...

If you are already very fit and active, you need to do a variety of impact exercises – ideally '50 impacts a day' against gravity, working in different planes on your body. This can range from brisk walking (**great for the spine**) to jumping around in a class. Strength training is **best for hips**. If you are more worried and less fit, try a gentler approach. Walking less fast, for longer, may be key.

To keep it simple I have summarised into three sections – for those of you who are already gym bunnies/regular exercisers let's call you 'already very fit'. For those of you quaking at the thought of any organised movement let's say you are the 'cautious' ones. I read a quote that said '**what seems hard now will one day be your warm-up**'. Buying some inexpensive 0.5 kg hand weights and working up to 1 or 2 kg in a regular routine may be the easiest, most effective change you can make for your health.

> ### Bone friendly workouts
>
> **Already very fit**
> 50 jumps a day
> 20min jog 3 times a week
> 50 steps up and down stairs
> Brisk walking (with or without lightly loaded rucksack*)
> Boxercise
> Aerobics
> Tennis
> Light weights
> Circuits
> Intermittent jogging
>
> **Cautious about exercise**
> Gentle walking to build confidence up to 30 minutes/day (with or without lightly loaded rucksack*)
>
> **Everyone**
> Squeeze tennis ball repeatedly
> Push ups against wall
> Stand on one leg carefully
>
> *posture friendly with 2 tins beans inside

The tennis ball mentioned is one of my favourite medical facts. When I was a student there were already studies on this – 'squeezing a tennis ball 18 times a day could increase bone density in the wrist' – a common site for women's postmenopausal fractures, called a 'colles' fracture. Because we simply don't do that complex squeezing action in daily life, this exercise is a superpower. I spent most GP consultations with my postmenopausal ladies asking them to keep a tennis ball by the bed. I wonder how many still do?

Looking at hips – a common site for fracture – **walking at a considerable pace** of 5 to 6 km/hour is preferable to slower walking in new studies but slower walking for longer may be just as good. Aim for 30 minutes a day minimum. **Running** is excellent only if you are capable of doing so. **Hopping** around in an exercise class although excellent for stimulating bone has to be considered carefully in frailer individuals where of course there is the risk of fracture itself. If you have a high fracture risk or, say, for example have had fragility fractures in your spine, sudden high-impact exercise like jogging or jumping is *not* going to be a good choice for you. This is something to be sensibly discussed with your doctor, nurse or physiotherapist. **Walking with waist-bound weights** has long been recognised to be a good weight-bearing exercise but they can be tricky to find, so using a comfy rucksack with a couple of bean tins may be easier. **Muscle-strengthening exercise will help protect your body by reducing the chance of falling, and the muscles will in turn act on the bone to help keep it strong**.

Yoga has shown benefits on bone density in some studies but more importantly may improve strength and stability to prevent falls. A brisk walk to yoga class and you are winning! Pilates and yoga are thought to both strengthen muscle around the spine and improve posture. Always inform your teacher if you have bone thinning or back problems. We know that some flexion poses on the spine may be detrimental in osteoporosis, so if you have a diagnosis seek a specialist instructor with knowledge of bone disease. Swimming and cycling don't show direct improvements on bone density (no gravity) but new techniques of looking at bone might suggest other bone benefits – that is more future science.

Let's not forget dancing – random movement and bounce – the effect on your body creates a stronger heart, muscles and bones. What's not to love? Dance while the tea is brewing... Make like a *Mamma Mia* extra! It's those little exercises that add up to improve your health.

Always endeavour to **keep your muscles strong.** They will naturally decline with age and it is one way of keeping us super active, healthier and energetic as the years pass.

How will you know if you have bone thinning?

You sadly might not. Osteoporosis is rightly called the 'silent epidemic'. It is thought that up to 30% of postmenopausal women suffer from osteoporosis and it is obviously becoming a more profound problem as we live longer lives.

What is osteoporosis?

Any bone thinning means that the 'honeycomb' structure of the bones is not as tightly packed as it once was. We say that the **bone mineral density** is decreased. If this is not too severe we call it **osteopenia**, but if worse it becomes **osteoporosis**. Rather like comparing the inside of a UK chocolate 'Crunchie' bar with an 'Aero' bar, the spaces in the bone material are larger the less dense the bone is.

You may not realise there is anything wrong until you are lying in a hospital bed with a **fracture** and the doctor tells you they suspect bone thinning from the X-ray. You might have a simple fall, *nothing attention-seeking like a ski jump*, and suffer a broken wrist or hip. Osteoporotic fractures in the spine may go unnoticed, but heal causing a change in posture, shrinkage in height and chronic pain. Apart from making you feel miserable this can obviously go on to affect your quality of life. You may lose height, your posture may change and your ability to go about your everyday activities will be affected. Some women may notice they have lost a noticeable amount of height since their 20s. A loss of one or two inches can be an early sign of undiagnosed vertebral fractures or osteoporosis. Keeping strength in posture is so important as we age for many reasons: we can move more easily, see where we are going and sleep without discomfort.

Getting a diagnosis

So, whether you consulted your GP because you have a family history and are worried, or you were unfortunate enough to have a broken bone and signs on an X-ray, you will be referred for a DEXA* scan. This usual 'gold standard' test is of the hip and spine. It is simple, painless and importantly not claustrophobic. It is currently recommended that DEXA scanning is limited to Caucasian postmenopausal women simply because the data behind the computers that interpret them is only created with data from this group. Results may be inaccurate for other groups. The radiation dose is very small. You lie on a bed in an open room (no tunnel) and the radiographer will explain to you that the robotic arm moves up and down, back and forth above your bed to record the measurement. The result is a 'T score' which will label you with either '**normal**' bones, **osteopenia** (less severe bone thinning) or **osteoporosis** (more severe). Osteopenia *does not mean* you have osteoporosis, but if untreated you *may* go on to develop it. This T score is then presented to your GP for action or not.

* Dual-energy X-ray absorptiometry

What about offers on bone scans through the post?

Sometimes patients are sent offers to have mobile bone density measurement, or it is offered locally through their hospital. This is often a wrist measure as it is a portable machine and may or may not be an accurate representation of what is going on in the hip and spine. It is *reassuring if it is very good* but there can be a grey area where it doesn't show the full picture of what is going on with your bones. Treatment for osteoporosis is not normally given on the basis of these portable scans alone.

I have a diagnosis, what now?

Do not be dreadfully fearful if the diagnosis of osteopenia or osteoporosis is made. The message from the hugely respected Royal Osteoporosis Society is to *keep moving and not be fearful of moving.* Fall prevention is the main focus. Your doctor has an integral role and will prescribe you specific bone medication and discuss lifestyle issues. Don't dismiss the need for medicine. The **Royal Osteoporosis Society** in the UK is a fantastic source of support and information, as is the **National Osteoporosis Foundation** in the USA.

Osteopenia

You will be given a calcium and vitamin D combined supplement by your doctor and lifestyle changes will be discussed with you. You may be referred for specialised physiotherapy or exercise education by your GP or a consultant.

Osteoporosis

Your doctor will talk to you in detail about this – here is a brief summary. Alongside lifestyle advice, as with osteopenia, you may be able to have physiotherapy or other exercise advice to help prevent falls and increase your strength. The NHS website has videos and information on this, as does the Royal Osteoporosis Society.

Medication

Most of these work to strengthen bones by slowing down the cells in the bone that break down old bone. They are called *anti-resorptive drugs*. Other treatments stimulate the cells that build up bone. These are *anabolic drugs*. Many of the medicines are once a week and some are even monthly or by three-monthly injection. Your GP and local specialists will have a specific protocol for these. They will discuss with you the risks, advantages and side effects, and a good source of information is the National Osteoporosis Society online resource. NICE guidelines are used by clinicians when making decisions about medication and osteoporosis.

Calcium and vitamin D supplementation

Despite recent publicity casting doubt on vitamin D for protecting bones this is not changing any guidance and the thoughts are that patients at risk with osteopenia or osteoporosis still require both vitamin D and calcium supplementation. It is important you have a supplement prescribed and monitored by your doctor. If you do suffer gastrointestinal intolerance with supplements, changing to a different formulation like a chewable tablet can make a large difference.

Women who have had breast cancer will need to discuss their bone health with their doctor. Often treatments such as chemotherapy or surgery will have reduced their ovarian function and oestrogen levels will be lower. Some chemotherapy may have had a direct negative effect on bone. This will often mean they are given vitamin D and calcium supplementation and should comply with this medication and consider similarly altering which formulation if not tolerated.

As a special treat for my readers my next expert specialist opinion is from Professor Dawn Skelton, Advisor to the Royal Osteoporosis Society and leading world expert in osteoporosis.

How aware do you think the average menopausal woman is about osteoporosis compared to a decade ago?

The Royal Osteoporosis Society has improved awareness, but fear is still massive and people think of 'brittle bone disease' and that they are going to crumble. We have a system of assessing risk that doctors can use (FRAX*); it uses the WHO online database and this only looks at Caucasians over 65 so is slightly limited. The ROS provides information sheets and videos of exercises and this will help greatly.

How much of osteoporosis is related to genetics and how much to lifestyle factors?

My gut feeling is that you can have good genetics and a bad lifestyle leading to osteoporosis, or poor genetics and a good lifestyle and still develop bone thinning. However, in the second group you *can* do a LOT TO MITIGATE IT AND POSTPONE THE POINT AT WHICH IT BECOMES A PROBLEM FOR FRACTURES TO OCCUR. Many women are diagnosed at the point of wrist fracture and then have medication or lifestyle change and do NOT go on to have a spine or hip fracture. Women need to know that they CAN move around safely with a more fragile skeleton and *avoiding falls* is the important point. We introduced a Fracture Liaison Service in Scotland which is now becoming national where we DEXA scan ladies with a low trauma fracture. This picks up cases early. We have had great success preventing hip fractures as women receive medication and exercise/lifestyle advice.

What would you advise for walking in the cautious and less regular exercisers who may or may not have had a diagnosis?

If you are not fit, you should not suddenly start brisk walking – as you fatigue you are more likely to fall as you lift your feet less. It is far better to build up from where you are now and listen to your body. Brisk walking may potentially do more to help but if not possible it is better to *simply do a longer walk*. For younger and fitter women obviously brisk walking is fine.

What would you like women to be more aware of given this chance to speak to them?

Sitting is a real problem. There is lots of research that although we are going to the gym and so on, we are sitting down watching TV after. We know that in younger adults after two hours of sitting there are cardiovascular marker changes in the bloodstream – this does not happen when you are sleeping, it is only when you are awake and not using your muscles. After two to six hours sitting this worsens. Now we are looking at the bone markers in these studies and future research may reveal we need to stand up often. Standing desks are not a gimmick!

Do cycling and swimming help our bones even though they're not strictly movement against gravity?

Cycling is good in that it strengthens muscle and maintains muscle strength but you do need impact to improve bone density. Cycling uphill does work but there is not much evidence for cycling on the flat. However, we are changing the way we look at bone. We have only looked at bone mineral density for 30 years and there is more to stopping a fracture than just BMD. Now we have a few very expensive machines – 'slow PQCT' (qualitative computerised tomography) – looking at the *actual structure of bone* in state-of-the-art research facilities – these are showing that activities that do not improve BMD may *still change the structure of the bone* and so far short-term studies are showing swimming and cycling may be helping.

Do vibration plates work for osteoporosis?

They only work if at the correct amplitude and frequency; Power Plate has an evidence base, but not other brands. There is a fact sheet on the ROS website and, of course, if you have vestibular or balance problems and suffer nausea and dizziness this would not be for you.

*FRAX – Fracture Risk Assessment Tool – questionnaire

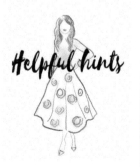

Helpful hints

Be mindful of your bone health and any family history

Eat a calcium, vitamin D and mineral rich diet and promote it within your household

Maintain a healthy weight

Stop or reduce lifestyle factors (smoking, excess caffeine and alcohol) that may drain your bones – achieve some lifestyle balance

Work 'bone-friendly' exercise into your weekly schedule at the level you can manage

Enjoy feeling happier and energised with stronger muscles from exercise

Ask for help and information from your healthcare professional if worried

Use online resources www.bda.uk.com and www.theros.org and www.nof.org

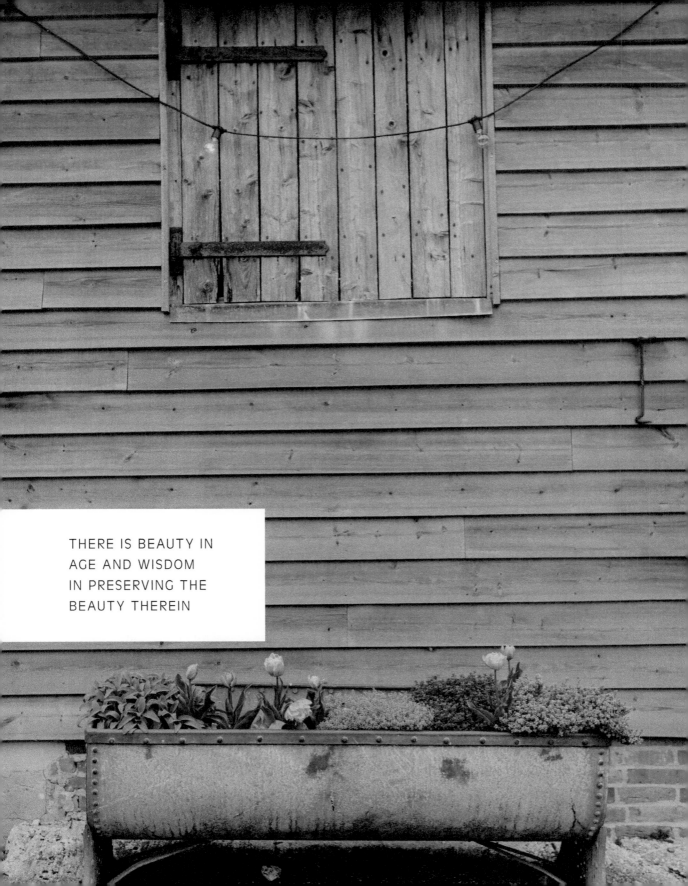

THERE IS BEAUTY IN
AGE AND WISDOM
IN PRESERVING THE
BEAUTY THEREIN

CHAPTER 13: MUSCLES AND JOINTS

MOTIVATION TO CHANGE BEHAVIOUR

How do you change your habits?

There is a lot of preaching advice (I hope) in this book that does not come across as patronising. I hope to remain real, and I am quite a buzzy, focussed person when I put my mind to something. Despite this, I can get stuck in ruts of unhealthy snacks/not exercising enough due to excuses, like everyone. However, recently this happens less as my habits have become 'just my life' and I actually feel FOMO* on my own fitness if I don't follow my own health advice at least 80% of the time. *Fear of missing out

How do I explain to you what you need to do? I value my writing because I believe if women understand why something works they are more likely to comply with it. That may not be enough for you. Here I am going to turn to my expert friend Dr Louise Pendry, Psychology Lecturer at Exeter University, to help you out. She has the secret. Two words.

Implementation Intentions.

What are they?

She explains that to form a successful habit, we need to create a 'When I will' type scenario. In one 2010 study, by Sheina Orbell and Bas Verplanken, participants were taught about the value of flossing their teeth. Half were then given the following information to help form an 'implementation intention'.

"You are more likely to carry out your intention to perform dental flossing every day if you make a decision about when and where. Most people perform dental flossing in the bathroom immediately after they brush their teeth at night or after breakfast. Write down where and when you intend to floss your teeth every day for the next four weeks."

In comparison to those who did not receive this information and have the opportunity to form an implementation intention, these participants were quicker to create automatic habits to floss regularly.

How do I end up doing an implementation intention myself?

So, once I get up (on a writing day) I will get my gym kit on and with the kids at school I am back home and straight on my exercise bike. That is my example and it works. **I set the time and the place. That way I am more likely to do it.**

Repeating this a few times a week over time it then becomes automatic with me. I lay out the kit the night before, I hang my keys up after the school run and take the keys to the garage, fetch my water bottle prepared on the worktop and go to the bicycle.

What happens if one day I plan to do this and then emails and life get in the way? Do I return to being a sloth?

Research by Philippa Lally and colleagues found that missing the odd event of this planned behaviour did not matter *occasionally* if you get back to it.

This I have found to be true and for the last year have easily maintained a regime of exercise three to five times a week.

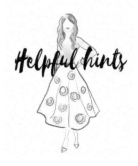

Helpful hints

Other triggers for healthy behaviour

Train with a friend – if you can't answer to yourself alone you may do better committing to someone else. Walking along the beach quickly before work suited my friend and me, and the joy from talking and laughing cemented the behaviour as a 'good thing to do'.

Keep the exercise or the new recipes fresh – alternate classes at the gym, change your route for running, keep challenging yourself with physical goals like different weights lifted.

Be accountable to yourself – some journal or document their physical progress – miles cycled, steps walked. If a fitness step monitor motivates you and puts you in healthy competition with your partner, then go for it!

Have a goal – maybe keeping up with your grandkids, maybe making your IBS better by nutrition changes – whatever – know why you are doing it and what you want to achieve!

MUSCLE AND HEALTH

Muscle is a silent worker; the relationship partner you take for granted. Unless it fails, you just assume it will always be there for you, uncomplaining and undemanding. There are 640 named **skeletal muscles** in the human body – more if you count the individual muscles bound together in groups. These are the muscles that move our bodies rather than, say, the heart muscle (cardiac) and blood vessel wall muscle (smooth). Most of us probably know the names of about ten 'bone-moving muscles' off by heart and otherwise pay them no attention.

Muscles make up about 40% of our body weight, and the strongest by the force it can emit is the jaw muscle with the pressure it can create on the molars. No jokes there about us chatty people having strong jaws.

In health we can control the function of skeletal muscles and they often exist in pairs with one muscle working in one direction and the other moving the limb the opposite way. For one muscle to work it has to contract and the opposite paired muscle relax. It's quite a feat and one we take for granted.

We have slow-twitch fibres in muscle for endurance activities and these can work for a long time without getting tired – like on an endurance jog. Fast-twitch fibres are for rapid movements as they contract fast, but they also get tired quickly as they use up lots of energy. Remember your first 100 m sprint at sports day when you gave it all you had?!

Muscles are important in keeping us upright, balanced and preventing falls. They work for simple tasks like rising from a chair to running marathons and achieving the perfect yoga pose. Use it or you will lose it is not such a blanket misnomer. We know that if we continue to keep muscles active, specifically with strength training in later life, we are more likely to keep our confidence, maintain mobility and most importantly our independence. Doctors can tell people to exercise to prevent falls but no one really wants to be told they are a 'fall risk'. Positive ways of embracing this mentality are to join a fun dance or exercise class, feel the good you are doing your body whilst you are distracted by the fun and social side.

Do you have to think of your muscles if you are only in your middle years? More and more evidence is emerging that by keeping muscles as strong as we can we conversely may reduce our chance of decline too soon. A fall can lead to a broken bone, immobility, infection and depression – many a GP has lamented such a fact, so let's start looking at what **you can do to prevent that now.**

Cynically, you age from the moment you are born. It is natural, inescapable, but as this book is trying to convey, how you age is flexible. The patients who have sat in front of me at 85 with the demeanour, smile, body of someone 15 years younger did not focus on the passing of the years. They made the most of each one and muscle was a huge factor. Chronic disease can have foundations laid in the young. If you are 40, smoking, excessively overweight and drinking alcohol daily, anyone can predict you most likely won't age so well. By exercising your muscles, you could start to change all of that. Muscle will work to move you, your aerobic function of heart and lungs will improve, your metabolic rate will rise, fat will burn away and the limit of breathing on your progress may motivate you to give up the ciggies in the process. All because you got out more and exercised those muscles.

We naturally lose a small per cent of muscle every decade as we age. We burn fat in our muscle and healthy muscle helps preserve a good metabolic rate. Muscle takes up less space than fat. Muscle never turns into fat or vice versa! Severe weight loss diets may mean we lose muscle, the metabolism slows and often we then regain fat but one does not turn into the other!

In the UK the health department of the government recommends all adults, 65 or over, take a minimum of 30 minutes moderate activity at least five times a week.

After the age of 50 lean muscle mass is lost at a rate of about 1% a year. We are not entirely sure why – muscle proteins maybe aren't made as efficiently as they are broken down, hormones change in balance, exercise may not be as effective? The term SARCOPENIA is used to denote loss of muscle mass or strength and ultimately leads to frailty and falls. Many studies have been done – they tend to show a loss of number of muscle fibres and also the number of nerves innervating them. *This will all be accelerated without a physically active lifestyle and balanced diet.* So you need to get moving and eat well from now. Never too early to start. In studies where people maintained muscle better there was a higher level of nerve *activity* in the remaining muscle. So, although the motor units (nerve and muscle junctions) of the muscle were reduced, the nerves were compensating in those who had done training. I told you, use it or you lose it.

Muscle and metabolism

Working your muscles will help you move, maintain strength in bones, regulate your sugar and blood pressure, and maintain a healthy weight. Muscle is not just a mover, it is the main protein (amino acid) store in your body, and if you suffer a disease where sources of energy are dramatically required fast, like in cancer, the muscle will provide a source of glucose. It is a primary site for glucose uptake and storage. Skeletal muscle is also the primary outlet for glucose disposal in the body and is therefore important in metabolic conditions such as diabetes.

In cancer, lung, kidney and chronic and acute infections, muscle mass can decrease drastically – we call this **cachexia** in medicine and it is a very important sign. There is more to muscle than lifting.

When we exercise our muscle, certain chemicals (namely myokines) are released that communicate with other processes in our body, so a small change in exercise can have a strong ripple effect in the body:

- stimulate metabolic pathways
- improve glucose uptake
- improve fat oxidation
- regenerate skeletal muscle

Thus you can see that exercise really can reduce the chance of non-insulin dependent diabetes, obesity and muscle atrophy. Use it or you lose it AND gain a whole load of complications.

If you can incorporate weights you are comfortable with in your workout and build up slightly under guidance you can reverse the ageing of the muscle. Your stamina and metabolism will increase and you will also burn more calories for some time after you put the weights down that day. Squats, jumps and lunges and good body resistant floor work burn a lot of calories as they use the large muscle groups together.

If muscle is working well, blood flow is better around the body and even your skin and libido can improve, what's not to love!?

Testosterone

This can be an emotive topic. Men have a decline in testosterone with age, as do women. Women produce testosterone in their ovaries and adrenal glands on top of the kidneys. Some women have low levels of testosterone as they go through the menopause and the ovaries produce less. The automatic reaction would be 'let's take some to replace it'. It is indeed used in an unlicensed form in the UK (the doctor takes responsibility for prescribing so usually only prescribed by a doctor specialising in the menopause) as a second line HRT, usually after oestrogen therapy (with or without progesterone as appropriate) has been prescribed. Not all women would need testosterone and it has to be given in the minimally effective dose to improve libido and possibly concentration but not cause facial hair growth and so on. Doctors are divided on this subject often, and it seems that in some studies the relationship between testosterone and libido is not always linear and can be very personal.

Our *naturally occurring testosterone* will stimulate protein synthesis and muscle growth. To combat this decline why not try progressive resistance training (PRT), recommended for men and women. As strength and endurance improve, the weight and the number of reps in exercise may be increased to keep stimulating muscle. This will increase or maintain your lean body mass. Having enough protein in the diet to sustain this is imperative and sources are of course meat, eggs, dairy, pulses and so on. Protein powders are readily available but as women our kidneys *can only handle a certain amount per day* so these tend to only be used when you are not getting adequate sources from diet. **Always try to get it from your plate.** If you are adding protein powders to smoothies make sure you are considering that the average-sized woman requires 50 mg protein and putting 30 mg into her morning smoothie may be pushing her over the limit for kidneys taking the strain. Many a keen body builder patient I have shocked by measuring their impaired kidney function whilst they were supplementing with high-dose protein powders. So innocuous, but if abused *so detrimental* to someone allegedly respecting their health and body.

Power in muscle is as important as strength. This will predict how fast and efficiently you move. Good muscles to strengthen are your leg muscles as these produce the greatest power when trained and will enable quicker bodily movements generally.

Resistance exercise transiently increases testosterone levels in women; chronic resistance training in women may increase testosterone levels generally.

Preserving function and independence is more important than anything else as we age. Posture and balance are key to this. Pilates helps many women retain control.

Joseph Pilates (German) made the connection between mental and physical health. He looked at other existing forms of exercise and in the 1920s opened a studio in New York where he taught his method that he initially called 'Contrology'.

Pilates as it is known now is a system of exercises designed to strengthen the body in an even way, focussing on improving core strength. This is usually done on a mat or using special equipment called:

- The Reformer
- Cadillac
- Wunda Chair
- Spine corrector
- Ladder barrel

Where such equipment is involved the instructor needs to supervise carefully, so this may be on a one-to-one basis or small classes.

Weights, stretch bands, gym balls and rollers can all be incorporated into a class.

There are pulleys and strings to provide resistance and support. Movement flows more than the static poses of yoga. The supportive nature means the exercise can be appropriate for people of all ages and ability and strengths. There are many reports of the health benefits but more research is always needed. Those practising it report:

- Release stress and tension
- Balance
- Mobility
- Flexibility
- Whole body strength

Some clients report improvement in lower back pain. Because the exercise is muscle strengthening it can help you maintain a healthy weight, but for losing weight the NHS website suggests combining it with other activities in your life. What will be important is your teacher and choosing a class that is relevant to your ability. Classes can range greatly in intensity. Always check with your health professional if you are injured or have other chronic health problems before starting a new form of exercise.

Let's now seek the wisdom of Frances Stephens, a well-known Pilates teacher.

FRANCES STEPHENS

www.francesstephenspilates.co.uk

What age range of women do you teach?

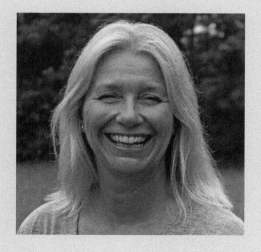

I teach age 44 to 90 currently. I have no more than 12 women in a class as I have to be able to move around the room and correct any mistakes.

Can you give me a rough idea of what ladies should look for when choosing a class or instructor?

They need to look for experience and that the class is well supervised and not overpopulated. They need to connect with the teacher personally and should have an opportunity for a meeting before having a trial class.

Do you think classes with The Reformer or other similar equipment are superior to those with mats and small equipment? Or can one get just as good a lesson without?

Yes to the latter. I use mats, large and small balls, bands and weights in my classes. Classes with larger equipment require close supervision by an instructor as well. Both can be as good as each other.

Is Pilates something that is easy to learn from a DVD or would you always recommend a class?

I think a DVD can be a great support to learning in a class once you have been taught techniques. I like people to learn initially in person.

How long do your classes generally last?

One hour.

Are there any contraindications to attending a class?

A good instructor will work *with* you and you must make them aware of any ailments or limitations.

As a practitioner and a Pilates regular yourself, what benefits can a woman over 40 hope to see after regular practice?

At 45, you would gain in terms of posture, poise and focus. You would become more aware of your health and breath and be more vital and strong. The other huge benefit of a class is friendship and social support – especially important as we get older. The talking that goes on in my classes is nearly as important as the class itself.

How regular does practice have to be to have a beneficial effect?

Once a week is good. I am a great advocate of functional work. This means that you have what we call 'nutritious movement'. I have studied the writing of Katy Bowman and she is a 'biomechanist'. We want to preserve our function as we age and keep moving well. Notice how you stand and move. So I include that in my classes – looking at how the movements we do every day can be optimised. How do you keep balance? Can you get up onto your toes easily?

Will one lose weight?

Not per se but you will be stronger and more toned.

What is the oldest age you have taught?

I have just done an annual review on one of my 90-year-old ladies!

Further reading recommended by Frances

- *Pilates for Life* by Lynne Robinson
- *Dynamic Aging: Simple Exercises for Whole-Body Mobility* by Katy Bowman

MY PERSONAL EXERCISE FOR KEEPING WEIGHT STABLE AND MUSCLES STRONG

I learned in my 40s that long schleps of cardio just did not work for me and probably raised my cortisol and kept a tummy bulge around my middle. I now aim for minimum of a 20-minute resistance regime up to 5 times a week – sometimes more, sometimes less. Ideally, have a professional work with you to create a safe routine and monitor for injury initially, and don't do what hurts or injures you. This is just my example:

- **Upper body:** weights, biceps and triceps work including warm ups and stretches. I sometimes combine this with leg work at the same time depending on my mood. A selection of the following which I mix up according to the video I am following (Jenni Rivett, Joe Wickes, Hot and flashy, MadFit) or workout I have read in e.g. Women's Health.
- **Abdo:** e.g. reverse abdo crunches, leg raises (alternate or together), plank, side planks, scissor crunches, bicycle crunches, plank with knee to elbow, push ups (total or from knees).
- **Legs:** e.g squat, squat holds, reverse lunges (forward lunges stress my knees).
- **Cardio:** e.g. mountain climbers, alternate leg crunches, walking with high knees on the spot.

I personally avoid leaping around to preserve my pelvic floor after two emergency caesareans and to protect my back. I find if I use a free tabatta timer on my phone I can choose the pace –20 to 40s exercise plus an interval of 10 to 20s between. If I am not feeling the burn or sweating I am not doing it right, but this is personal and what I find works. The fat goes and the muscles strengthen without building up, the clothes fit and I have more energy.

Read more about losing weight at any age in my blog:
https://drlouisewiseman.co.uk/the-one-thing-a-woman-over-40-might-need

Yoga is similarly excellent for posture, strength and bones when performed correctly. It helps many women in menopausal time to decompress mentally and physically. As with many women I have found many benefits from yoga and would urge you to seek out a highly trained teacher near you if you think it might be what you need.

PRESERVING JOINT HEALTH

Joints are simply where two bones meet. In good health they are covered by articular cartilage which helps them move smoothly across each other and keeps our movements fluid. When the cartilage breaks down over time, accelerated by injury or damage, then joint disease can develop. If due to wear and tear, we call it osteoarthritis. Extra areas of bone can develop to compensate, called osteophytes. Doctors sometimes look for these in examining, for example, hands to see if arthritis is caused by osteoarthritis rather than a disease process like rheumatoid arthritis.

Osteoarthritis (OA) is of course ubiquitous. In the USA 13% of women over 60 have knee osteoarthritis. In the UK numbers quoted are around one in five adults over 45 years. The symptoms are:

- Joint swelling
- Tenderness
- Stiffness
- Sometimes locking

The resultant decreased ease of movement can cause disability and reduced quality of life. There are a myriad of medicines and physical therapy that can help but in order to give yourself the best chance of dancing and walking, even dashing for the bus with ease, start thinking of protecting your joints now.

Rheumatoid arthritis (RA) is a progressive inflammatory disease of the joints with specific features beyond the scope of this book – not just related to wear and tear. Obviously a rheumatoid sufferer can suffer this alongside osteoarthritis.

Don't strain

A good place to start is to try to do things the easy way for your body, not the quick way for now. If pulling a garden trolley takes two hands don't try and fudge it quickly with one. It is cheap to buy a silicon or rubber disc to help you remove tight lids from jars so don't strain your hands repeatedly while young.

Avoid over-extending your joints. Be mindful of your body, and when things hurt take notice.

Joints can hurt from excess activity – a day gardening/ a new workout regime/joint damage – or if your joints are not great your ligaments can become slack and this puts more strain on the joints and muscles.

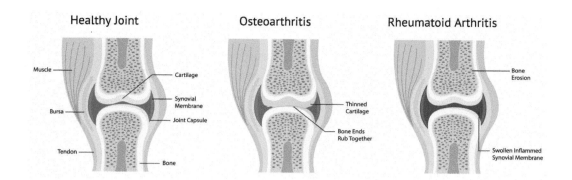

Healthy Joint — Muscle, Cartilage, Synovial Membrane, Bursa, Joint Capsule, Tendon, Bone

Osteoarthritis — Thinned Cartilage, Bone Ends Rub Together

Rheumatoid Arthritis — Bone Erosion, Swollen Inflamed Synovial Membrane

Simple steps

Use your hip or shoulder instead of your hand to close a drawer or door if your smaller joints hurt. Hug larger objects closer to your body as you carry them. Carry bags on your forearms if your hands and wrists are sore.

The human body has a surprising capacity to repair itself but our joints are still fragile. Cartilage that has worn away does not grow back. We know that weight is a great contributor to osteoarthritis. This is more applicable in the knees than the hips. Somehow weight seems to be more of an issue on the joints for women than it is for men. You can directly reduce your risk by shedding pounds if you are overweight. One study showed that when a woman loses 10 pounds her risk of knee OA halves!

If you are a keen runner there are many benefits to your health and it would be wrong to tell you to stop. If you have started to develop arthritis, maybe try substituting one of your runs for a jog on a forgiving treadmill or swap for a cycle or some gentle weights. If you have previously had an injury your chances of having joint pains later in life are increased.

Keep muscles strong to stabilise the joint. Quadriceps and hamstrings are both important as you want the joint to be supported both sides. We used to think it was just the quads. It stands to reason that if your quads, hamstrings and abdominal muscles are stronger, your hips have to do less to support your body weight. Strong quads may help compensate for a deficient knee ligament. Stretching properly after a workout helps, although studies have not found direct relationships between flexibility and reducing arthritis.

If your gait is awkward or painful on walking long distances seek the chance now to have a Physiotherapist/Pilates expert observe and teach you how best to correct it. Our bodies are always compensating for any weaknesses over time. Remember, hip pain may actually be felt in the knee so if you have problems consult your doctor to actually get a diagnosis of where a problem is and make a plan. Often exercises recommended by physios start as pool training so the water supports joints.

If your knees and hips are already a problem, then floor abdominal exercises may still be possible. Light hand weight routines and swimming and yoga will be good. All with advice from an expert and tell your class teacher of your ailments.

If you are generally fit and want to start future proofing your joints now, consider:

Cross-training – this can mean a variety of exercises in the gym or doing something different to your normal sport – it uses different muscles from the ones you are used to. This will give your body balance and stimulate your mind.

Flexibility work – think yoga, tai chi and Pilates.

Aerobic exercise – start more gently with lower intensity if needed.

Stretching exercises – you must stretch your muscles back after exercise and this can encourage a long lean look.

Exercises with reduced impact – cycling, walking and swimming are easier on the joints; swap for indoor cycling or a stair climber if needed.

Weight training – muscles are kept strong and this aids in joint stabilisation. It is really important to work with a trained professional at the beginning of a new regime as injuries can be just as powerful as the gains from work like this.

Here I bring in the expert opinion of a doctor who keeps moving AND motivates other women to move and run!

SPECIALIST INTERVIEW – DR JULIET MCGRATTAN

Former GP until 2019, Juliet worked as a **Champion for Physical Activity for Public Health England** from 2015 to 2019, delivering presentations to healthcare professionals about the evidence for and use of physical activity in clinical care. Working as a freelance medical journalist since 2012 she is currently the resident health expert for *Women's Running* and *Outdoor Fitness and Adventure* magazines as well as writing for various other online publications. Juliet's blog – **www.drjulietmcgrattan.com** – encourages everyone to have active lives.

Her first book, *Sorted: The Active Woman's Guide to Health*, won first prize in the BMA Medical Book Awards in the Popular Medicine category in 2018.

She is the Women's Health Lead and a Master Coach for **261 Fearless**, a global non-profit using running to unite, empower and educate women around the world. She is also the founder and director of the 261 Fearless Club UK Community Interest Company.

When did you start running and why?

I tried in 2000 and hated it. My knees hurt and I always felt so terribly out of breath. I made all the classic mistakes of going too fast and too far, too soon. I started properly in 2008 after my third child was born. I knew I needed to get fit, wasn't happy with my body shape and wanted some time to myself. We lived in the country with no classes or gyms nearby and running from my front door was really the only thing I could see I could fit in. I was spurred on by the local 10k race and made a pact with myself to run it the following year. I did and by then I was smitten.

What benefits do you see in yourself and the women around you?

Running can be transformational both for body and mind. Achieving something you didn't think you could do, whether it's your first mile or first marathon, is incredibly empowering. You quickly gain confidence in your ability and marvel at what your body can do. Running has so much to give. The therapeutic thud of your feet on the ground as you run solo provides a welcome headspace. The company of a running friend, when you find you're solving each other's and the world's problems, turns even the worst day into a good one. Running gives you self-esteem, experiences, adventure, health and the most amazing friends.

How do you think running activities can help women through the perimenopausal and menopausal years?

This is a great time to be running. The physical benefits of running include bone and muscle strengthening and we're all aware how bone and muscle mass decreases rapidly during the menopausal years. If you enjoy running then you'll want to do it regularly and therefore experience all the health benefits of exercise including a reduced risk of major diseases such as heart disease, type 2 diabetes and certain types of cancer. The risk of all of these increases with age, so running can be a great way to counteract that risk. Equally important are the mental health benefits. When hormonal changes are causing mood swings, anxiety and general misery, then running can be an escape. The feel-good endorphins that flow round your body after exercise are very powerful and can change your day. There's also the opportunity to join a running club, meet new people, push yourself out of your comfort zone or just enjoy time running mindfully on your own with nature.

Do you think injury is more common with age and how do we combat that? Do you think joints suffer or improve with stronger supporting muscles?

We know that repair processes slow down a bit with age so older runners just need to allow more time for recovery. It's when you rest that the repair and strengthening happens, that's when you actually get fitter. Skimping on recovery time can lead to injury. I believe that muscle-strengthening activities help to protect joints and should be part of every runner's routine to help protect their back and knee joints.

The other thing that happens with age is that reflexes, co-ordination and balance all deteriorate; this can definitely lead to more injuries. I really notice how hard the older ladies in my running group find it to stand on one leg. They think I'm mad when I tell them that they should do it every night, when they brush their teeth, and then try to do it with their eyes closed!

Do you think there is an age when women should stop running?

Definitely not. You should stop when you don't enjoy it or don't want to, or can't do it, whatever age that is.

What would you say to someone with no contraindications who wants to start running as a form of fitness over the age of 40?

Do it! But do it right. Learn from my mistakes and don't just go out and think you can run. After a few metres you'll be gasping for breath and heading home. Find a 'Couch to 5k' beginners group or use the NHS app to help you gradually build up from 30 seconds of running with walking in between. Go at the speed of chat (preferably with someone you can talk to so you can actually chat), even if that means you are only shuffling along. If you're at that pace, then you can maintain it for longer; speed will come later. Turn up to your local parkrun; you will find a warm welcome and you can walk it all if you want to. Reach out to the running community on social media, they are full of encouragement and support, and think about joining a local running club that has a specific beginners section. It'll take time but I guarantee that you will amaze yourself and you will feel so proud of what your amazing body can achieve.

See more of Juliet in her personal interview in The Women section.

CHAPTER 14: FOOD IS LIFE

Food is essential for life. Like sleep and water, it is imperative to keep our cells living and our bodies breathing. We have developed a bizarre relationship with food. The more developed we have become the more artificial and synthesised our food can be. The medicine in this book is back to basics and this is what is happening with food. We think we are advanced in snapping up books by glamorous writers and foodies, telling us to cook fresh and use 'food from the earth', but that is how our predecessors automatically functioned. *We need to be told* to re-evaluate our dietary and culinary attitudes. *We need to be told* to eat from the soil, as though it is novel and ground-breaking. Our ancestors were *breaking and tilling the ground* without colour hardbacks to show them how.

I would love to say I was the junior doctor who prepared her seed snacks and packed her lunch to get her through a long A & E shift. I would love to say I lived early married life astounding my husband with nightly prepared French cuisine. That was not me. I was nurtured by my mother with home-cooked foods, appropriate treats, and I learned a healthy relationship with food. However, student and doctor life meant that *fast and convenient* became my 'vitamins', the *hospital canteen* my 'kitchen'.

Food is fuel and we run well on it. We can run on the most processed, easy to access 'petrol', but at some point our engine will be clogged and our efficiency impaired. You can 'get away' with a lot when young but we are realising that the cards you are dealt, in terms of genetics and inherited disease, can be affected by what you fuel your tank with. *The earlier you can start refreshing your body with proper nutrition, the greater your chance of avoiding or delaying the*

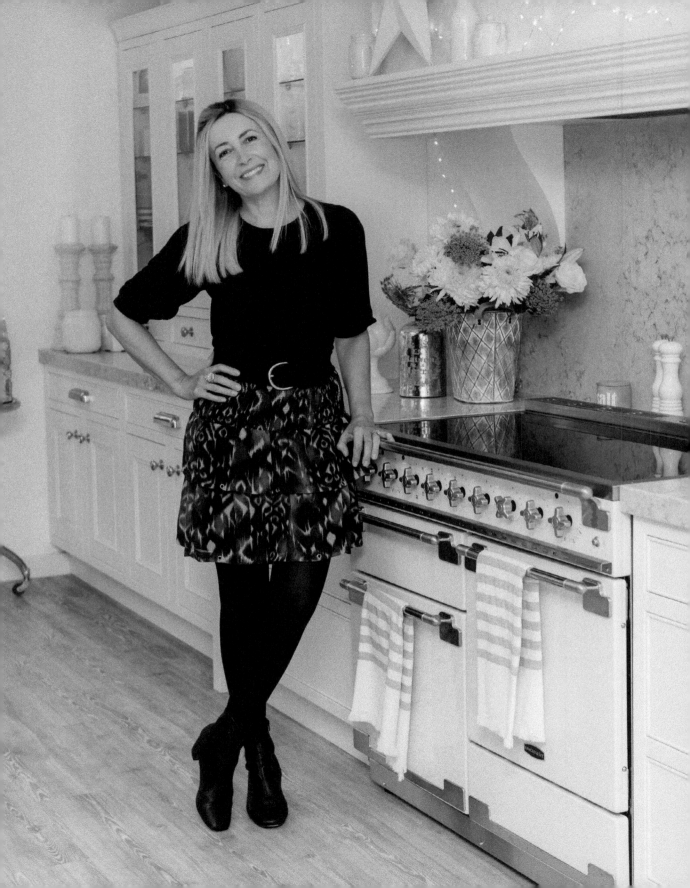

chronic diseases our parents dreaded – mature onset diabetes, obesity, cardiovascular disease, dementia, osteoporosis... Our forgiving bodies will serve us adequately, full of white carbs and useless fizz, but *some of us* can end up craving *more and more* of those quick fixes while the mineral and vitamin supplies dwindle. This will leave you **frazzled, overweight, lethargic and depressed**.

There are many 'food books' on the market and many 'diets' available to investigate online. Many of them work, some long term and some short term. Some are fantastic real food books that will become your best friends, providing nourishing meal ideas. If they are extreme, fast and severely restrictive with no science basis, then the evidence is usually that within 18 months of stopping an extreme 'diet' you will have regained the weight and *possibly up to a third more as well*. This is what doctors are taught about 'yoyo dieting'. Simply I ask you to evaluate the process and to seek not to follow a 'diet' but to find a 'lifestyle choice' that provides you with **all the food groups** that you need and that is **sustainable**. A couple of paid sessions with a qualified registered dietician or registered nutritionist may change your life forever.

You will not 'stop and start' with a lifestyle choice, it will become *part of your life*. You will start to automatically make those healthier choices and not feel deprived. Many a talk I have started with the words '**Life is a system of choices**'. Unless you are a very young child YOU are in charge of what passes into your mouth. In the past, I could devour a family pack of chocolate biscuits unhindered whilst watching TV. I was rather good at it. I now choose not to do it. That is a lifestyle choice, *not a diet*.

Life is also about balance. If we are told not to do something we automatically seek out that one thing and 'treat' ourselves. We reprimand internally then say 'Oh, just this once'. That makes us feel rubbish after the fancy cake – we have failed, we are failures, *I am a failure*. Then we crave that very thing again.

TAKE AWAY THE REPRIMANDING AND THE GUILT.

"That fancy cake was a welcome treat sitting with my friend in a café chatting about our worlds. I savoured it, I was mindful of it and I don't regret it."

Then the cake is no longer such an issue.

How different does that sound? **Can you have your cake and eat it?** In balance. Some of us can't just limit ourselves to only one piece, so we have to make decisions about that too.

In my interviewing process I spoke to many women, and maybe less than 20% were happy and *fully compliant* with **100%** healthy eating. For those particular ladies, keeping a healthy figure was part of their work and they did not go through phases of poor eating and self-admonishment. The rest were either healthily in balance or *self-critical* of their food intake. Aiming for, say, an 80/20 balance seems a healthy attitude to have – all hail those who can live virtuously without considering otherwise.

It can be confusing to look at your weight and know what is good for you. Seek out the advice of your practice nurse. A helpful tool is measuring your waist and height in the same unit, e.g. inches. If your waist is more than half your height, then this could be an indicator of 'early health risk'. Fat around our waist is more harmful than, say, subcutaneous fat around our thighs, as central fat may indicate 'visceral' or more internal fat beneath wrapped around our organs and this implies a higher risk of cardiovascular disease and diabetes and so on. For this reason, apple-shaped women with a relatively larger tummy may have higher risks to their health than being more pear-shaped. All must be taken into account with your general health.

Should we count calories?

Let us consider two best friends in their 50s, Gretchen and Nancy. Gretchen is super organised in that effortless way that some women are, but not obsessive. She finds that by having an awareness of healthy **calories and using an app or a diary she maintains her ideal weight for her. Eating out and choosing food is not an issue. Her best friend Nancy loves cooking for everyone and trying out new recipes and only cooks fresh, never counts a calorie. Both women lead active lives although they have a completely different approach to food. Both women are healthy with a figure** they are happy with **and good body parameters in terms of percentage fat, body mass index, waist to height ratio and so on.**

Which way of life is correct?

Either is great. We do know that when things go to extremes problems arise, with eating disorders and food obsessions. We all socialise around food and, if you have concerns, this can *mean socialising while eating becomes difficult* so you may in turn choose to isolate yourself.

We know that energy expenditure and energy intake have to be in proportion to not cause huge weight gains and that we often manipulate this with dieting. The content of what you are eating however, I BELIEVE, especially for women over 40, needs to be healthy. Once you ditch the excess refined sugar your tastes change and everything tastes better. You can then trust yourself more to make healthy decisions and *crave the healthier foods*. Following someone else's generic diet that is not tailored to **your body**, your needs that day, your hormonal state, your age and specific energy requirements, may be like trying to fit a square peg into a round hole and is literally exhausting. Make sure food is your fuel and there is **good stuff on your plate**. That is what we must start with for our best life.

Falling off the wagon

Trainers, scientists and foodies alike have been keen to tell me that we must not remonstrate with ourselves at the slightest hint of unhealthy eating. If you create healthy habits and patterns, but then slip a little, you can always return to it **if it worked for you**. We tend to be a little 'all or nothing' but there is something reassuring about being *flexible* in our mental relationship with food.

Do I practice what I preach?

I was a good 'mum cook'. Birthday cakes and weekly bakes and spaghetti bolognese – I was your girl. However, I needed to up it a notch. On my quest for 'better health' for all the family

I decided to ditch the packets of anything too processed and go for it raw. I armed myself with recipes from Allrecipes, BBC Good Food and Joe Wicks and made a pact with the children. I would try a different 20-minute recipe every day for 21 days. I didn't have time to faff.

The deal was, if it was a good recipe I would laminate the printout and put it in a file. Crunchy parmesan-topped salmon and homemade sweet potato wedges – laminated – tick! Better than fish and chips from the freezer any day! Twenty-one days passed and only two recipes were rejected.

My job was done. We had winters with less colds and coughs and my cooking was no longer laughed at. Small triumphs add up to big wins on the health front. I now find cooking and preparing food a solace, a mindful time. Cooking with love – who knew?!

What do you NEED to eat?
Carbohydrates, proteins, fats, water, smaller gems called micronutrients (vitamins and minerals) and phytonutrients (antioxidants obtained from plants). If you get the balance right *your body will start to respond.*

WATER

Essential for metabolism, movement of substances in and out of our cells, balancing bodily processes, regulating temperature and maintaining circulation. There is general advice about how much we should drink but there are variations in this in relation to demographic group and climate, so one size does not literally fit all. For babies and children, the fluid requirements are weight-specific and fluid balance underpins a large amount of paediatric medicine. Babies at birth are literally 70% water and by the time we are elderly this will have dropped to about 55%.

If you don't drink enough, you will suffer constipation, kidney stones, urinary tract infections, even chronic kidney disease and so on.

Thirst

We recognise thirst as a dry sticky mouth and the *feeling* of thirst. This can be accompanied by tiredness, poor concentration, headache, dizziness and fainting. Some astute menopausal ladies will be thinking this comes in line with the menopausal symptoms that some women describe – **how much of this is worsened by the water lost in sweat during hot flushes and the changes in thermoregulation (body temperature regulation) that occur? Keep the water at your side to help.**

For most UK women up to 80% of our water comes from fluid intake and the rest is from food – think of soup, fruit, vegetables, salad. Our environment and activity will obviously affect needs. If you dehydrate yourself with excessive caffeinated drinks and aren't getting enough water, literally *each skin cell will become dehydrated as will your brain that is doing the thinking for you.* We are not designed to live without water so start there. Calculate what you need in a day and fill up that portable BPA free cup and make sure you get through it. If you ever bottle fed a baby, you would have been meticulous calculating how much fluid you gave them in a day. Apply the same obsession to yourself for a couple of days to develop a healthy habit and you are set for life. It's not rocket science, but when your body is craving a snack fix ask yourself first if you are thirsty and cross that baby off the list. Your urine should have a good strong stream and be almost clear and not offensive smelling – if it looks dark and you are otherwise well your first thought should be that you may be dehydrated.

The very young and the old often have problems responding to cues to drink so need to be reminded, but we can simply be **too busy to think**. One small serving a day of fruit juice, which could be diluted with water for the sake of your teeth and maybe for a healthier option, is possibly enough and will contribute to your fruit and veg intake as a serving. My personal choice is to not have fruit juice as it feels rather like liquid sugar and I prefer to obtain it from solid fruit. The odd fruit juice or smoothie is wonderful but remember that drinks do have calories too, something I saw clearly in patients I cared for, fitted with gastric bands, who cleverly bypassed the effect of the band by gaining extra calories from liquid 'nourishment'. Also, if you are watching your weight maybe enjoy eating that fruit and *all of its fibre* for your gut.

Alcohol will make us pass more urine and become more dehydrated. Try to drink water or 'non-sugary soft drinks' alongside alcohol. See later on for recommendations on alcohol.

The UK government advises 1.2 litres (six to eight glasses) of water a day and the USA guidelines tend to be eight glasses of 8 oz size per day (1.9 litres). Glasses can vary in size obviously! We know that when the weather improves, the guidance is to increase our fluid intake. Work out what is best for you to keep you feeling well, your urine clear or very pale, and your body energised based on your requirements that day. Many UK experts would advocate nearer the USA amount if you are an active person.

Signals from the brain help regulate water intake, and in some studies having less than 1.8 litres intake total body water a day has been shown to start triggering messengers in the body to promote thirst.

THE FEMALE PLATE

It is impossible to prescribe a perfect meal for every day, as we thrive on variety and our needs fluctuate. Good scientifically based recommendations include the Eatwell Guide or the Mediterranean diet. My strong belief is that the Mediterranean diet and way of life is becoming more relevant as we look to what makes us potentially live longer with less chance of disease. It is not just the food content of it but, as you will read here, the entire way of living, socialising, the very essence of belonging to a valued community and the sense of purpose and involvement this purports.

Very often what is thought of as a normal diet will consist of up to 65% carbohydrates. We must remember that carbohydrates are **not** all bread and pasta, and that green veg, fruit, potatoes, legumes, wholegrains, rice and wheat also come under this umbrella. All carbohydrates break down to sugar molecules eventually and this causes the pancreas to release insulin, and sugar then either passes into the liver, muscle or fat. If you run on sugar highs and lows, when it drops you will feel you need a snack, and then the fat burning you should be having between meals switches off.

I asked Dr Suzanne Barr (Registered Dietician at Imperial College) what the ideal plate would look like. There obviously is not an exact 'ideal plate' – this depends upon many factors – but her suggestion in line with global dietary guidelines and the Mediterranean diet is:

HALF VEGETABLES/QUARTER CARBOHYDRATES/QUARTER PROTEIN
This is also illustrated well in the new Canada guidelines (see references).

Many protein sources are not just meat and fish. Tofu, tempeh and edamame all originate from soya beans, and contain iron, calcium and other vitamins and minerals. Lentils, chickpeas and green peas also pack a protein punch. Quinoa and oats contain some protein. As you will see from the Blue Zones studies later, reducing the amount of meat in our diet may help our chances in the longevity lottery.

Women need B vitamins for all the body's energy processes and thyroid function. Getting your five veg a day (and steaming veg not to lose B vitamins) and watching not to have excess alcohol reducing our B vitamins is essential (see alcohol chapter).

Women need iron. We obviously have higher requirements than men premenopausally and these can drain our reserves (see hair loss chapter).

Women need magnesium. We can often neglect to eat magnesium-rich foods – essential from our teens all the way through – get this from green leafy veg, nuts, fish, wholegrain bread, brown rice, meat and dairy. Iron and magnesium are essential for fighting fatigue and giving us mental reserve. There is also research to support magnesium in prevention of migraines in chronic sufferers – something to discuss with your doctor. More on magnesium in my sleep chapter. I am not going to recommend Magnesium supplementation in a blanket statement here as it can cause dizziness – d/w your doctor. I have discussed the value of magnesium in the form of Epsom salt baths. A couple of handfuls in a bath can be a great soother mentally, and help exhausted muscles too and aid sleep – great perimenopausally or at any time! Skin absorption is thought to be extremely efficient.

Good fats. Gone are the days of low-fat advocates; we need healthy fats – monounsaturated and polyunsaturated – for our mental health and balancing our hormones. They help the good cholesterol and lower the bad cholesterol and hence reduce the risk of stroke and heart disease. Good examples are olives, nuts, seeds, fatty fish and avocadoes. What we want to avoid are trans fats such as those found in some fried foods, crisps and so on. We also need to reduce the portion of saturated fat to a maximum of 10% of our daily calories – this is found in red meat, butter and whole-fat dairy.

Omega-3 are a type of polyunsaturated fat that are really good for us – protecting mental health, protecting against heart disease, helping reduce inflammation in our bodies (arthritis and skin conditions) and keeping our mood good and our energy high. We find these in oily fish, tuna, halibut, eggs, chia seeds, brussels sprouts, spinach, kale and beans.

Olive oil is great as extra virgin on a salad or normal olive oil for cooking.

What is a real Mediterranean diet?

I love the advice given by Younger Lives (lifestyle specialists in staying younger, healthier and happier) – www.youngerlives.com – as it transposes into an easy list you can stick to your fridge. As a scientist I want numbers and lists – as an amateur cook I need this kind of guide, so it works perfectly.

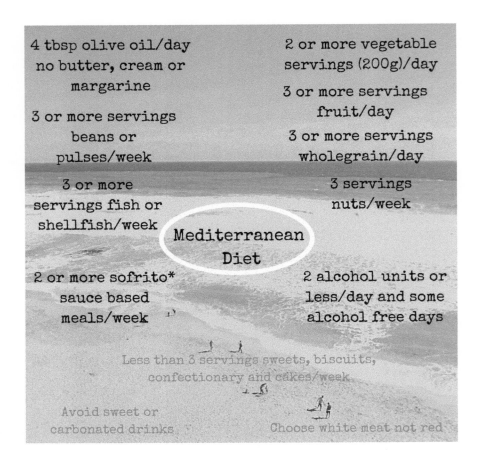

4 tbsp olive oil/day no butter, cream or margarine

2 or more vegetable servings (200g)/day

3 or more servings fruit/day

3 or more servings beans or pulses/week

3 or more servings wholegrain/day

3 or more servings fish or shellfish/week

3 servings nuts/week

Mediterranean Diet

2 or more sofrito* sauce based meals/week

2 alcohol units or less/day and some alcohol free days

Less than 3 servings sweets, biscuits, confectionary and cakes/week

Avoid sweet or carbonated drinks

Choose white meat not red

Let's find out a little more about www.youngerlives.com.

*Sofrito is a tomato-based sauce. There are many culture-specific versions of this, e.g. with tomatoes/onion/garlic/olive oil/peppers/paprika. Garlic and onions are thought to have a lot of beneficial properties – not least on the immune system via the gut.

Dr Holly Whelan BSc Biology, PhD Neuroscience, Fellow of Royal Society for Public Health; Dr Mark Cobain BSc Psychology, PhD Neuroscience, Fellow of Royal Society for Public Health

Younger Lives are health & wellness behaviour change experts. They specialise in converting complex health science into simple programmes that help people live healthier, happier and more fulfilled lives.

Mark has worked in healthy ageing, heart health and behaviour change research for over 20 years and was the inventor of 'heart age', a personal risk communication tool.

Holly has worked in health and social marketing and behaviour change for over 20 years. Their unique combination of the science (neuroscience and behaviour change), along with the consumer understanding and business insight, makes them perfectly placed to create programmes that help engage and improve people's health & wellbeing as well as support businesses in *'doing well by doing good'*.

Younger Lives have worked with many big names across the globe, including Bupa, Movember, Unilever, Weight Watchers, NHS, AXA, Singapore Heart Foundation and Cleveland Clinic Abu Dhabi, as well as developing their own bespoke behaviour change programmes to help people live longer, healthier and happier lives. One of their lead programmes is an online course that helps women 40yrs+ transform their lives so they can immediately start to feel years younger and live their best lives. This expert course is based on years of research and guides women on what they personally should do and why, as well as providing them with simple, proven behaviour change techniques and skills that they can use every day to achieve the life transformation they want.

What message could you give the readers of my book who are maybe 'not feeling so confident' in themselves to make a change and feeling they are 'too old' to gain better health now?

The first message is that it's never too late to start making changes that will improve your health, happiness and quality of life. There are amazing stories of people who have completely changed their lives after years of maybe not being perfect. The key thing to remember is your body is an incredible machine – it is able to repair itself and get stronger with the right care and lifestyle. You only need to take a look at the many success stories of people being able to lose loads of weight after many years of being overweight, or women taking up running in their 70s, or people completely turning their lives around after illness or difficult periods such as divorce or trauma. Research backs these individual stories up, and even shows that the right lifestyle can improve and prolong the lives of those living with serious health conditions too – so it really is worth the effort whatever your situation.

The second message is we can gain personal confidence in making change by starting small and establishing simple healthy habits, one day at a time. Everyone who made a change started at this point. For example, by adding a piece of fruit to our breakfast every day or going for a walk after dinner every day we start to create a new lifestyle one day at a time. Our goal should be to find easy, repeatable things that we can build into our lives which turn into healthy habits that we do without thinking.

Please explain to the reader what the role of Younger Lives is, for example in a corporate setting.

There are two ways we work with corporates:

1. We help corporates develop their own behaviour change programmes as specialist consultants.
2. We offer corporates scientifically validated behaviour change programmes to help them support the health and wellbeing of their employees and also their consumers.

What do you think makes you unique and successful in changing your clients' patterns of behaviours and lifestyle?

The key to a healthy and happy life is all about having the right behaviours and positive attitude.

However, *keeping* to the right behaviours is not always that easy because of how our brains are wired (the neuroscience). For example, from an evolutionary point of view our bodies are programmed to crave fat and sugar, when it is available, so we can deal with times of famine – which is really not that helpful in today's world of being surrounding by unhealthy food 24/7! Another problem can be our own personal history and the identity we have built up over many years, which can lead to damaging habits that we are not even consciously aware of and are very difficult to break – e.g. I am stressed so I need to eat this chocolate (comfort eating), I need and deserve a few glasses of wine when I get home to wind down after a hard day at work (self-medication with alcohol), or I am a red-blooded man who eats meat and doesn't like vegetables (identity).

A behavioural approach is therefore needed to help create the right motivation and practical conditions to support people to make sustained changes.

A few examples of the behavioural approach are:

1. Personal identity – how do you see yourself, where are you now and where do you want to be in the future and why? Getting this right is critical for maintaining long-term motivation.
2. Whilst information is helpful, too much can also be overwhelming and doesn't necessarily lead to action. So a behaviour approach is about helping people understand where they want to start and why, and then putting very practical plans in place to make this achievable.
3. Finally, constant feedback and rewards are important for behaviour change to stick. Tracking progress and celebrating small wins is critical to ensure that behaviours are maintained and

ultimately become part of your identity and not even conscious over time.

Do you have any long-term data to know if clients stick with healthy behaviours long after their work with Younger Lives?

A clinical trial of heart age in a workplace setting in Spain – this showed that having a heart check-up and presenting patients with their results in the form of a 'heart age' leads to an increase in motivation, a desire to make changes and a significant improvement in health one year later. An independent trial of life age by Imperial College London in 2018 showed a reduction in life age, so the body improving, reflecting huge improvement of parameters in terms of body weight, nutrition and physical activity.

What does the future hold for Younger Lives?

We are always updating our thinking and products based on the latest science and everything we have learnt. Our **life age product** reflects the latest science, and we are launching a new online-taught programme specifically for women who are looking for practical help in how they can stay at their very best in their 40s, 50s and beyond.

In the workplace, we are working on supporting the older worker and people going into retirement, as well as helping people with their levels of personal energy so they can feel and be at their best at all ages.

Thank you to Holly and Mark, who are at the forefront of behaviour change.

Now, why do we get hungry?

Focussing on sugar, our blood sugar drops 90 minutes after a meal and this can lead to a hunger sensation. We often grab the carbs for a quick fix. Before this happens we need to reassess what we are eating. Following the list below should reduce these sugar lows:

- a good grounding of green carbs (vegetables), giving our gut a good microbiome
- fibrous carbs for energy
- protein for cell and tissue growth and regeneration
- good fats (see skin chapter) for brain, nervous system, hormones and immunity.

If we don't get enough this leads to weight gain and, many believe, inflammation. A diet of unhealthy, sugar and saturated fat laden food will lead to what we associate with middle age – the muffin top, puffy congested faces, skin breakouts, bloating, low energy and low mood. *More seriously, diabetes, cancer and cardiovascular disease may be more likely if we are not feeding our bodies well.*

Why are sugar levels essential and why can excess sugar become harmful?
The pancreas releases insulin in response to the body taking on sugar and it has a crucial role in helping us dealing with that sugar. Hence if the insulin is inadequate or not working well diabetes can develop. Our blood sugar is normally maintained at a certain level and insulin manages it so that the **correct level supplies the brain**. If you consume up to, say, 500 calories of your intake as sugar (from carbs) then the *liver stores this as glycogen*. If you consume more (up to 2,000 calories), the *muscles store this as glycogen*. Any excess needs to be burned off. If you can take glucose up into 'storage' in your body easily, we say you have a 'good insulin sensitivity'. If you do no exercise and have a very sedentary life, the sensitivity of your body to insulin weakens. Add to this a high sugar diet and muscle CANNOT remove glucose from the bloodstream so effectively and this leads to a high blood sugar.

> *GLUCOSE NOT USED BY THE LIVER OR BRAIN BECOMES **FAT** CELLS AS
> TRIGLYCERIDES. In other words:
> *SUGAR NOT USED FOR FUEL BECOMES FAT.

Visceral fat within causes insulin resistance and eventually non-alcoholic fatty liver disease (NAFLD). Insulin resistance eventually continues to develop into type 2 diabetes and metabolic syndrome.

Fruit should be respected and consumed as it is, allowing benefit from the fibre and antioxidants and so on. If you want to have the ease of a smoothie in the morning or as a meal replacement, consider making it full of healthy fat/fibre/greens and only a small amount of fruit if needed. So, half an avocado, chia seeds, greens, banana and so on. I like to add a nut butter for a protein buzz.

If you are eating healthily and focussing on increasing the greens side of your plate for more gentle energy release from healthy carbs, then you will be burning fat between meals, not gaining weight, sleeping better and losing weight as you sleep in a healthy way. If your blood sugar is in balance *you* are more in balance.

There is a very complex collection of chemicals and hormones controlling our hunger. Some finer points regarding them:

- Sleep increases leptin (the satiety or satisfaction full hormone) so lack of sleep makes you eat more. Omega-3 helps leptin production.
- Obesity might mean ghrelin (released when the stomach is empty to get us to eat) doesn't reduce when the stomach is stretched. White carbs and sugar increase hunger without stretching the stomach lining. Protein does stretch the lining, so should be eaten at every meal to make us full.

- Stress in females raises cortisol and belly fat – excess exercise may have this effect. Manage it through relaxation and meditation.
- Excess carbs and fruit sugar lead to excessive insulin – exercise conversely aids insulin sensitivity in muscles. Omega-3 lowers our fasting insulin, and magnesium in our food raises our insulin sensitivity.

Prevent sugar swings by eating good protein, good fat and fibre-dense carbohydrates.

Eating cake and sweet treats is linked to dopamine release and we get into the addictive phase of emotional eating, not eating for nutrition. Insulin when it is released can hang around for up to eight hours; it takes sugar up into the body but stops fat burning and your sugar will eventually go low and you will crave to eat even more. Gradually you may develop insulin resistance. So think about your daily habits and your sugar.

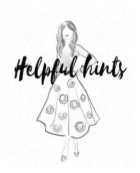

Helpful hints

Meal plan weekly, don't shop hungry, snack plan if that is your downfall

If having breakfast focus on protein, good carbs and fibre

Have **fruit raw** more often than juiced

Break cycle of bingeing, self-loathing and repeating

Recognise that food can be an **emotional crutch** like alcohol

Check your **water intake** is healthy

Consider reducing caffeine slowly – known trigger for headaches and migraines and in some women breast pain – some women find ginger and lemon teas and similar help with replacing sugar cravings

If you can't do without snacks have healthy ones available – unsalted almonds, brazils, try spreading a date or apple slice with unsweetened peanut butter

Evaluate any **intolerances with a professional, not by guesswork.** If appropriate, seek advice for meal plans and nutritional needs from a dietician, fully qualified registered dietician or registered nutritionist.

What do we know about portion sizes?

We live in a bounty of a world when it comes to food, and portion sizes have increased. You may read that we allegedly eat less off a blue plate, and obviously distracted eating causes us to eat more anyway, but do we really know what good portions are? A good portion of oily fish (salmon, herring, mackerel, sardines) would be the size of a pack of cards, white fish (cod, plaice, pollock) the size of a cheque book, a matchbox size of cheese gives you a good calcium and protein dose, pasta as a tennis ball size, or potatoes as a computer mouse size give you a good carb dose of energy. What is the relevance of 30 g? Well, 30 g is a handful of nuts or the weight of a good porridge breakfast uncooked. You would need 80 g of fruit or veg to give you one of your five a day roughly. What you might find reading this is that we all need to consider increasing our fruit and veg portions and lowering some of our starchy carbs. Again, something to discuss with a dietician or read further about.

Do you need supplements?

Always better from your plate but see bone chapter for reasons for vitamin D as a supplement. The doses in multivitamins are not tailored to the individual and one size does not fit all. We do know that something like folic acid is essential and thus many countries' policy to add it to the flour (soon in UK) and the recommendations for supplementing in pregnancy in the UK. Many water-soluble vitamins if taken in excess may be urinated out. Fat-soluble vitamins A, D, E and K can be harmful IF TAKEN in excess as they can't be peed out and will accumulate.

What's the coffee story?

The only warning in this book about coffee is that an excess of three or more cups a day can have a negative effect on bone density. Many studies though have researched the benefits of java. Unless you have excess and suffer palpitations, anxiety or lack of sleep, there are many good things: reduced incidence of Parkinson's disease/incidence of new cases of type 2 diabetes (can worsen existing diabetes)/liver cancer; and coffee has a good burst of antioxidants. There was also found in a women's study to be a reduced incidence of depression. Arabica beans evidently have positive effects on the brain, and robusta on the risks of heart disease and diabetes. Read more current research if you can as I have a feeling that new facts will constantly emerge. Remember oodles of cream and sugar cancel out the benefits.

What's the deal with processed meats and meats in general?

According to the experts I spoke to, the evidence of inflammation from meat was limited as it is difficult to eliminate effects from other parts of the diet. Sticking to lean meat that is non-processed and avoiding calorific red meat and fatty meat seems eminently sensible. Nitrites in sausages and bacon that are processed with them (as preservatives) have more evidence of links with bowel cancer. Plant-based diets are emerging in studies as being extremely healthy in many cases as long as they are balanced.

Let us now look at the nutrition we provide the body within the context of the perimenopausal years. I am delighted to have interviewed Jackie Lynch and she gives many pearls of wisdom here based on her own professional experience.

JACKIE LYNCH

Registered Nutritional Therapist
Founder of WellWellWell clinic in London
Regular writer in the national press, guest
expert on TV and media (e.g. Channel 4's
Superfoods). Author of *The Right Bite: Smart*
Food Choices for Eating on the Go **and** *Va Va*
Voom: The 10-Day Energy Diet
Host of The Happy Menopause podcast
The Happy Menopause **book coming soon**

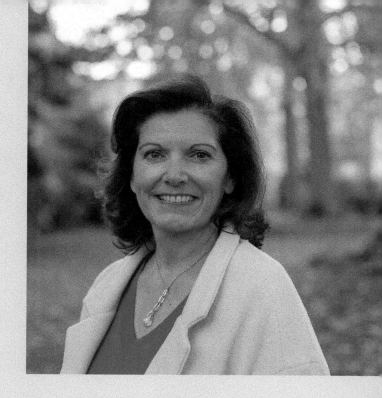

Tell me about your career to date please, Jackie, and how you came to set up your clinic.

My first degree was in French and I moved to France after I graduated, living there for 12 years. I learned a lot about food then, because of the French passion for simple and delicious home cooking. I remember being completely shocked by the aisles in supermarkets dedicated to ready meals, when I moved back to the UK in 2000.

I worked in the sales and marketing of intellectual property, which involved TV and film, publishing and product development rights for brands like *Teletubbies*, S Club 7, *Noddy*, *Mr Men* and Agatha Christie. It was a busy life and a role that I loved, which involved a lot of travelling, and by 2001 I was running a large global sales and marketing team.

I was inspired to completely change direction in 2005, after I went on a health retreat in Morocco with a company called In:Spa – after just a few days of a wholefoods diet and plenty of fresh air and exercise, I felt like a completely new woman. I genuinely hadn't realised how tired and stressed I'd become and was amazed what a difference the right food could make in just a short space of time. By the following year, I'd given up my job and embarked on a four-year journey to study nutritional therapy.

I graduated in 2010 and launched my **WellWellWell nutrition clinic** in West London. My specialist area of interest is female health, in particular the menopause, because there are so many ways that the right nutrition can make a big difference to the health and wellbeing of women in midlife.

As well as my clinical work, I like to spread the word about the importance of nutrition for optimum health through my workshops, my nutrition blog, the books I've written and my latest venture which is The Happy Menopause podcast.

What would be the pattern of events for a client coming to see you for the first time; maybe she is 50, feeling exhausted, starting symptoms of menopause and working a part-time job with a family?

There's usually a specific symptom that will trigger women coming to see me, and in many cases they won't associate it with the menopause, unless it's something very obvious like a hot flush. Women in their mid to late 40s can be assailed with a range of symptoms like fatigue, low mood, increased PMS, heavy periods or flooding, headaches or skin issues, but they often don't make the connection with the menopause because they're still having regular periods.

All the women I work with have one thing in common – they have a huge amount on their plate and are usually exhausted and stressed, even if they won't admit it to themselves. One of the biggest challenges I have is convincing women to look after themselves as well as they look after everyone around them!

Why is it so important that we gain our nutrients from our plate and not just a vitamin jar? Do you think vitamin D might be a reasonable exception?

Because vitamins and minerals are designed to work in synergy – there isn't one food that only contains vitamin C or zinc, for example. All the food we eat, both animal and plant sources of food, contain a broad range of nutrients which work together to keep us fit and healthy. There are far more than you might imagine, if you consider all the protective plant compounds with very long names that most people haven't heard of. While there is an argument for using supplements where therapeutic support is needed, this should be on top of, *rather than instead of,* a balanced diet, because diet always has to be our starting point. It's also important to take into account that certain minerals act in opposition to each other, so a high-dose supplement of zinc, for example, could knock out copper, which may lead to anaemia; too much sodium affects potassium, and so on.

Vitamin D is so important to our health and wellbeing that it's produced by the body through exposure to sunlight. While it is found in some foods like organ meat, oily fish or dairy, the amounts are tiny and I do think everyone should be supplementing vitamin D, especially over the winter when the rays from the sun are too weak for us to make vitamin D. People who use high-factor sunblock, cover up in the sun or are unable to leave the house should be using vitamin D all year round.

Your writing very much focuses on evaluating our symptoms and tracing these back to a possible deficiency of nutrients in the food we put in our mouths. Do you find women have an 'aha moment' when you point out how powerful this is?

Sometimes my clinical work is a bit like being a detective. When people come to my nutrition clinic, they submit a health questionnaire and a food diary in advance, so that I have time to review it, look at the clues and start to make the connections between the symptoms they're experiencing and the food that they're eating. While they understand the theory when I explain the connections, the real 'aha moment' is when they apply the advice to their diet and start to see a tangible improvement in their symptoms. There's nothing more rewarding than that for a clinician!

What advice would you give to the 55-year-old, naturally past menopause lady struggling with her midriff and finding her favourite clothes no longer fit?

Abdominal fat is a real challenge for postmenopausal women, because the body just wants to hold on to it. The fat around our middle has a specific hormone profile and can produce oestrogen, so the body thinks it's doing us a favour hanging on to it, which makes it very challenging, because the body will always win in this situation. There's no point in going on a super-strict diet, because it won't affect the abdominal fat if your body thinks you need it, so you need to take a step back. As our ovaries stop producing oestrogen when we approach the menopause, the adrenal glands are programmed to produce small amounts to keep us fit and well. However, the adrenals also produce our stress hormones and, because many menopausal women are pretty stressed, this reduces the production of oestrogen, which is why the body tries to store it on the belly. So, for me, the first step is to focus on a diet and lifestyle which regulates levels of stress hormones. As they reduce, the adrenals can take over the production of oestrogen and you will find it much easier to lose that abdominal fat.

What do you think about the phrase 'you can't out-train a bad diet'?

It's not a phrase I'm familiar with, but I can completely see the logic. An intense training regime doesn't give you a free pass to health. It might mean that you're slim, but that's not the only parameter for health and it's very important to know what's going on inside the body. Visceral fat can gather around the organs, even if you're not carrying external fat, and this can be very dangerous. Excessive levels of sugar can cause any number of problems, such as diabetes, anxiety, digestive problems and neurotransmitter imbalance. Overtraining can also increase levels of stress hormones, which is never a good thing.

What would be the main messages you would give to a woman dealing with menopause naturally and how nutrition and lifestyle could moderate any unwanted symptoms?

I'd say, if you only do one thing, balance your blood sugar, because just by doing that you will improve your energy, your sleep, balance your hormones, regulate your weight and reduce anxiety. That solves a lot of issues in one go! Losing caffeine and alcohol can make a huge difference to hot flushes. Make sure you eat real food, because it's so much more nutritious than processed food. And finally, take the time to be good to yourself – rest, relaxation and daring to say no, so that you don't overload yourself, will make a huge difference.

How motivated are women when they see you, and if they start eating well how long before that reaps results in their energy, happiness and zest for life (plus ability to fit into their jeans!)?

They're very motivated – by the time they've made the effort to reach out, many women are at the end of their tether, and they really want to get back on track. As to how quickly diet and lifestyle will make a difference, it will largely depend on the issue we're working on and the underlying causes. I work with people who are seeking support for a wide range of health concerns, but I'd normally expect to see an improvement within 8-12 weeks.

Certainly Jackie has given us great food for thought and you can listen to her Happy Menopause podcasts at www.well-well-well.co.uk – and you might spot a doctor you know on there!

CHAPTER 15: LONGEVITY AND BLUE ZONES

HOW WHAT YOU EAT AND HOW YOU LIVE COULD MAKE YOU LIVE LONGER, HEALTHIER AND HAPPIER

You may be an aficionado of the term 'Blue Zones' or you may be a Blue Zone 'virgin'. Whichever you are, as a woman over 40 you need to familiarise yourself with the concepts and what they can do for you.

We are all fascinated with the idea of living longer and better. This often consists of looking at our parents or elders, crossing our fingers and resolving to get fit when the bulge stops us doing up our favourite skirt. Winging it just won't cut it if you are looking for your best life.

In 2004 Dan Buettner, an explorer and *National Geographic* writer, commandeered the term Blue Zones. He had investigated the five zones in the world where people lived the longest healthiest lives. These were the areas where the rate of residents living to their 100th birthday was up to *10 times greater* than the general population of the US! We have now been using the term Blue Zone for 15 years. These 'magical' places actually hold the science that can unlock our understanding of why some people live longer. No, you cannot take a magic pill as there are no guarantees, but that life roulette wheel could do with some science to make it work more in your favour, so read on.

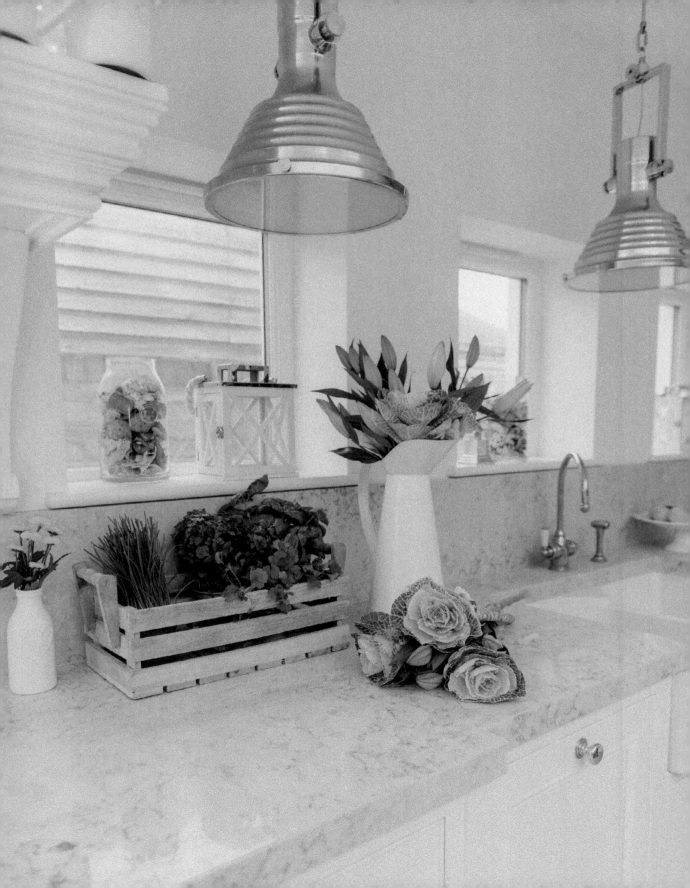

The five places called Blue Zones are Sardinia in Italy, Okinawa in Japan, Nicoya Peninsula in Costa Rica, Loma Linda in South California (Home of the Seventh-Day Adventists) and Ikaria, an island in Greece.

You think you will just follow your parents' path? Think again. Studies have shown that *around* only 20% of how long a person lives is down to genetics. Scientists have been looking at the genome for the answer as to why some live longer but your lifestyle and environment seem to play *a much bigger role*. Let us look at the features of each Blue Zone and then a summary of what the takeaway points might mean to you and your life.

I have not focussed on the dietary content of each area as this might tempt you to latch onto an individual dietary component as a magic answer to longevity. No, that is not appropriate for this book. Each area lives on:

Seasonal food and has good vitamin D levels from sunlight

Fresh produce grown on the land – fruits, vegetables, cheese from local farming stock, etc.

We know that **plant-based eating may have an anti-inflammatory effect** and that **fish** is such a valuable component of any diet.

The content of the Mediterranean diet in terms of prebiotics, probiotics and supporting the gut microbiome is therefore strong (I will explain all this later). More importantly for this book *that is not a recipe book* is the WAY OF LIFE, of living, eating, belonging and **having a purpose** to get up for in the morning.

Having a purpose.

Think about that last phrase and how it applies to you, especially if you are past the chaotic frenetic years where you had no choice but to be busy with many 'purposes'.

Volunteering and socialising also give purpose.

SARDINIA

In this mountainous island, the work is mainly as shepherds. Generations work together and the elders in the community have an active role in advising authorities, so they feel included and listened to.

OKINAWA

There is a close-knit social network amongst women, called 'YUIMARA', where neighbours and relatives check on each other daily. Residents practise HARA HACHI BU – reciting this phrase before a meal, reminding them of mindful eating by stopping when 80% full.

NICOYA PENINSULA

Life is about community, different generations living together, growing food and cooking together. If you live alone, you are visited regularly by your neighbours. Happiness is a goal.

LOMA LINDA

This area is the residence for the Seventh-Day Adventists who believe that maintaining their health is a way of honouring God. The population here is 10 times as likely to live to 100 compared to the general US population.

The Adventists strongly believe in taking care of the body that God gave you. They pray before eating and their faith encourages them to want to do good and volunteer, as they want to have a meaningful purpose.

IKARIA

There is a relaxed sense of time – the residents *own it rather than it owning them* – and a festive spirit (expressed through dance and song). *The aim is to dine slowly with family and friends; the locals are mindful of satisfying the stomach.*

Summary of Blue Zones and you

Are you inspired reading this? How do we apply this to our own lives?

Let us look at the general message:

A plant-rich diet is one that will protect cells and hormones from inflammatory injury or 'damage' and calm down your stress (cortisol) response. If we lose the ability to repair the body quicker than we damage it, then it fails, or ages. Overall, the Blue Zones tend to have meat on average five times a month. This is a little different to the old 'meat and two veg' daily model.

It is not for this book to advocate what you should eat, and meat/fish intake is a personal and often moral issue. It is becoming achingly clear that one needs correct protein intake and that correctly sourced fish that is not contaminated is potent (a tin of sardines is great for your bone calcium – see bone chapter) but if veganism is for you do it well with strong protein and calcium sources. We know that colourful foods are invaluable for us – kale, spinach, chard, grapes and blueberries all have polyphenols and resveratrol that act upon the longevity genes in our bodies. We need these antioxidants to top up our 'anti-ageing' bank.

The **active lifestyles** of the Blue Zones in many ways are not conscious decisions but natural and endemic to their way of life in order to function. If we relay this back to our own lives, some of it may have to become a conscious change – we do not have a flock of sheep to tend so are not active every 20 minutes by default. Getting up from the desk or going out to do a run must be a conscious decision. One study showed that every hour running adds another seven hours to life. We know that group sports (that are social) reduce stress alongside encouraging fitness. We also know that walking is fantastic for us. Blue Zone residents *have to walk* in many cases; we choose to use transport or cars. Think where you could use your legs and, even better still, where you could use stairs.

Social eating is not the same as eating with your TV. Mindless snacking (that may even be emotional eating depending upon your choice of boxset!) leads to us eating more and not responding to normal cues of when we feel full. We also might simply associate TV watching and snacking as a combined reward, a habit that is quite easy to break.

Valuable take-home lessons from the Blue Zones

The sense of purpose and having a meaningful life figure high in the Blue Zones and this is one to really be assessed as we age, children leave home and we retire either from paid work or that of being a parent. Life without purpose can become insular and our social contact time can dwindle. It is not a coincidence that Okinawa has a strong social connection between women and they live longer, or that in Ikaria everyone eats together and savours it. **Mindful connections and mindful eating are imperative**. Women survive longer after disease such as breast cancer if they have social connections (see my friendship chapter).

Volunteering is good for the soul.

Close family ties can be a luxury afforded to few and you may not have a choice in this matter. If family are near, see them. Intergenerational contact benefits all ages (see chapter on the psychology of ageing).

Being able to **relax and play** are vital in all these communities. Relaxation could be introduced by bringing your book to work to read quietly at lunch if you have no company, or meditation. We know that having fun is integral to a happy life. Laughter has strong physical benefits. No prescription can override this.

CHAPTER 16: GUT HEALTH, FRUIT & VEG AND THE ORGANIC QUESTION

We know now that gut health is so integral to EVERYTHING.

We know that exposure to nature and the soil is natural and that our sterilisation of home environments and excessive use of 'antibacterial' products has an impact from a young age.

Your immunity, your happiness, your skin and your hormonal system all communicate more than previously thought with the gut.

Scientists have done extensive work on the gut microbiome. What is that exactly?

The microbiome is the collection of genome (or genetic material) from all of the microorganisms in the gastrointestinal tract.

The microbiota is the collective community of microorganisms living in the gastrointestinal tract. There are 100 trillion microorganisms in the gut. There are all different types – what we call: fungi, protozoa, helminths, viruses, along with bacteria.

The gut lining gives us protection from our food, and the organisms within it help with our immunity.

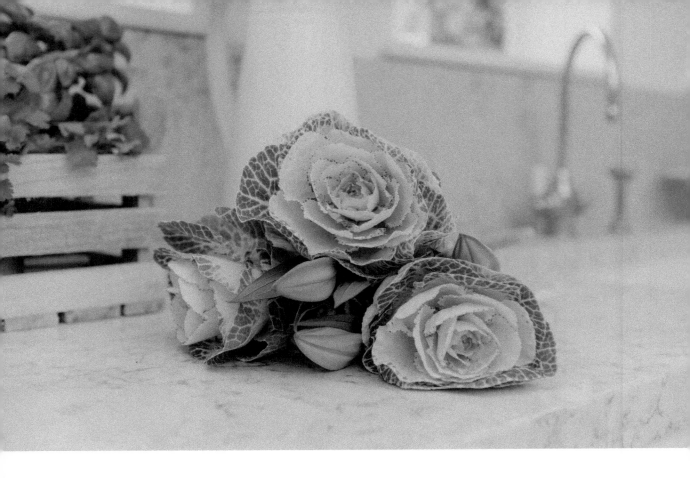

From the moment you are born you suddenly start being colonised by bacteria, and twins born at the same time will acquire different bacteria. Those first few years are integral to our health later on. This microbiome is something *you never really know, never see or feel but might be influencing your general health, mood and food choices you make.* It is this same gut microbiome that will affect how we respond to certain patterns of eating and why one diet will not work for all. Our 'bugs' control the calories we absorb and provide vital enzymes (chemicals to accelerate chemical reactions in our metabolism) and vitamins and keep our immune system healthy.

Plants like artichokes, leeks and asparagus for example are prebiotic and great for the gut. Prebiotics are simply foods containing undigestible fibre that the health bacteria in our gut thrive on.

Probiotics are the healthy bacteria and we find these in yoghurt, fermented foods like kimchi, sauerkraut, kefir and so on. Making kimchi which is full of fermented vegetables and contains pre- and probiotics is an easy way to help yourself. Kefir, which is fermented with goats' milk, has been proven successful in reducing some skin disorders such as eczema and psoriasis in some people – in our house it underwent a successful small trial against hay fever – but these are all things where you need to *read current research and find out what is best and relevant to you*. Making fermented products yourself is an inexpensive way of reinforcing your healthy microbiome; not everything has to be expensive to work. Another point of interest is that the way we clean vegetables may remove a lot of the fibre products and prebiotics. The old wives' tale that the goodness is in the skin is still relevant. Advice can be that soaking veg in water with some bicarbonate added may be better for retaining the prebiotic component and removing fungicide and pesticide – better than just scrubbing the goodness away.

Good bacteria produce chemicals that help protect our gut lining, fuelling the cells here and help many processes in the body and brain including making you happier and potentially more resilient. Potent stuff!

INTERMITTENT FASTING

This is not an eating book or diet book so I will only lightly touch on this. For years we were taught as doctors that breakfast is essential in the early moments of our day to kick-start our metabolism and that without it our body thinks we are in starvation mode, cortisol rises and we cling onto any fat we have. Thus skipping breakfast might encourage a slow metabolism and further weight gain. There is now more evidence that intermittent fasting may help *some people in losing weight*. Women and men may respond differently, as may individuals.

An important point here is that no diet is 'one size fits all'. I have women of all different body shapes explaining their struggles and successes to me at the end of my talks. Some women respond better to some strategies than others. Nutrition science is very much moving into personalised recommendations these days. I would still advocate that breakfast is essential for children and those working out of home as it is the most convenient time to eat before leaving the house and without it there may be a longer period of starvation.

Time-restricted eating – as in consuming all our calories within an eight-hour window – can stimulate something called SIRTUIN genes. The levels of sirtuin in our blood serum can be a marker of our frailty – as in if they are low the person may be more frail. There is exciting future science in these studies.

For those in whom intermittent fasting works in reducing weight gain and so on, it may be related to the circadian rhythm of their gut bacteria which themselves could benefit from periods of fasting. This is another interesting concept in future science. Intermittent fasting has some interesting effects on the brain as well. In the time without a constant supply of food and glucose the brain has to 'modify or become plastic' in the way it works and this is good for it being able to cope in slightly more adverse conditions. It encourages adaptation and can help to prevent cognitive decline, shown in some studies.

A simple rule that encourages health is not to eat in the four hours or so before bedtime as in this resting time we are not able to use the excess energy, and in theory it would follow that it would more likely be laid down as fat stores. If you were to combine this with, say, intermittent fasting in the 16/8 pattern, so eat within an eight-hour window, your breakfast might be delayed. My own trial of it simply meant that after a few days I did not wake starving for breakfast and my sleep was better as I was not stimulated by sugars nor had discomfort digesting my food after hours. Because there were less hours in the day for eating meals my snacking basically stopped and I was mindful of packing the most nutrients into my meals. I have not done enough personal research to advocate for all but there is plenty to read out there about this topic. It seems men and women may respond differently and in some women it is not so helpful for weight control anecdotally in all cases.

Basically we are not all the same and common-sense healthy choices should prevail, and not extremes.

Why snacking is not always a great idea
Read my interview with Jenna Macciochi at the end of this chapter.

What do herbs, dark chocolate, fruit, vegetables and coffee and tea have in common?
They contain polyphenols. Dietary polyphenols have many beneficial roles in the body. By their activity in the gut and on the gut microbiota they can:

- improve obesity and diabetes
- reduce blood pressure
- improve our lipid or cholesterol profile
- have anti-inflammatory properties.

And so they generally have beneficial effects on cardiometabolic disease and colonic cancers, majorly via their action on the gut microbiota. Research has shown that flavonoids (a subset of polyphenols) can help with eczema. Many herbs have been found to be beneficial – for example: black pepper, cayenne pepper, ginger, oregano, turmeric (and curcumin), etc.
Whilst it is helpful to health to reduce salt, you can see why it is great to use herbs for flavourings and whole body health. Think about what you can add to your cooking to bring it up a notch with health-boosting properties.

YOUR FRUIT AND VEGETABLES

There is a large amount of discussion about organic versus non-organic. I think you have to do your own research and come to the conclusion of what is practically and financially correct for you. It is important to focus on eating seasonally and, if that isn't enough, consider the role of frozen vegetables that may retain many more nutrients than those sitting in your fridge for a week. Get to know the local farmers and where the food comes from. Ideally of course grow your own.

We all are increasingly aware of the need to include a large amount of fruit and vegetables in our diet. Fruits and vegetables are essential components of a healthy balanced diet; they provide nutrients, vitamins, minerals and fibre. The value of complex carbohydrates such as these in our diets far exceeds any nutritional content of carbohydrates in processed food.

We need to be eating good-quality produce that contains high levels of these components and that looks appetising and is pleasing to taste. It seems that the recommendations from the government and Department of Health are related to an ideal world where five-a-day has become ten-a-day and, rather than embracing this, the general reaction was one of disbelief and then a dismissal of the whole thing. Some die-hard nutritionists could be heard saying 'Well, try to aim for more a day and see how you go'. This almost seems the logical argument.

Finance is a large part of this. The amount of fruit and vegetables to feed a family of four all fulfilling the recommended quotient would be quite large. Do bear in mind that the cost of ready meals per week is also potentially large. If we could all return to the 'good life' era where we could grow our own vegetables, then the cost of this would be reduced. We do not live in that kind of world for the most part. If you grew your own you would not be spraying pesticides and you would know the evolution of your fruit and vegetables personally from the state of seed to fruiting plant.

My grandfather made mini greenhouses for all his veg from old windows, the frames painted a glorious sparkling white. We had our own apples and so on, and various tomato/raspberry plants still make their way onto the windowsill of my parents' home. There was, at that time, no awareness of organic and non-organic produce, and we just knew that if you grew it yourself it might taste better. As time progressed and the larger supermarkets came into their own, prices would compete, and now you might find the longevity of the fruit's life will vary.

I think you have to make your own decision. I have spoken to experts who think that organic food may be unsustainable and others who think just eating fresh from local suppliers and buying regularly is the easiest solution. Others like Yvonne Wake have advised me that organic is an investment in our future health. We know that organic food can contain higher quantities of antioxidants. You will probably have already come to your own practical conclusion about what is right for you long before you picked up this book. Simply considering fresh, frozen and regular small purchases will be a good start, whether or not you are choosing organic. I will often try to buy organic and if not possible will look for fresh supplies. There are theories of certain items being more valuable as organic and some less to worry about (the concept of the dirty dozen and the clean 15 I really like, but that is for you to look up and discuss. Experts have varying opinions and different countries have different pesticide use).

Why fruit and vegetables per se?

A recent study in 2017 by the American Heart Association looked at a specific health measurement – peripheral artery disease – in other words, circulation in the body and its relationship to fruit and vegetable consumption. There is already well-documented evidence that fruit and vegetable consumption lowers your risk of coronary heart disease and stroke, but the circulation in the peripheral arteries of the body had not been looked at in so much detail. The study was done by lifestyle and medical questionnaires on a huge number of subjects (more than 30 million) and 64.1% of those studies were female. The circulation was measured at two points, as is common in measuring peripheral circulation, and the results showed that those people eating three or more servings of fruit and veg per day were 18% less likely to have peripheral artery disease.

Interestingly it was found that the subjects were more likely to eat fruit and vegetables daily if they were:

- female
- increasing age
- never smoked
- currently married
- physically active
- increased income
- frequent consumption of fish, nuts and red meat.

You may find yourself, dear reader, in some or all of these categories so I may be preaching to the converted. There are of course many more studies to be done as mentioned by the American Heart Association in their paper but it really does augment the importance of our mothers' words *to eat your fruit and vegetables*.

The American Heart Association recommends eating eight or more fruit and vegetable servings per day.

The UK NHS website has some really helpful information too on this very subject. It refers to 350 studies that were looked at in a major review (for the scientists reading, it was a systematic review and meta-analysis) that sparked the discussion about the amount of fruit and veg needed. The studies found the association with benefits in health but could not prove cause and effect by their nature.

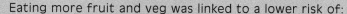

Eating more fruit and veg was linked to a lower risk of:
- Cancer
- Stroke
- Premature death
- Chronic diseases
- Total cardiovascular disease
- Heart disease

The results definitely showed that the more you increased intake, the more additive the effect on your health. The tendency, reading this, is for me to think I must eat more, and really the study has succeeded if that is our impression.

Good foods for good health

Coronary heart disease
- Apples, pears, citrus fruit, fruit juices
- Green leafy vegetables, beta-carotene like carrots or sweet potato, vitamin C rich foods

Stroke
- Apples, pears, citrus, carrots, green leafy veg, pickled vegetables

Cardiovascular
- Apples, pears, citrus, carrots, green leafy veg
- Butternut

Total cancer
- Cauliflower, broccoli

All cause death
- Apples, pears, berries, citrus, cooked or raw vegetables, potatoes, green leafy veg, salads

So, my general impression is that the old adage of 'an apple a day keeps the doctor away' has more and more truth to it now. There is research that stewed apples are especially good as rich in soluble fibre and increase the level of good bacteria.

245

Of course, the information gained, you could argue, can have other factors at play – those who eat more fruit and veg may be more likely to exercise, drink less alcohol, not smoke and so on.

In conclusion, everything in life is about balance and moderation and we tend to realise quite rapidly what makes us feel and look better. A little amount of effort and planning can mean that the hurdles to change to healthier eating disappear, and our bodies will thank us in return.

Cook fresh, and savour food, with sensible portion sizes and defined mealtimes within the day.

I am really privileged to have interviewed a real expert in the science of our gut health, amongst a myriad of topics – the immunologist Dr Jenna Macciochi.

DR JENNA MACCIOCHI

www.drjennamacciochi.com
PhD Imperial College, Immunologist and Lecturer at the University of Sussex.
Author of 'Immunity: The Science of Staying Well' released 2020.

"My research looks at nutrition and lifestyle in shaping our immunity. I also write for media and consult for brands. I grew up on a farm in rural Scotland and we lived pretty much farm to table. My mother was a professional cook, so I quickly learned the kitchen basics and a love for cooking. After having my twins in Zurich prematurely and them being placed in NICU, I totally lost my confidence and never thought I would work in my profession again. I joined a local postnatal fitness group and this became a beacon of hope, helping me through the postnatal fog. The instructor suggested I become a personal trainer. I qualified and worked in the fitness industry until we decided to move back to the UK."

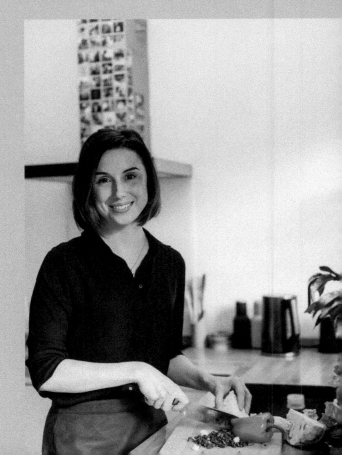

Main female role models?

My mother. She entered a close-knit rural farming community marrying my dad. She also continued to work in catering. She taught me the basics of cooking and my dad taught me the basics of growing and caring for plants. When my dad was diagnosed with cancer Mum threw herself into supporting his health with diet and lifestyle. Mum also inspired me with her interest in beauty.

My PhD mentor Professor Clare Lloyd at Imperial College is probably my biggest inspiration. She and her colleagues were extremely proactive in making changes in academia to support women in science.

What exercise do you do?

I cycle to and from work, five miles each way. This is like a 'moving meditation'. Calisthenics twice a week and Reformer Pilates weekly. Occasionally I join a circuits class in a local studio and I do weights at home.

What is the immune system?

It is not, in fact, one thing, and it's not in one place; it's a whole galaxy of cells and molecules incorporating multiple cells (known as white blood cells or leukocytes), organs (such as lymph nodes, bone marrow and spleen), molecules (called cytokines) and their collective array of biological functions. Your body's borders act as the first line of defence. Skin presents a physical barrier. The mucus membranes that line your natural openings, e.g. mouth, nose and vagina, make and release substances that create a hostile environment for or attack and destroy invaders. These physical barriers are as delicate as they are protective. To understand the immune system is to liken it to a castle. A fortress with many layers of defence, from skin to first-line warriors to special forces, all working as a team. Your microbiota, the collection of bacteria and other germs that live on us and in us, are part of this.

Immunity is far more than fending off coughs and colds. Its protecting every inch of our body *all the time*. And we don't even notice it. It works with our metabolism to detect what we have eaten. It heals us when we damage something. It's even our main cancer surveillance system. Our immune system recognises challenges from our environment and signals from our emotions. In fact, scientists have started to consider it a kind of second brain – a specialised network of bio-sensors designed to pick up information from within and around the body and relay that information to the brain, where it can motivate us and manipulate us to behave in specific ways. We now know there is an intimate link between our immunity and mental health. It is not often that one body system touches so many aspects of human biology in both sickness and health.

But there is a lot that can go wrong, from autoimmune disease and allergy, to mental health problems and metabolic issues – even cancer. Immunity underscores our health. For women it's important to know that our unique hormonal situation means we have quite a different immune set-up from men. Science has proven that man flu is real! Men do indeed have a weaker immune system but our feisty immunity means we are more likely to get autoimmune diseases; 80% of autoimmunity is in women.

What are the main lifestyle elements that support a woman's immune system?

Accept that it's normal to get a few colds each year. There is no way to boost your immune system singularly. Washing your hands and steering clear of infected people is your best bet. We all must get **sleep** sorted. Amazing things happen to your immune system while asleep. Second, **stress**. Women are more likely to be working and still doing the lion's share of housework and childcare. Stress in the short-term sense of running for your life is helpful but constant stress erodes our delicate defences.

A lot of our immune system is formed from day zero, at birth, and we know a lot of research is coming forward about our gut microbiome developing as our gut gets colonised in our first days and years at an astonishing rate. If someone is, say, 55, is there anything that is reversible about this? Is it too late?

Really interesting question and one that I cover in my book. Much of our immunity is built in the first five years of life as we become colonised with microbiota. First from our mother, which is why vaginal birth seems to be better for health (no judgement, my preemie twins were C-section which saved their lives). Next is breast milk which is a creamy bacterial soup that really starts to seed our guts with the right bugs. Breastmilk also contains special fibres that feed the right gut bugs and this just hasn't been recreated in formula.

But it's never too late to start. Take care of your gut health with a diet full of diverse plant fibres (we should aim to eat 30+ different fruits and veggies per week. If you are not eating a lot of fibre, then you may need to build up slowly). Probiotics may help, especially if you have had a lot of antibiotics. Otherwise with diet, protein is really important as we age and I'd recommend an omega-3 supplement and check your vitamin D levels regularly. Get yourself in a strong sleep schedule, waking and sleeping at the same times every day for your circadian rhythm. Take care of your stress and start doing regular physical activity.

What proportion of our immunity is down to the genetics we are handed and what is due to our environment? (This may motivate some women to change.)

Genes are important but environment matters more. Our environment and behaviours can manipulate our genes by turning them on and off – this is called epigenetics. Nurture is a much bigger part than nature. The metaphor used by scientists is: 'Your genes load the gun, but environment pulls the trigger'. A little immunity TLC from time to time can, for most people, keep all components functioning more smoothly. Immunity is not fixed but continuously nurtured by our encounters and adventures. It is shaped by our changing emotions and surroundings, responding to how we live our lives. Our immunity even has the capacity to learn and develop a memory. Collectively this plethora of influences determines at any given point if we get sick and for how long. The human 'exposome' is the exposure equivalent of the human genome. The exposome represents a concept that incorporates the complex exposures we face and subject our biology to throughout our lives, including infection, our diet, lifestyle factors and social influences. It also incorporates how our bodies respond to these challenges.

Much of what I have written about in my book is designed to 'reduce inflammation' within the body. What are the results of chronic inflammation in our body? Do we really lessen our odds of cancer by protecting our immune system or is it just bad luck if we develop it?

Yes, and no. On the one hand the best way to avoid chronic inflammation is to not over eat. Overconsuming food is proinflammatory; even the act of eating is mildly proinflammatory. Stop snacking because all the marketing messages tell you to. Even if it's 'healthy' food. The other triggers of chronic inflammation are vast and many: smoking, elevated blood sugar or blood lipids, stress, lack of sleep, many over-the-counter medications and prescription medications, carrying too much body fat. Chronic inflammation causes damage to our delicate tissues all over the body. But it is slow and insidious, and we may not notice the effects until decades down the line. We now know that inflammation, above telomeres (see genetics chapter), is the main driver of ageing.

Cancer is a wide range of diseases with a common characteristic: something goes wrong in the way the cells regulate growth, and this results in uncontrolled cell growth. This happens deep in the cell's genetic material. Cancer is somewhat a matter of odds – an unfortunate by-product of the way evolution works. While there is much evidence that exercise and healthy living can reduce the risk of certain cancers, reducing is not preventing. You cannot remove all risk. Lifestyle can have a huge influence on the risk of cancer overall. And of course because our immune system is also the main cancer surveillance system, it's important to take care of our immunity from that perspective too. Not all cancers have known lifestyle components although some do. Even with the perfect diet and lifestyle you are still at risk of getting cancer.

Much of the evidence for longevity not only comes from the quality content of food, but also the social nature of enjoying it. Is any of this linked to the immune system?

Yes, I like to talk about the food prison: the way we imprison ourselves in a restrictive way of eating because we feel it is clean or virtuous. But really we feel miserable, cut off from social connection because our perfect diet is incompatible. Those feelings can actually stress our immunity, and reduced endorphins from enjoying food can impair our immune system.

'Leaky gut' is a very current buzzword and used as something to define illness almost! Can you explain why our gut leaks and why some of it is helpful to our bodies?

For digestion purposes, humans have developed a very complicated and highly specialised digestive system. Our digestive tract is delicate, a fragile barrier that is just one cell thick. This is where gut health comes in. Your gut works hard to absorb nutrients whilst keeping out undigested food, bacteria and potentially harmful things we might end up swallowing. Most of the time, this gut barrier remains intact, with tight junctions separating the gut contents from the rest of the body. Our microbiota rest atop the gut's mucus layer at a safe distance from the intestinal wall. Any bacteria that wind up too close get wiped out by our own potent antimicrobial poisons, while our immune cells *lining up along the gut* also play an important role in keeping our microbiome in peaceful coexistence with us by making sure they stay on the right side of this delicate border. On the other hand, this barrier must be at times open to enable absorption of essential fluids and nutrients from our foods. This is normal, this is leaky gut. It happens every time we eat, to a certain degree (hence why snacking all the time is probably not a good idea). Bits of bacteria and food from our gut enter the blood causing a transient inflammation. Our immune cells all over the body are presented with bits of food and bacteria, which have potential as triggering danger signals. Now, let's be clear: leaky gut is a normal physiological phenomenon. In most people it's not an issue. Our gut barrier integrity fluctuates throughout the day depending on what we do and what we eat. Meals heavy in saturated fat or fructose and poor in fibre exacerbate the whole process. **The newest studies show that the bacteria in your gut microbiome play an enormous role as gatekeepers of leaky gut.** Balanced and well-fed healthy microbiota reinforce the integrity of the gut, protecting the sanctity of the body. We now know that fibre is the key to controlling our gut barrier, minimising the damage caused through the act of eating itself. This is because short-chain fatty acids (e.g. butyrate) ensure the firewall can work properly. When your gut microbes don't produce enough butyrate, you might experience symptoms attributed to leaky gut. When we eat a fibre-deficient diet our gut microbes starve, which impairs this peaceful relationship. Eating a very large meal or a meal heavy in excessive fat (particularly saturated fat) or fructose (fruit sugar, in the absence of adequate fibre) is a known factor. Hyperglycaemia – prolonged high blood sugar – found in poorly controlled diabetes and high cholesterol can also compromise the gut barrier. Specific nutrient deficiencies include vitamin A, D and zinc which are super important for the gut barrier.

Thank you so much, Jenna.

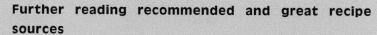

Further reading recommended and great recipe sources

www.bbcgoodfood.com, www.allrecipes.com

Joe Wicks book series

The Midlife Kitchen by Mimi Spencer and Sam Rice

Va Va Voom by Jackie Lynch

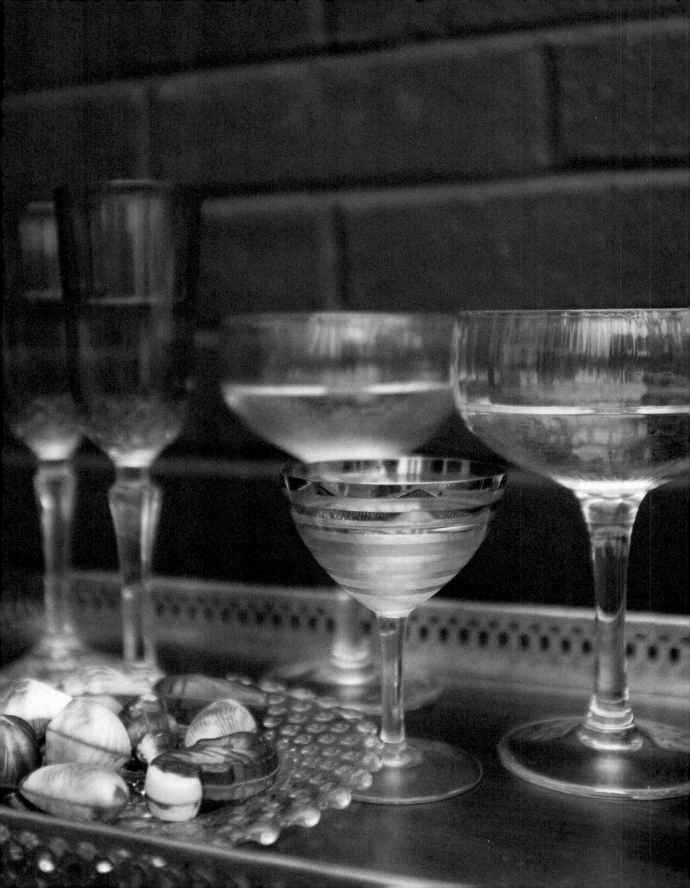

CHAPTER 17: ALCOHOL AND THE FEMALE FORM

Sitting down with a glass of wine at the end of the day has become a socially acceptable pastime and most women tend to look to their friends for acceptance of behaviours. You may see that sentence as either threatening, true, or you may be disparaging of the army of middle-aged wine drinkers.

My own opinion is that your decision on this should be a personal one and not 'shoved down your throat' by someone else. I love a drink with my friends and family. I love a party but find at this stage of my life, if I do not drink for weeks, I feel brighter, sharper, better. If you are drinking throughout the week have a look at the pattern of what you do and whether it is really just now 'habitual'.

There is great value in socialisation around drink and we cannot discount it. There is a balance to be had. There is great joy in enjoying your favourite drink. Conversely, we are often seen as 'not being fun' if we don't imbibe. You obviously can have total fun without alcohol.

Many women I interviewed were keen on the winding down effect of wine at the end of the day – often daily – but not keen on the widening effect on their waistlines.

The imperative value of a 'girls' night out' with or without alcohol is incredible support for women who feel they may be struggling alone.

ARE YOU AT THE BOTTOM OF YOUR LIST?

If women are drinking above the weekly allowance (currently 14 units a week for women) the alcohol will be having quite an effect. Often just the slow drip of a daily regular intake is enough to have a strong overall effect on the body. Although numbing the anxiety and relaxing you at the end of the day it will ironically be causing more anxiety and depression the next day and dumbing down your reaction to life.

ALCOHOL AND ITS BENEFITS

There is a well-known protective effect of alcohol against ischaemic heart disease (IHD). In men the risk of IHD can be lowered if a man drinks seven units of alcohol per week allegedly. However, if the units consumed climb, then any advantage will be outweighed by unwanted effects on health. There is a lot of debate over studies that are often themselves linked to the alcohol industry.

However, chronically increasing your intake makes the risk of some other nasties rises significantly:

- Accidents
- Strokes
- Liver disease

After smoking the risk of cancer from alcohol is a major player. Heavy drinking increases the risk of brain haemorrhage and so on.

A doctor's assessment of your alcohol intake can highlight problems, but having been a doctor I was aware that some people would think of a number when calculating their drinking history and then maybe halve it!

Work out how many units of alcohol you, on average, drink in a week.

https://www.drinkaware.co.uk/understand-your-drinking/unit-calculator

After working out how many units of alcohol you consume you can look at the facts. In the UK extensive work between 2013 and 2016 led to the Chief Medical Officer revising guidelines for safe drinking in those who choose to drink.

Weekly drinking guidelines apply to adults who drink regularly or frequently, i.e. most weeks. The Chief Medical Officer's guidelines for both men and women are:

- To keep health risks from alcohol to a low level it is safest not to drink more than 14 units a week on a regular basis.
- If you regularly drink as much as 14 units per week, it is best to spread your drinking evenly over three or more days. If you have one or two heavy drinking episodes a week, you increase your risk of death from long-term illness and from accidents and injuries.
- The risk of developing a range of health problems (including cancers of the mouth, throat and breast) increases the more you drink on a regular basis.
- If you wish to cut down the amount you drink, a good way to help achieve this is to have several drink-free days each week.

The newest research altered some opinions further and importantly for women, the following:

- That the net benefits from small amounts of alcohol are less than previously thought.
- That drinking alcohol increases the risk of developing a range of cancers. The Committee on Carcinogenicity recently concluded that 'drinking alcohol increased the risk of getting cancers of the mouth and throat, voice box, gullet, large bowel, liver, of breast cancer in women and probably also cancer of the pancreas'. These risks start from any level of regular drinking and then rise with the amounts of alcohol being drunk. This was not fully understood when the last guidelines were drawn up in 1995.

We also know that the calories from alcohol may replace calories that would be taken from nutritious food. Vitamins, especially B vitamins and minerals, may be less than brilliant in more serious drinkers and **not having a great balance of these may make your menopause more arduous. I found some historic papers relating some mineral deficiencies to worse symptoms of hot flushes and so on – something that there still needs to be more research on, this just emphasises the importance of a good diet at this time.**

If your liver is busy metabolising alcohol it stands to reason it will be less efficient at dealing with other processes in the body – dealing with nutrients and hormones and so on.

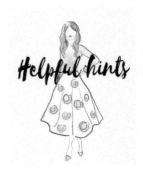

Benefits of reducing alcohol:

Reduced sugar cravings as blood sugar stabilises

Reduced calorie intake from alcoholic drinks so possible weight loss

Reduced cravings for processed foods

Increased control of emotions

Quality of sleep improves – more rejuvenating sleep

Skin may look brighter, less congested, less broken blood vessels appearing, reduced symptoms of rosacea (there are obviously many other causes of rosacea)

Improved libido

Helpful hints

There are of course blood tests that can be done to attain some hold on whether you are doing damage to your body, but often the regular drinker can function quite successfully as they have developed tolerance. **Also, a clean set of blood tests is meaningless if you know in your heart your drinking is affecting too many aspects of your life.** I was always careful to not reassure patients too enthusiastically if their liver blood tests were returned from the lab normal – the body has a way of compensating and managing intake for so long and then the equilibrium can *suddenly flip* and the liver won't cope anymore with no apparent warning. I have friends who are functioning alcoholics and other than their high alcohol intake there are no outward signs of any problems. It is only when you scratch the surface that problems with anxiety and weight issues and so on are discussed, which may of course be alleviated by reducing the number of glasses of wine. Not to mention how it may exacerbate all the symptoms of your menopause and become a risk factor for breast cancer in this age group.

Look at what happens with wine, when the drinking becomes excessive:

You have a drink.

Have a small drink and your liver metabolises it to water and carbon dioxide, which you pee and breathe out. Your body hangs on to the antioxidants in the wine and the carbs from beer. You metabolise the alcohol and it produces fatty acids. These are stored as triglycerides (fats in the liver) until they can be used.

Have a few more drinks and a spate of bingeing.

The triglycerides that the liver is hanging onto are building up. The liver can't cope with them all.

Those triglycerides cause inflammation, liver cells die, scar tissue develops and cirrhosis may occur.

Add in to the mix some unhealthy eating simultaneously with a load of processed red meat, refined carbs (Christmas dinner anyone? ;-)) and some fat and you might end up with non-alcoholic fatty disease. You can't see this until it's too late.

It is reversible until it gets to the cirrhosis point – give up for a month, like dry January, and those fat stores and the inflammation in your liver can reduce. Reducing your body fat by 5% could reduce your liver fat by 30%. It is all this unseen fat along with visceral fat that means the *slimmest person in the room is not always the healthiest.*

If you have read all of this and feel somewhat motivated to reduce your drinking or even stop altogether a few tips may help you. The last thing I want is to be patronising and prescriptive. I am not teetotal, I just want women to be mindful of their drinking and their motivation for it.

Anyone for a habitual Pinot?

This unbelievably is not supposed to be a patronising statement. If you see a drink as a reward at the end of every day **do you limit it to one**? In many of my patients/friends this would creep up to half then a full bottle, and they are soon cascading into multiples of the recommended weekly intake for women.

CAN YOU SET YOURSELF RULES?

My rules to my patients were at least **three days off in the week** to allow liver recovery and so on – ideally four or five. *Can you* just have one drink? Can you change the drink to low alcohol? If you can't then have more days completely drink free. See the benefits in your clarity, waistline and bank balance if your habit was previously strong.

Having a healthier drink as an alternative, like sparkling water (sparkling water can make reflux worse but I couldn't find enough evidence for it affecting bones like other fizzy drinks – all in moderation), elderflower cordial, diluted iced juice and so on, can 'as kindergarten-like as it sounds' break that routine of pouring yourself a drink once the kids are in bed or your partner is home. Pour it into a special glass with ice to clink. We are very much creatures of habit and our minds constantly associate different actions together. Just like smoking often goes along with having a drink, having a moment of rest and peace may be associated with popping a cork.

I will leave you with one thought. Can you easily not drink for the next two weeks? If you think you cannot, then ask yourself: why?

If you can, then do it, and tell me how you feel after!

Resources
Alcoholics Anonymous, NACOA (National Association for Children of Alcoholics), SMART recovery
www.drinkaware.co.uk,   https://www.nhs.uk/live-well/alcohol-support/, www.alcoholchange.org.uk

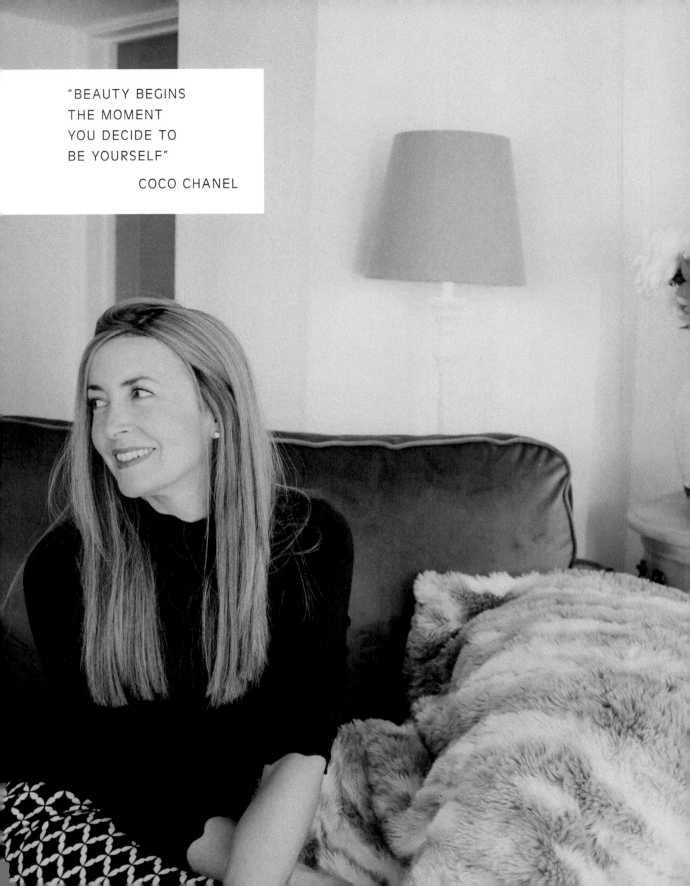

"BEAUTY BEGINS
THE MOMENT
YOU DECIDE TO
BE YOURSELF"

COCO CHANEL

CHAPTER 18: PSYCHOLOGY OF FASHION, BODY IMAGE AND THE FEMALE STATE

I have voiced on social media for a long time my opinions about pressure on girls (and boys) these days, which translates into strain on women as they pass through midlife and beyond, forever increasing in a world that salutes appearance and form above depth and intrigue.

SHE IS SUCH A PRETTY GIRL

As children, girls are often led to understand that appearance is to be prized and is a means of gaining approval. Many of the women I spoke to could clearly remember being praised for appearance by their elders, and equally as many recall the lack of emphasis on appearance and looks. Some saw this as rejection, some not. The latter group did then definitely grow to be more confident adults. If there was an emphasis on sports, fitness, outdoor sports, riding and so on, then body image seemed far healthier – that was my anecdotal impression. If this 'appearance-related praise' is a driving force in younger life, then we in turn act in ways to reinforce this as we get older and we seek approval and self-validation by 'improving' or 'optimising' our outward appearance. I will not dispute that I would give my parents a fashion show whether it was a new hand-me-down from my cousin or a birthday present dress – was this love of fashion or seeking approval? As young as the age of two there is also an ability to see possessions as **part of us**, to enhance us, and this is where clothes could come in.

As we go through puberty the effect on our body image strikes a different chord between boys and girls. Boys actually reach nearer to the 'masculine muscle ideal' as pubertal changes *increase muscle*. In many developed countries the ideals for women are still sadly associated with 'skinniness' and thus young girls *when gaining size around breasts and hips* are naturally moving further from what is seen as 'the ideal'. If we contrast this to the times of the 1950s and Marilyn Monroe we see a large unfortunate shift. Indeed, what proportion of real women will actually fit into the silhouette of what we see as ideal slimness today? Naomi Wolf wrote in 1991 in her book *The Beauty Myth* that only one in 40,000 women fit the actual ideal body shape required to be a model. If it is actually almost impossible to attain, then we are on the back foot from the start with no end of diets or exercise allowing us to reach that subjective goal. There is a changing movement of embracing curves but this has a long way to go to filter down, and of course much of this is augmented by surgery. Femininity will always be associated with beauty and not just brains. Social media influence surrounds us with the 'ideal model type'; 'perfection' is reinforced even if the airbrushing is on someone's phone app or with selfies taken at a jaunty angle.

We are programmed how to see and judge beauty

Sadly, from a young age, being overweight or not fitting societal norms of facial appearance has negative associations in our society, and the goodies and baddies in fairy tales are depicted very differently in terms of size and objective beauty. Watching even computer-generated cartoon films now in Ultra HD brings this home just as vividly as when we read those same fairy tales as children from books. Rarely is the heroine anything other than beautiful and the enemy 'unattractive'. Just take a moment and think of this. This calls into question much debate around our attitudes to facial or other disfigurement and totally stereotyped impressions deduced from appearance. There is much work to be done with embracing acceptance. Social media is of course perpetuating the 'beauty is queen' ideal, but then what is beautiful to you? We know children respond to 'beauty' but how much is from what they have *learned*?

Be you, your beautiful self

I want you to start thinking of *beauty as health* and, by maintaining and improving your overall health, you are achieving beauty which will be smiling back at you in the mirror. I actually started this book with the working title of 'Beauty Inside Out' but then saw how this could be misinterpreted. I was not writing about symmetrical textbook beauty. The antithesis of this self-acceptance to me would be the young girls visiting their cosmetologist with an image of a star that they wish to copy in terms of features, filler and facial profile – the 'face off the peg' model. How desperately sad that in seeking beauty they are seeking the image of another, *not the one they were born with*. At extremes the facial features of the young become one bland canvas, all similarly tweaked, possibly extreme in real-life encounters but judged as the norm on social media images. Again, though, we all want to fit in.

If you have something done, do it for you

I am NOT, as you might have misinterpreted, slating the plastics and injectables industry. Far from it. I think there is a good time and place for mature women to do what they want in a safe environment to make them feel good. Who knows, I might be writing a book in ten years about the safety of interventional treatments! If you have been distressed about something all your life and you **do something about it**, there are great gains psychologically. I have close friends whose lives and self-esteem have been revolutionised by a single procedure. A boob job can be transformative with a great surgeon. Botox for that number 11 frown you hate might get you smiling again. **As long as** one has prior accurate assessment by a qualified reputed medical or surgical **clinician** and full psychological support so that the outcome is good *for you personally*. You need to be understanding of the procedure and the risks and make sure the clinician is on the correct register and ideally recommended to you or you have seen examples of their work. Do they listen to you and your needs? This will be as true at 20 as it is at 50. Do the young of today always have this true motivation for interventional surgery or do they just want to belong to the manufactured group? The growing rise of poor management of those with body dysmorphic disorder is a real problem, and our preoccupation with that 'first impression or Insta-pression' will only exaggerate this.

The effect on teenagers and eating disorders

As puberty hits, awareness and hormonal changes coincide and boys and girls can become extremely vulnerable to negative thinking. Risks of eating disorders in girls (and sometimes boys) increase at this time. Social media is coming in between the ages of 10 and 15, when girls are most vulnerable to outside influence, and this will change the way they cement their self-esteem and self-image if uncensored. We know how formative these years are – every woman I interviewed could remember clearly her idols as a teen, whether it was Kylie Minogue, Twiggy or Margaret Thatcher. We cannot blame all of the poor body image on social media. I knew two girls growing up whose lives with anorexia and bulimia started with one hurtful comment from a school 'friend'. One of those victims was in my family and has suffered a lifetime of turmoil since. We ALL need to be super aware of language we use around children of both sexes as they grow from a young age. Many of my interviewees recall with great clarity the detail of their mother's diets, and they then either repeated this pattern or swung the other way so as not to comply. Everyone thinks their family is normal. Talking about 'feeling fat', 'clothes not fitting', 'going without food', 'losing weight' is common language at the water cooler in the office but not so great when overheard by your seven-year-old. **Food needs to be seen as nourishment, life-giving, not associated with the words 'deprivation' or 'reward'.**

I shall now step down from my soapbox as we need to practise what we preach and embrace the power of food to enrich our lives, and our children will learn that from us seamlessly by example.

NOW TO US OVER-40S

Why not represent us at our age accurately, and also the variation in women's sizes as you will see on the street? The value of the anti-ageing market is huge worldwide. We know that women respond better to marketing with real images.

Should we be fighting this ageing?

Because of our vulnerability and the negative connotations of ageing we are sitting ducks to the 'advertising world', and there is immense power in this industry to play on our vulnerabilities to make us want to delay ageing. *My approach would be: please, please give us the products, advertise them with integrity, on real-age women, but drop the nomenclature and give us some positive words: vibrance, health, vigour – cream to make me look like me* only better*!*

So where does the quickest method of transformation and manipulation of image come in alongside makeup?

The life-changing power of clothes

We all wear them, and the concept of fashion and being in line with current trends is a great psychological debate in itself. Who decides what is fashionable? Why do some decide to follow, and how do some set the trend? Since being a young girl I was fascinated by the potency of an item of clothing to elicit joy and change my mood. I was also frustrated by the desire and hankering after clothes I simply could not afford.

You may be in the indifferent camp. We all have to wear clothes for the sake of common decency, and thermoregulation, but can a woman who has never paid attention transform how others see her, more importantly how she sees herself, with a new interest in sartorial elegance? We have all seen makeover programmes where the poor unsuspecting victim is photographed make-up free in sweatshirt and tracksuit bottoms and then is revealed *dizzyingly glamorous* in teetering heels and a fitted dress. Is this frivolous and superficial? I really think not and I don't think the power of looking at ourselves in a new light regardless of our 'chronological' age is worth dismissing.

We culturally value appearance, so clothes are an integral part of that. For fashion, social media is highest on the list of influence at this time and is being manipulated by brands to maximally exploit this. It is powerful stuff. 'Click-throughs' to purchase sites set up by the savvy influencer are lucratively feeding into our obsession with 'wanting that new look yesterday'. If we are constantly looking at accounts of people we see as 'better than us' it can be really demoralising. It is such a true but abhorrent concept. My advice: if comparison is the thief of joy in your life and some accounts make your heart sink with envy and despair, then *mute them on your account or unfollow* and they won't be influencing your day with a deflated sigh.

Seven seconds to a first impression

Clothing and appearance are closely interlinked. We all know that inevitably we assess someone generally in the first seven seconds of seeing them, we ourselves have to be quick to make a first impression. We often imagine how others see us – a kind of external eye – and we think we are being judged – you may remember feeling this as a child. I remember excruciating pain looking back on how a bully saw me at school because I did not have the expansive wardrobe of clothes that her mother bribed her with. Fast forward to adulthood and we can still experience self-doubt in a group of women when you get the sideways glance up and down. We often interpret it as derogatory, but is it? It could be curiosity, admiration or simple comparison, it *may not* be negative, but we often default to that assumption. Girls compete, women empower. If only always.

Love a girl in uniform

Uniform can be very levelling and take away the stress of fitting in and conforming.

For more than two years at work I was in 'scrubs' or 'greens', and to some extent *loved the neutral nature of this and the fact that one didn't have to decide what to wear.* I remember one esteemed consultant teaching me and commenting on the array of bracelets up my arm. There was little else one could do to personalise the green pyjamas other than maybe a dash of lipstick. This was my stamp of personalisation.

Aside from how we see ourselves or think others see us, what do we feel in our clothes? Clothes may serve a purpose – be suitable for us to perform a function like gardening, doctoring, travelling. The way you dress will be influenced by the phase you are in in your life. There has to be a practical element. In my GP years the order of the day was smart, neutral clothes. Then I was at home starting to write a novel, living on a building site as we renovated our house. I admit I sunk into the 'school-run mum' bracket. I don't mean that in a derogatory way. The school run can be a jaw-dropping fashion parade – yikes! Somehow I always wanted to look like I had not made too much effort but still wanted to look good. Go figure!

The power of your clothes

On a serious note you *can feel different* and more engaged depending upon what you wear. The phrase 'dress up and show up' can also work for us at-home workers! You may actually feel more efficient and clever in corporate gear rather than those slouchy pyjamas. You may even perform better. (I am sitting at my desk as I write in a pinstripe suit, and if you believe that then start questioning your faith in everything you read!). Similarly, if you go to the doctors' you don't expect the GP to be in cut-off jean shorts, sliders and a cropped top... just sayin'.

I wanna be in your gang

You may remember the feeling from childhood of wanting to belong. We want to belong to a group, we want to be *similar*. Add in to this, though, that we want to actually differentiate ourselves within this group and stand out in some way. *This was always me when I was young.* I remember, later on at med school, discos with some crazy psychedelic print black and white jeans – what was I thinking*? I wanted to be different but similar.*

The mean girls' ethos of belonging and looking down on others can be diluted and filtered into other groups in life. We do tend to gravitate to those with similar ideals and tastes, it is human nature. We hunt in packs. On your social media you may have a large girl gang devoted to your fashion choices. How wonderful is that... or is it a pressure, and is it conformation in the most dislikeable manner – which way do you feel?

Fashion is immediate identity, stated clearly in our dress. We need real women reflected in modelling, but they are vastly underrepresented in terms of race and size and disability.

Let's get chemical, chemical

Dopamine on our brains rules most things we do: how we eat, shop, have sex, seek out pleasure and so on. Shopping for clothes is a complex beast with this. Sometimes the anticipation of a purchase of clothing or accessory is as great as the purchase itself. It drops rapidly after, maybe linked to guilt, and then reinforces the need for a repeat dopamine buzz; the fact that this chemical could persuade you to part with hundreds of pounds for one handbag has to be considered. Are we for real? On the other side that bag may give pleasure and quality for years and years to come and look the right type of smart that we want, so no judging...

Fashion and the female form still deserve applause (aka, shake that booty)

No doubt, just as when we were young girls, many of us want to wear clothes that present us in the best light – a flattering fit, maybe a heel to enhance the silhouette. I would just regard this as the fun and drama of fashion and hope no one takes this away from me. Fashion week in any city and the excitement of runway shows are the epitome of this. As I interviewed Maria Grachvogel in her atelier, I marvelled at the drape and cut of the beautiful separates majestically displayed around the room. Fashion is marvellous, miraculous, majestic and most exciting. What you do with it is entirely up to you, and ain't that just the best?!

I need that bag

New designs and images in fashion can stimulate the brain and that pesky dopamine drive. That watermelon design handbag edged in glitter catching my daughter's eye last summer in a fast fashion shop was the same as any adult fashionista let loose in the shoe room of Harrods. I know because I interviewed a couple of wondrous people there and deliberately arrived early so I could just soak in the glittering atmosphere. The novelty of the new can make dopamine sky high and this fuels the ever-changing world of fashion. My experience of decluttering with a stylist was emotionally charged. Like many women I tend to develop emotional attachments to clothes. I might remember that 'my mother gave me that' or 'a friend and I bought one together' and then I keep them for nostalgia purposes long after their wearing days are over. This *can* be exciting when fashions come full cycle and items can be regenerated and recycled.

Impulse buyers make quick purchases to fill a hole in their life, create an image they are trying to obtain or elevate themselves socially. Whilst reading Professor Carolyn Mair's book, *The Psychology of Fashion*, I came across a formalisation of this state. If your repeat buying becomes detrimental (debt, lack care in other areas of life) it can become **chronic buying disorder**... Anyone? I thought so. I believe this must be perpetuated by bargain cheap clothing, and then ethical questions about production come into play. The guilt and remorse can release dopamine again and lead to more buying behaviour. Taking clothes back reduces the economic strain but may perpetuate the whole cycle on repeat. It may be linked with other mood disorders or erratic eating.

That dress, what price?

Add in to the mix the political and moral dilemmas of clothes manufacture and there is more to our quick buying fix than meets the eye. Environmental damage from manufacturing methods and inhumane labour adds up to *not such a pretty dress* on the disposable sale rail. Ignorance is bliss and has been for so many years but now consumers are questioning their own morality in supporting the industry; just like palm oil in our diets we have to set our own moral compass and decide what is acceptable to us. If you have a plethora of unwanted clothes you have to take steps to change a repetition of behaviour.

Let us pause here and hear from Carolyn, who is a world expert on the psychology of fashion.

PROFESSOR CAROLYN MAIR

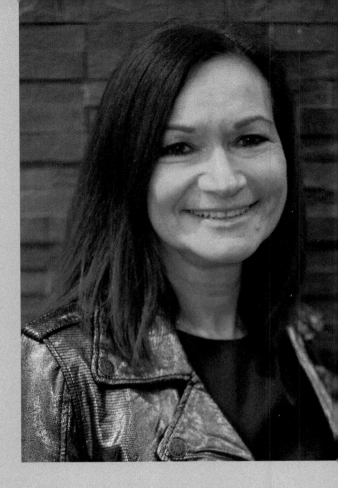

https://psychology.fashion/
Twitter @Carolyn_UK
Instagram @psychologyforfashion

Carolyn is an award-holding freelance consultant specialising in the psychology of fashion. She works with educators, global clothing brands and media outlets. Her extensive career history includes:

- *Bachelors in Psychology and Computing*
- *Master's degree in Research Methods in Psychology*
- *PhD in Cognitive Neuroscience*

Until 2017, Carolyn was Professor of Psychology for Fashion at London College of Fashion where she established the Psychology Department and pioneered the first-ever degree programmes to apply psychology in the context of fashion. Prior to this she was Professor for Applied Cognitive Psychology at Southampton Solent University. In her early careers she was a graphic designer and teacher of English as a foreign language. When her children were small, alongside being a homemaker she worked as a novelty cake maker, soft furnishing designer, portrait artist, mural painter and dressmaker! Carolyn's mother was a great role model in terms of resilience and strength growing up, and the younger Carolyn loved the style of Twiggy, Maudie James, Julie Christie and Faye Dunaway.

Do you think there is a more negative influence on teenage girls these days with regards to body image and self-esteem?

Definitely, I feel very strongly about these issues with body shape and self-esteem. Fashion imagery is around us 24/7 now; it used to just be in magazines and on a billboard years ago and that was enough.

What do you think can be done to emphasise positive body image through the 20s and 30s for women particularly?

We need to feel beautiful in ourselves. We need to realise earlier on that not everyone is going to be considered physically beautiful to everyone, but we can all be beautiful beings. We can learn to appreciate what we can do and what we can contribute. Our bodies are more than objects to be gazed at; we feel better about ourselves when we appreciate what our bodies, and minds for that matter, enable us to do. Beauty should be considered an aspect of our self; you can be beautiful in different ways.

Have you seen fashion being used to heal? Can you give me any examples (e.g. I am aware of the Look Fabulous Forever UK campaign)?

The 'Dress for Success' campaign in the USA and 'Suited and Booted' in the UK, helping people dress for an interview so they can return to the workforce. This can help them feel confident that they can do the job, because they're dressed appropriately. It also can boost their confidence and self-esteem.

What do you think a mature woman in her 50s, 60s, 70s or 80s should feel and gain from her clothes in an ideal world?

I totally dislike rules over 40, 50 and so on. These 'milestones' are arbitrary. On holiday I will show my legs and arms more. I think a woman needs to be dressed so that it *contributes to what she is doing*. She needs to feel comfortable. As we get older we care less, which is probably just as well as we have far less choice.

Discuss the abhorrent phrase 'She dresses too young for her age'! I hate that! What is too young for your age?

Beauty is inside and out, irrelevant of age. The way you behave, your mannerisms, and you can have modernity in the way you are in life and your engagement. What we wear is up to us, but we need to be aware that it says something about us which might not be what we want or expect.

Care of appearance can be linked in medicine with mood – anhedonia. A lack of interest in anything can be strongly linked with depression. Do you think colour is important for mood with clothes? Do you think dressing generally can influence mood?

Have you read the study where men and women are dressed in red T-shirts and the photographs shown to observers and they are asked to rate their attractiveness? The people wearing red T-shirts are rated as more attractive, but then the photos are changed to monochrome and the rating is the same. The researchers concluded that wearing the red T-shirts made the subjects FEEL more attractive and that is what they radiated in the photographs! There is really no 'psychology of colour'. Colour is a property of light hitting an object and being absorbed or refracted. How we perceive colour depends on what it's next to, in front of, etc. Context matters. There is however, of course, *psychology of colour in context*. Cultural influences and socialisation in our younger years influence our psychological attitudes towards colour such that we can believe a colour represents a particular emotion. The power of belief is really strong.

What do you think the massive overexposure of self/body in the young generations implies for the future?

This means there's too much emphasis on how we look. In many images the women/models are simply standing or sitting staring blankly into the camera asking to be looked at. This objectifies women, suggesting they have nothing to offer other than the way they look. I think it is not going to go away. We need to educate younger people to respect themselves and their bodies more.

Do you think clothing will forever be linked to status or do you think we will get to the state in the future where really less is more?

I think we are turning to look at what is ethical and sustainable more now.

Have you ever personally been involved with any government incentives/legislation related to fashion?

Yes, I attended the all-party parliamentary group in fashion and textiles sessions, which were interesting, but the missing link is understanding how to change behaviour. It's not enough to tell people they have to. Psychologists understand how to support people through behaviour change. They can also help with trend forecasting as they are trained in analytics. This would reduce overproduction and, consequently, it reduces waste. It's a mystery to me why so few sustainability activists and fashion companies have understood this.

Read more about Carolyn's work in her fantastic book *The Psychology of Fashion*.

The positive psychology of getting dressed beautifully

Just as we may put our makeup back on after a period of illness, we also may dress to cheer ourselves. After hard times or disease or operations that affect our body confidence, being able to dress in a way we wish can be invaluable. Such a valuable resource in the USA for women returning to work, the **Dress for Success** campaign; and in the UK for men **Suited and Booted**. The '**look and feel fabulous**' campaigns for makeup and clothes for those with breast cancer emphasise the morale-boosting effect of taking care and time over make-up and clothing. Many might be immune to this but as a fashion-interested woman I think it is drastically powerful. I also think that dressing for the job is a boost to most, and if you love the corporate look for your job then go for it; if you love the eclectic style you have developed and honed into your 50s that is *your smart,* who should tell you otherwise – who would have the audacity?! We also tend to dress in a style that resonated with us in our formative years, maybe the first time we were independent and living away from home, making lifestyle decisions including clothing. I realise I am naturally drawn to the plain separates worn by Meg Ryan in the film *You've Got Mail* but I didn't realise the extreme coincidence until re-watching the film 20 years later with my daughter in 2019. Meg looks like she has my wardrobe.

Beware when you see that glorified item in the shop whether you *really* love it, will it *really* love you and does it earn a place in your wardrobe moralistically, sartorially, and can you afford it? If you can't, then walk away and leave the dopamine buzz for something that won't load you with guilt and debt. Have courage to be yourself and recycle and shop your own wardrobe. Visit preloved or vintage stores like me darling friend's www.willowandeve.com. Look at your own style influences. Every woman has her own style. Now, what's yours?

Working with a stylist

> "Dress shabbily and they remember the dress; dress impeccably and they remember the woman"
>
> **Coco Chanel**

I interviewed Nicky Hambleton-Jones, a well-known UK stylist, for my book in early summer 2018. We connected on Twitter and I wanted to know what made her tick. I had watched her show *10 Years Younger* when we were both more than 10 years younger. I was thrilled and a little star-struck when she agreed to be in my book. Fast forward a few months and I became Nicky's paying client for a fortnight '**for the sake of my book**'! I was to have my wardrobe interrogated and decluttered by Nicky and her colleague. My mother (a fashion designer before having me) was slightly incredulous regarding the idea – "What do you *need* that for? What *exactly* are they going to do?" My friends were either envious or scared for me. I was quite blasé until about two days beforehand, realising after a *significant* declutter that I still couldn't shut the doors on my two wardrobes. Nicky and Alyson turned up looking beautiful, accessorised and styled.

The Stylist, the Doctor and the Wardrobe

We started in the bedroom. They opened the wardrobe doors and started taking out the first rack of jumpers and laying them on the carpet.

"Start with these." Nicky looked at me and I looked at her. I breathed shallowly.

"What, try them on?"

"Yes, everything."

After the fifth beige jumper and the agreement we really *could not keep any more* just for the 'comfort pile', I saw I had been living in beige. Where had that girl gone? Where was the sexy mum who had fought to regain her pre-baby figure? I write that tongue-in-cheek but you catch my drift. I *was drifting* in a sea of beige waves interspersed with flashes of grey.

Emotion should not be so associated with clothes but of course it is.

With some hilarity I divulged to the stylish stylists that I had a 'dress for cleaning'. They looked at me utterly flummoxed.

"Doesn't everyone?" Evidently not.

I was heady with excitement as we met the next week in London, home of my student days. There is only so much you can read about shopping so let's stop there. I emerged with a fabulous selection of separates, a dress and some textured belts. All to complement what I already had and inject some excitement back.

Let us pause here to talk about life events and dressing. You dress to impress when you are young, you can be daring and frivolous. You can waft around Bond Street in vintage suede and chunky heels and look fab (I am so sure I did!). You have babies and are just excited to have a muslin to cover your jumper at the appropriate moment. Your work clothes may become a library of what you *should* project. I never gave up on clothes – my bank balance and love for a sale is testament to that – *but I did give up seeing what I could be*. Life is busy, and dressing takes a back seat.

Getting make-up on is a grand triumph (one I achieve every day). **Getting dressed is a practicality**. But **NO**. As I watched the movement of the swishy green skirt in the mirror during my trip with Nicky, NO, it's not a practicality, it's the icing on the cake. I look different. I look more 'dressed' and I look more *like me. I may even look younger*.

What I essentially learned is to *look* at yourself properly. Look at shapes that suit you and those you hide within. Keep some of the hiding clothes for comfort days, but focus on what makes you *feel good* and then sort out what you already have in that category at home. Be ruthless discarding or recycling/selling what you won't wear. If you feel guilty then sell or donate it and someone else will love it rather than buying a new item. Shop your wardrobe, wear your 'young' stuff – who is stopping you?

The real determining factor is to **try everything on.** You are dressing for you now, not the you when you have lost three dress sizes. We tend to have a notion whereby we keep clothes for when we are:

- Thinner
- Happier
- More daring

With all you have read so far I hope you see that **today is now. You are you, and you are important.** Are you going to look back at the age of 85 and say: "I am so glad I kept/never wore that outfit because I just didn't have the courage" or "Wasn't it fabulous that I had a wardrobe of clothes that never fitted me in my 50s? Life was a catastrophe every time I opened the wardrobe door!" You have one life – dress for it.

Is colour mood altering?

If you believe in it. Dressing can differ so much between individuals; we view darker colours as more slimming. Colour can change the reflection on your skin tone and the impression you create. Entire careers have been created by 'having your colours read' and seeing what is *supposed* to suit you. For the rest of us, might we use colour to our advantage to flatter and invigorate?

As I discussed with Professor Carolyn Mair, there actually is no 'psychology of colour', only in context. Our socialisation and the way we were brought up influences our psychology in reaction to colour. Colour is simply a physical property of light refracting off an object and is influenced by texture and the surrounding colours and level of light.

We all have a different relationship with colour, shaped by our surroundings, culture and beliefs. Since I was young I dreamed of living in a large white space and now live in a house virtually completely decorated in grey and white. Some cultures however believe white to be the colour of mourning. Colours like red, orange and yellow are said to evoke feelings of warmth and comfort, but in a different setting hostility and anger. Cool colours like blue, green and purple can calm you down but can be linked with sadness. This is ALL from your cultural upbringing and entrenched beliefs.

Could colour heal you if you are sick? This seems a ridiculous notion, or is it? A red tablet has a greater placebo effect than a white tablet. Red can make you react with greater speed and force, hence the use in danger signs. Blue lighting can reduce crime in certain areas... The list is endless and full of great points for discussion. *All of this is related to what you have learned in your life.*

However, colour is personal and we may not all see the same colour the same way. Colour-blind individuals can feel colour differences by energy vibration, and we cannot separate our younger years' influence from the direct emotion we now feel.

Manipulation of the colour effect can be used in advertising – almost subliminally influencing us. Just like colours can evoke a first impression of a website so can colours influence how people see you. We know you only have one chance to make a first impression.

One thing I learned from the wardrobe experience was **don't overwhelm** yourself. **Don't overwhelm** by keeping too much in your functioning wardrobe so that you cannot see what you have.

I met a 90-year-old lady in Vancouver airport, with the most stunning facial bone structure I have ever seen, her red lipstick immaculate as we discussed all the excitement of American politics waiting for our respective planes. For me she showed that age had no boundary when it comes to fashion, style and beauty. You see Iris Apfel on an advert. You catch Carmen Dell'Orefice on a billboard. You don't dissect their age, you just see fabulous icons of style and femininity.

CHAPTER 19: FRIENDSHIP AMONGST WOMEN

Our concept of friendship will mature and evolve as we age. In the playground we can weave in and out of friendships like girls dancing around a maypole. To find a 'best friend' at school is treasured and rare – you can be stuck in a 'three's a crowd' scenario and segregated according to who is current flavour of the month. Were you the confident happy girl whom everyone flocked to and who never had a shortage of 'besties' to name? Were you the wallflower who hid in the corner but bloomed late as a teenager and surprised everyone? The great thing about entering adulthood and leaving home is that you are thrown into a new environment and can redefine yourself. You can fake the confidence or just smile your way through, until you feel as comfortable as you look. You will have learned by then what a friend truly is. You may look for her, without realising, in those you meet.

I was bullied at school – a flippant comment, you say, attention-seeking and overstated. No, I don't overstate the impact. Four years of manipulation and my confidence shaken, waiting for approval, seeking it from an unkind 'classmate'. I grew up quickly. Life lessons were learned. I promised myself when I escaped her clutches that I would never allow myself to be treated in that way again. *They pick on the nice girls who try to please.* After that my friendships were healthy, immense fun; we all learned about life together, about real living. We made mistakes as teenagers and young adults, we compared, encouraged, wept with laughter and sadness together. You probably take some of these friends into adulthood like I do and they may be integral to your life today. They may form a segment of your conscience (What would * * * * do?), your reference point. You may be separated by oceans yet you recall their words, your chats at bizarre moments, as *every* person you have let in **that dear and that close** was there by *choice*. You can choose your friends but not your family. Friends are the family that you choose.

Friends could be the very opposite of you in personality or achingly similar. You may share life experiences. You may bond over happy moments or outpourings of grief when there is nothing wise to say that will suffice. Your silent presence will be enough.

You know your female friends do you good, you know the time passes in a flash whether it is over a bottle of wine, a coffee, a walk or a 'girls' weekend'. You know you are likely to leave their company refreshed and invigorated. Maybe they told you about a new product or exercise that you in turn want to try. We are influenced greatly by our friends, those we spend most time with. We are also influenced by our virtual friends. We see that girl online, whom we have never met; she looks cute in those trousers so we buy some. She tries that face cream – we want to be *like her* so we try it too. We want to belong and be part of a group. For this book though, I speak of the friends who have sat in the same room with you.

Watch a lot of therapists at work and they will be employing professional techniques to be like the very best, listening, encouraging friend. If you have a friend who naturally behaves like this, you will tend to seek her out when you are in need of practical advice. She may even be that friend who tells you things you just don't want to know, who makes you face up to cold hard truths. You will go back to her because you respect her honesty and insight.

We look for friends who mirror a part of ourselves. We look for trust, reliability, loyalty, empathy, shared humour, shared beliefs and morals and above all fun. If loyalty is broken or morals digress far we feel broken just as with a romantic relationship ending. We feel cheated that we held that friend so close. We maybe hold our friends on pedestals too high and take our differences too personally. We should not assume we are cut from the same cloth. What journey has she travelled to get here, with you, today? The perfect friend is one who does not judge. Life is complex, and if it is draining you and making you anxious you leave it be and move on.

One of my friends sensibly compares friendship paths to a train journey. We are on our own route and some people jump on the train for a bit; they may get off at a station along the way, they have a different path to travel. Others will stay on for the long haul with us. Some who depart may get back on at a later point then stay with us for the rest of the life journey. We have to assuage the guilt that arises from friendships that were just not meant to be and caused pain.

Focussing on the beneficial effects of female friendship, we know that many women state that their friends are of paramount importance to them as they pass through their lives. In a coffee shop I struck up a conversation with a lady in her 80s. She was concerned that she had left her husband at home with her daughter that morning after his recent illness, so she could travel to town to meet her close friend. She had not missed her friend's birthday in 30 years and explained they always met, every fortnight, for their own happiness. Having time away from being a caring wife, to regenerate her internal batteries, was *so important* to her. With her friend they felt like young girls again. In reclaiming those few short hours of friendship, this lady was happier and recharged for her role as loving wife. We all too often feel we have to be martyrs but in taking time for ourselves to be with our friends we may become better parents, partners and daughters.

Gradually the world is finding proper medical evidence for things we probably knew were likely to be true, **linking friendships with improved or maintained health**. The Nurses' Health Study at Harvard which started in 1976 collects all kinds of information about female health. One of the findings was that the more friends a woman has, the less likely they are to develop physical impairments as they age and are more likely to lead a contented life. Not having friends or confidants was as detrimental as being overweight or smoking. Other studies have shown that social isolation after severe illness such as breast cancer or after the death of spouse can impair health in women. Being socially integrated with family and friends is *protective of our health*. Men and women may, on a biological level, handle stress differently. An infamous study showed how women join together in times of stress. When we are stressed our cortisol (natural steroid) and adrenaline are raised and we in turn release oxytocin to calm us down. Men release far less of this than women. The oxytocin drive *reduces stress and enhances affiliation* – in women's cases this can lead to seeking out female friendships and nurturing them, which has great benefits for health. This downregulated stress response in women produces relaxation and strong affiliation (friendship bonds) and may help to explain why women may live 7.5 years longer than men. It also means that booking in that catch-up with your friends is **essential not trivial**. And you thought oxytocin was just about breastfeeding and orgasms! (My favourite line in my talks!) The female body and mind are truly remarkable!

Working at and investing in friendships could be one of the loveliest and most important ways of improving your health. No prescription involved. Most of the women I interviewed spoke fondly of their female friends and the important role they play in their lives. We may become more discerning about whom we let into our close circle as we age, but new friends can be just as important as old friends, especially if they are very relevant to our current life situation and can support and encourage us to get the best from life.

Returning to Jane Fonda and her insightful quotes: *"It's my women friends who put starch in my spine"*. I could not have said it better.

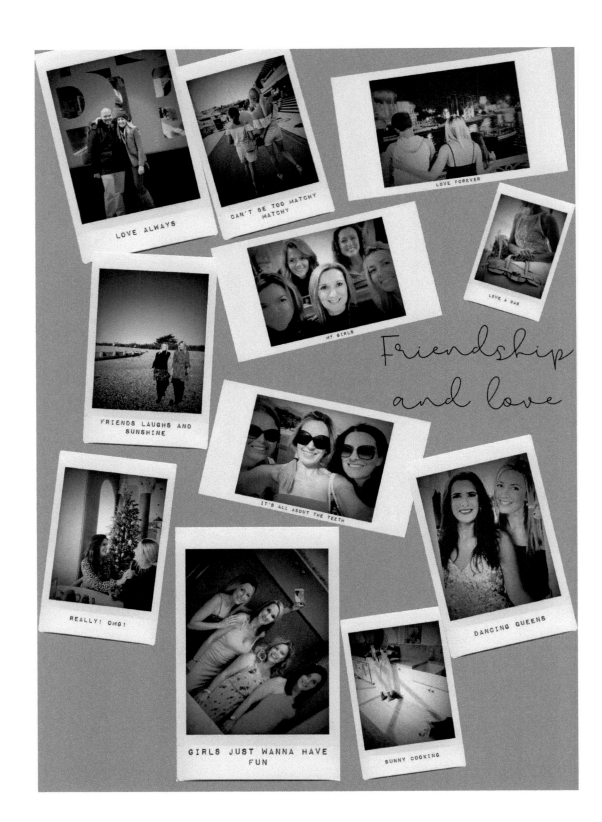

CHAPTER 20: SLEEP

 Sleep is what good dreams are made of

Sleep is a complex issue. The ultimate lifestyle accessory by choice not necessity. No matter your age, social status or bank account, investment in sleep is a basic human need. You cannot purchase, delegate or avoid it. This ubiquitous beauty boost and nourishment for your being is there for free if you want to take it. Along with water and warmth we have different needs for sleep as our lives progress.

Shift workers and young parents become obsessed with their shuteye bank. Sleep needs vary between individuals based on physiology, age and health. If you don't get the correct sleep *for you,* concentration and mood suffer, energy and motivation are sapped. Chemical changes mean your immune system comes under threat, weight may increase, libido and even fertility can decline. Ability to concentrate and retain information worsens and relationships and self-esteem will not be enhanced either.

After a bad night your behaviour may be altered. You may choose to miss your exercise that day and crave sugar and processed foods, thinking they will give you the buzz you are missing. There is no quick fix to replace sleep. Medical studies differentiate between true **insomnia** and **sleep problems**. True insomnia is a case for a doctor's appointment.

As a small child I woke early consistently, much to my parents' incredulity and exhaustion. Naturally, in the teenage years, our sleep cycles alter slightly and we tend to be awake later and

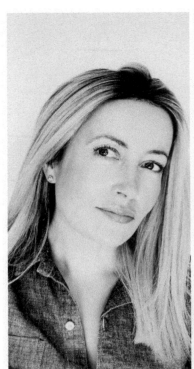
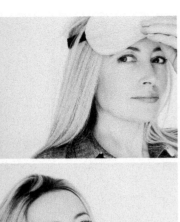
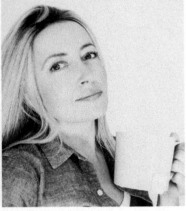

SLEEP PROBLEMS- DO YOU RECOGNISE
YOURSELF?
-taking a long time to drift off
-drifting off then waking with an overactive mind
-not sleeping long enough
-not waking refreshed
AROUND HALF OF AMERICANS AND A
THIRD OF EUROPEANS MAY HAVE 'SLEEP
PROBLEMS'. IF THIS IS YOU, PLACE SOME VALUE
ON ADDRESSING IT. THERE ARE GREAT
BENEFITS FOR OVERALL HEALTH AND
HAPPINESS.

naturally lie in, given the chance. As a medical student I learned to abuse the gift of sleep that I had previously taken for granted. Late-night chats, London nightclubs, contrasted with intense periods of study and zero socialising, meant we learned to burn the candle at both ends and then some. This only partly prepared us for our lives as junior doctors, sometimes working more than 100-hour weeks before rules about shift work and working times were established. The excitement of the white coat and on-call bleep to carry soon faded as the intense experience of being awoken from a short slumber in the on-call bed became reality. As the years passed and responsibility increased there was still no quick fix for managing deprived sleep. As we were running on adrenaline, it was sometimes decided as a team that we would stay up if it was likely we would be called again – was it worth even trying to sleep?

Fast forward to having children and my massive obsession with sleep resurfaced. I read every book about routines and baby whispering, and indeed my children did sleep through by eight weeks. This was instigated by my determination as a sleep-deprived doctor *to not go there again*. Do you count the hours you have slept or mentally keep a tally? How is your sleep now? Be honest. Like many things in life it is not completely *quantity*; quality is important too. Mine has improved greatly with some simple measures.

What is sleep?

Sleep is a state of unconsciousness but your brain and bodily functions are still active. The muscles and nerves are generally relaxed. The body responds to various cues and produces a complex group of hormones that then trigger sleep. In that sense one can understand how we can manipulate the onset and quality of sleep by our behaviour.

Healthy sleep cycles between three deepening stages of non-rapid eye movement (NREM) sleep (N1, N2 and N3) and rapid eye movement (REM) sleep. About 90 minutes after falling asleep REM sleep occurs and is the stage when most dreaming happens. Anyone who has observed their dog or child sleeping will recognise this fascinating stage of sleep well. We think this is when our brain stores information for memory. In the non-REM stages our breathing and heart rate is slowed and also our blood pressure lowered. If you are in the N3 deepest stage of this sleep it is more difficult to rouse you. In a healthy night's sleep there are three to five periods of dream sleep a night. At this time, you may have a fluctuating heart rate and involuntary muscular jerks.

Three-quarters of the way through the night is the lowest 'nadir', or deepest sleep. If you are exposed to bright light just before or after this point it can greatly disturb the timing of your 'circadian rhythm' (more below).

BASIC SLEEP HYGIENE

Not the shower before you slip between the sheets, this term originated as a recommendation for professionals to give poor sleepers. It reflects our society that we need to *consciously create a routine to sleep* – generations ago slumber would have beckoned after a working day with exhaustion and no electronics to keep us awake.

TIMING and ROUTINE

We have a **circadian rhythm** – a 24-hour sleep/wake cycle – a complex system influenced by light exposure and chemical pathways. It tells us when to feel awake and when to become sleepy.

Why is jetlag a problem?

Jetlag reinforces the news that we have a natural rhythm. Travelling eastwards is notoriously more difficult as we tend to still feel wired and awake when we should be winding down in our new destination. Drinking plenty of fluids, getting into the meal timings of the destination country and exposure to morning light in the new place can all lessen the effects. As someone who has travelled a lot back and forth across the Atlantic with my children, I know as a parent that the 'getting them to bed' part for children when back home in the UK can be a nightmare. Winding down for bed and maybe giving a couple hours' leeway on normal bedtime can help, and then gradually reduce this leeway over a few days. A warm bath and regular prompt mealtimes back home can prevent the family routine dragging the jetlag out longer than necessary. It usually takes a day for each hour difference, but travelling abroad for longer will make the effects more potent. If you are travelling for a short time, on a business trip or quick break, rising early in the western destination (maybe 6am starts) and making the most of the days may mean that when you return home you almost reduce the time difference from five hours to three.

Does sleep make you happier?

We are happiest when adhering to *natural sleeping times.* There is a link between worsening mental illness and poor sleep. Control your routine and mental health symptoms may improve. Management of sleep is often a priority for clinicians in management.

How much shuteye are you getting?

There are countless anecdotal stories of prolific leaders requiring only a few hours' sleep a night chronically. Most adults need seven to nine hours' sleep – research suggests that alongside deficient sleep, excessive sleepiness in the day may also predict some disease. This is often because of deficient quality of sleep at night. As a ballpark, sleep requirements are:

Age	Number of hours sleep required per 24-hour period
Newborns	16-18
Preschool children	11-12
School-aged children	10+
Teens	9-10
Adults	7-8

This may be an overgeneralisation. Maybe men require an hour less than women (that's my argument for a lie-in!) and as we age we tend to require less sleep and may wake earlier. The elderly still require sleep at the same level but can sleep poorly due to different ailments and be roused earlier. Teenage sleep routines, unguided, would naturally involve later to bed, later to rise. Some forward-thinking communities in the world alter their college hours to reflect this.

If you have an isolated bad night's sleep it is best to think positively and realise that, undisturbed, you should regain 100% of the deep sleep and 50% of the light sleep the following night.

Consciously *enjoying* the process of beauty regimes before bed may subconsciously prepare you for slumber.

Waking at the same hour helps our sleep routine – a lie-in bizarrely does not assist body clocks long term. Interestingly, in a sleep clinic many patients believed that the weekend could cancel out any problems created in the working week. The consultant Dr Peter Venn was keen to point out that one extra hour a night was an entire extra night's sleep a week!

Power nap or not? Scientists suggest that a nap under 30 minutes can be useful if tired, as long as there are four hours to go before bedtime so it doesn't interfere with sleep.

ENVIRONMENT

Body **temperature** needs to drop slightly for sleep. The ideal room temperature is 16-18 degrees – above 24 and we get restless. Ironically, wearing socks to keep extremities warmer helps some drift off. Try it and see if it helps you, although you may feel the need to remove them later in the night.

If you are suffering menopausal flushes, consider cooler bed covers (maybe a different tog rating to your partner) and looser clothing that may wick away moisture. Nancy and Eileen at www.cucumberclothing.com identified this night-time discomfort as a real problem. They have incorporated the use of sustainable fabrics that help solve the issue for menopausal women, breastfeeding mothers, and those going through breast cancer treatment, thyroid problems and so on. Basically for *any lady who gets hot*. Their anti-crease fabric lasts six times as long as cotton, and its antimicrobial properties remain strong after washing and no ironing needed. The fabric is produced in an eco-conscious way. What's not to love?! These ladies are impressive in that they have turned a problem they encountered into inspiration for a business idea.

You have to recoup the fluids lost in sweat at night, especially at menopausal time, in order to avoid headaches next day. See menopause section.

Light keeps us awake. Blackout blinds are not just for babies. Be like Audrey Hepburn and try a silk eye mask loosely fitted around this delicate area. The act of wearing the mask signifies 'sleep mode' to your brain and may prevent early morning light waking you. My sleep quality has massively improved since using one and I do get in quite a panic if I mislay it, much to my husband's amusement. A glowing alarm clock must be moved if stopping you sleeping.

Blue light emitted from electronics is a new threat. Scientists are still collating evidence to understand the effects on humans. The power of the blue light from your phone 'conveniently' taken into bed at night is worrying. The light tells your body it is *still daytime* even though the owls may be hooting. Your body reduces its melatonin (the natural biological marker of night time). **Your circadian rhythm is then set later than it should be.** The fact that scientists are studying whether there is going to be a future link between eye disease and blue light is a concern. The melatonin our brain produces at night is needed to regulate many processes in our bodies – cholesterol, sugar, calcium regulation, recovery of the nervous system and removal of waste products from the brain. Many processes that we would consider *anti-ageing* in the body are performed during sleep. Hunger and other hormones are regulated. *Reduce sleep and you are literally ageing faster.*

Significantly reduced melatonin reduces protection from breast, prostate and other cancers. Put your tech into *night (dimmed) mode* and remove electronics from your sleeping area. **It only takes a cheap alarm clock to replace your phone in the bedroom.** Stop the tech at least 90 mins prior to bed. Your love life and sleep may benefit, plus consider the sleep-inducing effect of orgasm!

A **pet** may disrupt sleep and cause allergies. If it is for your reassurance, establish where the pet sleeps. If you are living alone and the pet is your only comfort, then sort a long-term solution. Allergies or scratching from a pet in bed are more detrimental than a pet sleeping on the floor.

Noise disrupts sleep for some, not others. 'Pink noise' is a range of frequency of sound, similar to the sound of running water, used in studies to stimulate changes in sleep waves and possibly also improve memory recall. This will all be explored more in future medicine but, for now, if you discover a calming soundtrack that helps you drift off, then that is the right one for you! Preferably not played on your mobile phone next to you!

MENTAL

Early morning wakening is a feature of depression and many sleep problems can stem from anxiety. In milder cases work on what you can control. *Journal or list your worries* in the evening to offload onto the next day. If it helps, **be a girl guide** and *prepare the night before* – clothes, your bag, anything to reduce your morning to-do list! Avoid horror films and similar before bed as they may stimulate your brain too much. I always have to watch something else after anything particularly frantic!

If you are waking in the night and watching the clock, maybe get up and make yourself a drink. Obviously caffeine free! The act of rising may lower your temperature, aiding sleep. Try 4/7/8 breathing – breathe in through the nose for a count of 4, hold for 7 and breathe out slowly through the mouth for 8. If that's too much and makes you dizzy try 3, 4, 5. The physiologist in me knows this works because it stimulates our vagus nerve (slows the heart) but the worrier in me knows this just relaxes. Find your own combo of slower breathing. If meditation is your thing work on a mantra that is calming.

PHYSICAL

Exercise within the day may aid sleep at night. Relaxing yoga helps some before bed. Stressful exercise *just before* bed may disrupt sleep by raising your cortisol and adrenaline levels. It is a matter of finding what is right for you and what can fit in with your own life, and we all differ.

Alcohol encourages drifting off to sleep but you are likely to awaken in the night and feel restless, thirsty or needing the toilet. You have less restful REM sleep after alcohol. You produce heat as you metabolise it so the sensation of burning up may prevent sleep.

Nicotine is a stimulant and smoking may dry out nasal passages and cause potential chronic inflammation of throat tissues, increasing snoring or disrupted breathing.

Caffeine effect will depend on your tolerance. Triple espressos at 9pm will leave all but the most ardent caffeine aficionados totally wired between the sheets. A reasonable rule is none after 4pm. If you are caffeine sensitive, then STOP at midday. Chocolate has caffeine but in much lower concentrations than coffee.

Spicy food – if you suffer indigestion, eating late will worsen symptoms. You often need to sleep with extra pillows to reduce symptoms. Spicy food tolerance may be different between individuals but it is not rocket science to avoid the strongest curry if you are susceptible.

LUXURY SLEEP HYGIENE

Food to help you sleep. In theory, magnesium-containing foods have a calming effect upon the body – sweet potatoes, nuts. Tryptophan-containing foods can help melatonin production – oats, turkey, tuna, hummus, bananas and yoghurt. The loading of carbohydrates warms the body then it subsequently cools. I don't advocate eating late as I believe it encourages weight gain but a warm bowl of porridge is sometimes recommended for those not sleeping of an evening!

The power of bathing and magnesium salts

Expert medical herbalist Katie Pande BSc explained to me how magnesium plays a vital role in the functioning of nervous system cells and many processes in the body. Magnesium salts are best absorbed through the skin so there has been an evolution in people using Epsom salts in the bath. Absorption through our feet is very effective so foot baths are often recommended by nutritionists to aid sleep. Try before bed and the cooling effect after warming may also aid sleep. Replace any fluids lost bathing with a drink of water.

Katie explains that **lavender** is a sedative to the nervous system and will relax nervous system tissues. As an aromatherapy oil it can reduce insomnia exacerbated by stress or anxiety. **Rose** and **camomile** in aromatherapy also reduce stress. Teas containing lavender, limeflower and other herbs are readily available, and just the simple act of brewing and then enjoying the tea can start your evening wind-down. Sleep pillow sprays are a practical way to use this science. I think they are great for what they do if you have no allergy to any components and also for being part of a subliminal routine that symbolises to you that bedtime is near.

Be aware that just because sedative **herbal medicines like valerian** taken orally are 'natural', they are still *powerful*. Discuss with your doctor the interaction with your other medicines such as beta blockers. Valerian increases deep sleep so needs to be taken with caution. You would not take it unless you were going to sleep, certainly not for driving, and if given sedative medicine by your doctor the combined effect might be too potent to be thought safe.

Melatonin is readily available in the US as a supplement. A slow-release version is sometimes prescribed in the UK to those over 55 with chronic sleep disorders. There is concern over prescription in the UK due to the drowsiness (driving) and whether it alters the body's response to natural melatonin long term so doctors are divided. There is less regulation of supplements compared to medication so doctors are cautious about what may be in over-the-counter supplements purchased overseas.

Silk pillowcases are kinder to hair and skin than cotton and less likely to snag on our hair or punish our skin as we turn. Many models I know have trained themselves for **back sleeping**. I myself have had little success with this! There are studies of how the folding of our skin as side sleepers contributes to *passive wrinkles*. This is truly horrific! Sleep therapists believe that we turn far more than we realise anyway within the night. Pillow density and shape may improve your ability to get your beauty sleep back prone. There are also beauty pillows made of kinder materials than the traditional pillows on the market. Trial and error to find your perfect 'beauty pillow' match may be key for you whether you are a side or a back sleeper.

When to see the doctor

Sleep clinics involve specialist doctors from different professions who work together to study and treat sleep disorders. They have the facility to monitor people overnight as they stay in the hospital for a sleep study and measure all the physiological parameters to calculate what is going on.

If **insomnia is an aspect of your mental illness,** then discuss this seriously with your doctor, and all symptoms may improve if sleeping is corrected.

SNORING

As female obesity rises so does the rate of women attending sleep clinics for breathing problems. Muscle weakness around the airway increases with age and the muscles relax as we sleep. Air passing through the smaller airway creates noise. Snoring worsens after alcohol or certain foods. Snoring on one's back may be stopped by sewing in a golf/tennis ball to your pyjama top to keep you sideways! *Losing weight is a first step.* A relatively small weight loss can have a significant effect on snoring, and in the clinics collar size is often discussed to motivate.

Snoring can also be due to jaw size/positioning/tongue shape and size/enlarged tonsils and so on. In some cases, an orthodontic plate to hold the lower jaw forward and the tongue away from the back of the throat can help. There is an over-the-counter version called SnorBan that is recommended by some doctors.

Sleep apnoea means breathing stops intermittently at night which can trigger dramatic falls in oxygen levels, leading to daytime drowsiness. Long-term serious implications are risk of diabetes, heart disease, high blood pressure and possible weight gain. Referral to a sleep clinic by your GP is essential. Wives often report their husbands' symptoms as stopping breathing then taking a deep compensatory gasp of air! Losing weight and lifestyle changes help. Patients may be treated with quiet machines providing humidified air under pressure by mask. (Funnily enough, the symptoms reported by wives of male patients in clinic that they had observed in their partners, were far more accurate predictors of the severity of the problem than vice versa but don't dismiss the fact that women suffer too.)

Less commonly, conditions arise as sleep disorders.

REM parasomnias. Someone acts out their dream, usually later in sleep, and this can involve swearing, shouting or physical movement. The patient usually experiences violent dreams.

These patients do have an increased chance of suffering neurological disorders later in life, such as Parkinson's, Multi System Atrophy and Lewy Body Dementia. Sleep clinics usually have a linked neurologist to investigate this and, in many cases, reassure patients.

Non-REM parasomnias cause sleep-walking and talking in children, resolving in teenage years. More seriously, adults may suffer, and it can lead to automatic activities whilst asleep – cooking, eating, even attempting sexual activity, which understandably can be distressing and frightening for the partner. These episodes occur as the brain is part asleep/part awake.

After sleep clinic assessment these can be helped by medication, treating any breathing problems, and cognitive behavioural therapy.

Restless legs creates an overwhelming urge to move the legs, or a crawling sensation. It may be described as a bothersome twitching, usually with no cause, but the doctor must exclude iron deficiency and kidney problems. Look at your medication and any other health problems such as thyroid disease to ensure these are all in check. Stopping smoking and good sleep hygiene will help (including Epsom salt baths) but sometimes medication is needed – drugs such as gabapentin (a controlled drug) or other sedating meds such as clonazepam are required.

True insomnia can arise from deep-rooted psychological and emotional issues. It can greatly benefit from talking with a clinical psychologist and receiving CBT.

Value sleep like a best friend. Give it priority and time and it will give back to you a hundredfold.

Here we reach the end of my academic writing.

Remember, you have one life, make it your best one.

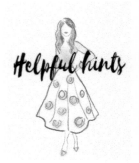

Helpful hints

Realise that change is possible at any age
Small habits create change – no need to be dramatic
Create mental space, time and fun for yourself
Allow peace, meditation and reflection to be valued as much as the busy parts of life
Connect with others – you do each other good
Friends are the ultimate blessing
Remember your plate, your gut and your brain are strongly connected
Movement and sleep are the bedrocks of life
Look forward to being the best you ever
As I said at the beginning, the secrets are eating well, exercise, relax, sleep, love but now you know why.

Now you don't need to just take my word for it. Here we have the words of some fabulous women that I know you are going to love. Welcome to the final stage of this BEST LIFE journey. Conversations from women around the world. Welcome to THE WOMEN.

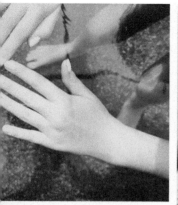

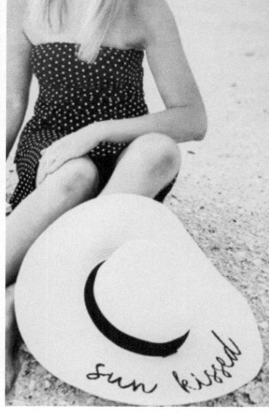

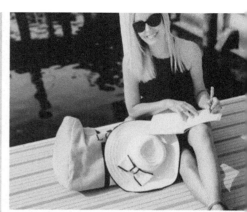

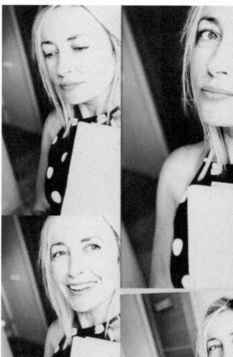

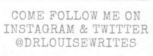

sun kissed

COME FOLLOW ME ON
INSTAGRAM & TWITTER
@DRLOUISEWRITES

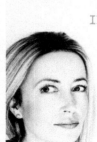

THE
WOMEN

"Listen with curiosity. Speak with honesty. Act with integrity. The greatest problem with communication is we don't listen to understand. We listen to reply. When we listen with curiosity, we don't listen with the intent to reply. We listen for what's behind the words."

Roy T. Bennett, *The Light in the Heart*

At the start of this journey I knew I had to write more than 'a book about women's health'. I needed to search deeper. Women have a silent fascination with each other. Young girls and fully fledged women all need role models throughout life, even if only to learn from each other's mistakes. Women need to support each other, then miracles are created. To incorporate this magic enigma of female experience into my pages, I needed to seek out some fabulous women. The women here did not know me three years ago. They have all warmly welcomed the unique concept of this book and have let me into their lives. I am proud to call many of them dear friends who will now be in my life forever. They inspire me, elevate my self-belief, yet they all have totally unique wisdom. Now I wish you the same motivation. Sit back, relax and let these women tell you about their own journeys with laughter, tears and passion. May it set you on an enlightening path of reflection about your own life and the future.

DISCLAIMER

All interviews have been given in good faith to share experience and belief. Any organisations or work mentioned are to place interviewees in the context in which they live and function and are not any form of paid advertising. Any recommendation of a product, supplement or way of life is an opinion of the interviewee *and not one that I or the interviewee take responsibility for advocating. I am not medically endorsing any of the supplements mentioned by including them in the writing.*

Any further exploration of websites or media mentioned is at your own discretion and in no way a recommendation of any purchase or activity. If you are thinking of changing lifestyle or taking a supplement, discuss this with your healthcare professional who knows you and your medical history personally: one size does not fit all. All opinions and recounts have been checked and authorised by the ladies involved to be released in this form and should be received in the generous spirit in which they were given.

ANNALISE FARD, 46

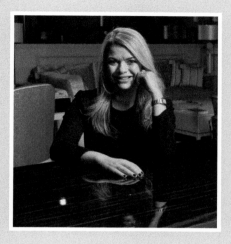

Director of Beauty, Fine Jewellery, Watches & Accessories at Harrods in Knightsbridge, London. Annalise studied American Literature and History at university. Travelling extensively afterwards and finding eclectic gifts inspired her to become a buyer. Previously she was a Buyer at Harrods, US Sales Director Bliss (owned by LVMH), Vice President Global Sales Bliss.

INTERESTS
Interior design, working out

MAIN ROLE MODELS
My maternal grandmother 'Nana' was a great influence, very strong and powerful. She managed domestic staff in hospitals and clinics across the region. My grandad had always supported her independence. When Grandad passed away, I naturally went to live with her – no reflection upon my relationship with the rest of my family, it was just to support Nana.

HOW AWARE WERE YOU GROWING UP OF BODY IMAGE AND BEAUTY? IS YOUR CONFIDENCE HIGHER NOW?
I think your body changes so rapidly when you are younger, and you are dealing with all of that. Confidence in myself, body, mind and soul probably came at about 18 years old. It must have been media and friends' influence making me feel less confident before that, as I had strong supportive family around me.

Much higher confidence now.

DID YOU HAVE STRONG INFLUENCES ON YOUR EATING PATTERNS GROWING UP?
I wasn't conscious of diets. Home cooking was not particularly healthy and we never really ate breakfast! Still some of my family have a biscuit for breakfast! Influences on my eating can be emotional. I adore carbs – not a sweet tooth but savoury.

WHAT IS YOUR OPINION ON THE MORE INTERVENTIONAL BEAUTY TREATMENTS?
I think it is a decision for you, yourself. You do what makes you feel the best. I have had semi-

invasive treatments only. I am very conscious that you can very quickly and easily go too far. Once you start having treatments you start seeing them in other women. I would rather they think 'she looks good for 46', not 'oh, she looks 39'.

FAVOURITE BEAUTY PRODUCTS
I love face masks: Meso Infusion Day Defence Hydration Mask (111SKIN) and Bobbi Brown Instant Detox Mask are two of my favourites.

SUPPLEMENTS
Phillip Kingsley PK4, Omega oil, Glucosamine, Vitadrip infusions by The Elixir Clinic at Harrods.

BEAUTY AND HOME ARE CONSTANTLY EVOLVING; HOW DO YOU KEEP AHEAD OF THE FIELD AND MAKE SURE YOUR KNOWLEDGE IS CURRENT AND IN FACT AHEAD OF THE MAJORITY?
Customers always come first. It could be trends that are evolving; they may share with us their knowledge of trends and that gives us insight. Layer on top of that the fact that Harrods is all about luxury and innovation. I am supported to do things differently and in a new way. I feel it is like 'running a ship' and I have fantastic teams of people working with me, with skill and efficiency. I am the one who has to have the long-term vision.

DO YOU HAVE A NATURAL INTEREST IN BOTH AREAS OF BEAUTY AND ACCESSORIES?
I can be in a meeting about the latest shade of lipstick one minute then looking at the next design innovation in timepieces! I am more satisfied and the business gets the best out of me when I am running at full speed – I just literally love it more!

WHAT IS THE MAGIC OF HARRODS?
I think the role of Harrods is to excite and inspire. The buying and the experience of being in Harrods should be enjoyable. I want to put the joy back into retail. We are so global, so we want clients to be able to touch Harrods from anywhere around the world. I want the shop itself to be a place you can come to have a truly amazing experience of products and brands.

TELL ME ABOUT THE WELLNESS AREA OPENED IN SUMMER 2017 IN HARRODS.
It very much speaks to the long-term future vision of beauty. My team and I travelled a lot for inspiration; this particular concept was very much born out of Asia. I call it 'integrative beauty' and it is all things brought together under one roof. I saw many amazing concepts on my travels but not presented in a luxurious environment. Clients enter through the holistic side, such as nutrition, then they might try the cryochamber, have a vitamin infusion. All the treatments should be supportive, e.g. if you lost 20 pounds in eight weeks with the Louise Parker method but stubborn fat is still there, you might consider cool sculpting for saddlebags and bingo wings. It is all about making the best of you, *not changing* you. Lifestyle changes that Louise advocates, like digital detox, turning off phones/iPad/TV and having a bath, will help your sleep and then in turn your metabolism and so on. She talks about eating beautifully, and that is me. I am meticulous in the way I enjoy food, setting a table to eat at in the evening rather than grabbing from the fridge. Louise supports all of this via her four pillars method. I wanted to combine all of this to make something wonderful that clients would want to return to and be loyal to.

WHERE DO YOU THINK WE STAND IN THE INTERNATIONAL FIELD OF BEAUTY?
I think in retail we are ahead in the UK. We have introduced a lot of Korean beauty and now it's all about J beauty – Japanese beauty. Our aim is to be the curators of the very best products. We have to maintain the trust that clients have in us of presenting the very best products from around the world.

CAROLINE NEVILLE MBE, 76

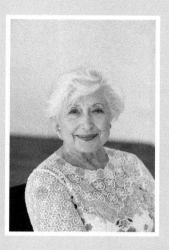

Founding member and President of **Cosmetic Executive Women** (CEW) in the UK, formed to educate and recognise women at executive level in the beauty industry. This involves an annual programme of supportive events and a philanthropic, health-promoting arm. Including the USA and French divisions, this involves more than 10,000 women. Founded **Caroline Neville Associates**, Public Relations Company in 1962, which 15 years ago was rebranded as her son and daughter took over, forming **Neville McCarthy Associates.** Caroline was chairman until it became **Aurelia Neville McCarthy Communications** after merging with another agency

"I write two columns on the industry in my spare time! I feel so happy to have such a rewarding second career at my age. Retirement has never featured in my vocabulary. As long as you have your wits and mobility, age is irrelevant."

TELL ME MORE ABOUT CEW.

We are equipping women to step up the ladder by creating a forum for them to have a voice. We **mentor, debate and network** and also **donate** annually to The Eve Appeal. I am the Patron of the **Get Lippy Campaign** with the charity uniting with brands selling lip products to donate £1 to the charity. I am working with them to raise the profile of gynaecological health to younger women to encourage them to attend for their smears. We are currently engaging with the government to raise the profile of our industry and also have an independent initiative called '**Cancer and Careers**' and have produced four books called 'Living and Working with Cancer' donated free to the public. We have a Young Executive Programme to nurture our future leaders. We have two high-profile awards annually – **Achiever Awards** for industry talent and **Beauty Awards** for creativity in product.

MAIN ROLE MODELS

Mother, my aunt and her husband. A school teacher who encouraged me to take my GCEs and shorthand and typing courses. I was always interested in fashion; I even made my own clothes from *Vogue* paper patterns. I really came into my own after school. My mother was smart and good-looking and I suppose I subconsciously followed her. I remember the night before going to the Coronation with my school, my mother gave me a Toni perm which I loved! I had a dress made from parachute nylon that I adored because it flared out when I spun around! I came into my own as the '60s came along and young people really set the scene. My Uncle George rose from local journalist to national, and inspired me to do the same. I worked as a secretary on the *News Chronicle* at 17, then moved to *Honey* magazine as a fashion department assistant. I had fallen on my feet. I had many successful female journalists as role models. I saw what success looked like and was highly motivated to be like my editor.

DO YOU COMPARE YOURSELF TO OTHER WOMEN?

I certainly don't compare myself to younger women. I am more interested in women of 50 plus and I love it when I see a woman who has obviously taken time and trouble to make the most of herself. It would be true to say I do not meet many other women of my age working! I consider myself to be very fortunate to have such a wonderful job.

I have always had confidence. I started a business at age 20, so confidence and belief in my ability was absolutely essential.

HOW DO YOU LOOK AFTER YOURSELF, BEING SO EDUCATED AROUND AND ENSCONCED WITHIN THE BEAUTY INDUSTRY?

I have regular full-body massages; I see this as maintenance of my body and senses. Facials are a must-have for me. I think my skin glows afterwards. I love reflexology. I need to be mobile and relaxed so these treatments maintain me. My brilliant hairdresser cuts my hair in a contemporary style. He advised me to let my natural white hair come through; I love it and so does everyone else who asks me who colours it! That makes me feel good.

"Being President of CEW, the leading organisation in the UK for women (and men) working in the beauty industry, is a very high profile role. I speak at events, appear on QVC. I am duty bound to appear as well turned out as I can. I think it's about being contemporary in my style; age is irrelevant."

DO YOU EXERCISE?

I walk a lot within my working day. I have four flights of stairs in my house. I don't sit down that much! Health is a priority for my husband and I. Walking more in Greenwich Park would be the one thing that would add to our healthy efforts!

YOUR ATTITUDE TO NUTRITION?

Every evening I will have fish and at least three vegetables. Other meals include plenty of fruit, nuts, salad, steamed veg. We gave up frying food years ago.

WHAT CHANGES HAVE YOU NOTICED SINCE 40?

Incontinence – my gynaecologist, whom I see annually, says it is my brain ruling my bladder.

I am generally happy with my body and shape.

Everyone's face goes 'south'... I have fared well due to genes, sun protection, never smoking, and regular moisturising and cleansing before sleeping. I have some age spots but they don't bother me and I am good at disguising them. Some of the problems that come with the ageing face can be dealt with by clever application of makeup. I tried Botox many years ago with an American dermatologist – at the time I thought it was amazing. In the last five years I did have light touch Botox treatments. I began being filmed for CEW events and thought I needed to erase my forehead lines. *Now I could not care less. I have earned every line and can live with them.*

HOW DO YOU FEEL EMOTIONALLY ABOUT THE PASSING YEARS?

Everyone is going to age. I know I am cherished by my husband and children, not for the way I look. Ageing gracefully is my objective. I am in a very happy marriage of 54 years. My children are proud of me. There has never been a better time to be an older woman.

WHAT IS YOUR OPINION ON THE MORE INTERVENTIONAL BEAUTY TREATMENTS?

For the industry Botox was a game changer. It did refresh faces, then it went too far with lots of immobile faces and bad work. Now there is a new reality. Light touch Botox treatments given by dermatologists are more the order of the day. But not for me currently.

Plastic surgery is for people with real problems. It's not a picnic. There are so many beauty enhancing treatments now, make sure you get a well thought of practitioner. It is a very personal choice.

TELL ME ANY SUPPLEMENTS YOU TAKE.

Vitamin D, B-complex, Turmeric, Trichocomplex by Philip Kingsley to help maintain normal hair, Absolute Collagen

FINAL WORDS

"As we stay in the workplace for longer, by choice or necessity, we must focus on keeping fit and keeping our minds active. There's no real secret recipe for success in this area; in my opinion, it's just luck. I find working in an office with young people exhilarating. I am not competing with them but we have a lot in common. We like the same beauty products, we all try to eat healthily, exercise, and we have lots of lively dialogue and fun in our office!"

CAROLINE NEVILLE MBE, 76

JO MOSELEY, 53

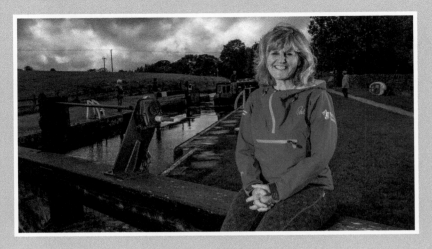

Photo credit Charlotte Graham Photography

Founder www.healthyhappy50.com; Twitter & Instagram @healthyhappy50
"My main work is for a structural engineering company. I also teach AquaFitness and speak about wellbeing and plastic pollution."

MAIN ROLE MODELS
My mum, who loved fashion and makeup and was a beautiful, glamorous woman. She was an incredible force of life in all her roles at home and in business. I think of her every day.

HOW AWARE WERE YOU GROWING UP OF BODY IMAGE AND BEAUTY?
Until I was 10, not very aware. I was called a tomboy for always playing outside. As I became a teenager I became very aware and absorbed all the ideas that being thinner was a good thing.

DID YOU HAVE STRONG INFLUENCES ON YOUR EATING PATTERNS GROWING UP?
Mum was often on a diet! And at the same time, she was a fabulous cook!

WERE YOU HAPPY WITH YOUR IMAGE AS A TEENAGER?
No, for most of my teenage years I felt very unsure of my body image and thought if I were thinner I would be okay.

WHAT WOULD YOU TELL YOUR 20-YEAR-OLD SELF AND IS YOUR CONFIDENCE NOW HIGHER?
"You are absolutely enough just as you are. Beauty comes in all shapes and sizes. When you talk about what you love and are passionate about, there is a special beauty that shines through. Believe in your values. Comparison will steal your joy. Practising gratitude now is a habit worth creating."
Higher! I have come through challenges and heartbreak that I thought would crush my spirit.

I am exploring new ideas and adventures. I have raised two sons of whom I'm so proud.

DO YOU COMPARE YOURSELF TO OTHER WOMEN?

I make a point of working hard not to, but admit sometimes I do.

DOES BODY IMAGE AND APPEARANCE MATTER TO YOU NOW?

How I look is part of who I am, but I worry so much less about what I look like and celebrate who I am. Moving joyfully in the sea and hills has helped me become friends with my body. When I catch myself in the mirror, glowing from a swim or paddleboarding, I feel I've found myself again.

DO YOU EXERCISE?

Aquafit, bodyboard, paddleboard, snorkelling, running, kettlebells, yoga, cycling.

YOUR ATTITUDE TO NUTRITION?

I love food and the whole occasion of eating. I especially like things that make me feel good – vegetables, nuts and beans. I love dark chocolate and peanut butter. I don't drink alcohol and never have.

WHAT CHANGES HAVE YOU NOTICED SINCE 40?

Changes to my menstrual cycle. Sun spots. Skin thinner, more laughter lines! I've had two frozen shoulders and plantar fasciitis, which aren't great.

HOW DO YOU FEEL EMOTIONALLY ABOUT THE PASSING YEARS?

Very grateful to be here as I have seen too many friends my age or younger die. I want to keep living life to the full and look after myself so that can be possible.

WHAT IS YOUR OPINION ON THE MORE INTERVENTIONAL BEAUTY TREATMENTS?

Not for me unless there was a real medical condition such as skin cancer.

HAVE YOU EVER HAD ANY BEAUTY DISASTERS?

A perm in the '70s!

BEAUTY PRODUCTS

Water, fresh air, exercise, cleanse and moisturise with plastic-free products.

SUPPLEMENTS

Vitamin D

SAM RICE, 47
MIMI SPENCER, 50

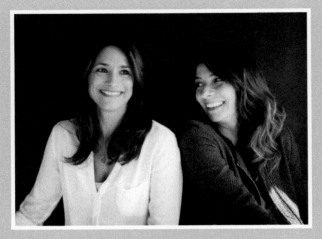

Sam and Mimi are authors of the cookbook *The Midlife Kitchen* (Instagram @midlifekitchen). Sam is a food, drink and health blogger (www.stealthhealthblog.com) and writer and has a monthly column called **The Mindful Drinker** in *Top Santé* magazine. She currently lives with her family in Singapore. Mimi is co-author of *The Midlife Kitchen* and a well-known journalist and writer.

SAM

MAIN ROLE MODELS

I have never really been one to have role models as such, although there are women I admire. As I've got older I've realised how truly amazing my own mother is. She is a highly intelligent woman who set aside her own academic ambitions to raise a family – seven children in total. In her 40s she went back to law school, gained a first class degree and practised as a lawyer until retiring. She absolutely embodies selflessness and unconditional love and those are qualities I deeply respect.

HOW AWARE WERE YOU GROWING UP OF BODY IMAGE AND BEAUTY?

As a young girl, not at all. As a teenager, I was into fashion and make-up but never felt any pressure to look a certain way – I spent my formative years living in Singapore so I was surrounded by people of all races and cultures and there wasn't one blueprint for how you should look.

DID YOU HAVE STRONG INFLUENCES ON YOUR EATING PATTERNS GROWING UP?

Diet was a non-issue; the women around me when I was growing up never dieted. We probably didn't eat particularly healthily, but people didn't concern themselves with it as much back then – it was the chicken kiev era!

WERE YOU HAPPY WITH YOUR IMAGE AS A TEENAGER?

Apart from a couple of dodgy haircuts, yes.

WHAT WOULD YOU TELL YOUR 20-YEAR-OLD SELF AND IS YOUR CONFIDENCE NOW HIGHER?

"Your life will be one big adventure – go with it!" Higher, I am less shy and I don't feel I have anything to prove to anyone.

DO YOU COMPARE YOURSELF TO OTHER WOMEN?

Not really, I don't feel any pressure to look younger. I meet so many confident, witty, experienced midlife (and older) women so I'm happy to be part of that tribe! Another thing to remember is that even if someone seems to be super-confident they might still be out of their comfort zone – the trick is to just take a deep breath and get on with it.

DOES BODY IMAGE AND APPEARANCE MATTER TO YOU NOW?

I exercise to stay a size that I am happy with; I do it for myself, no one else. I eat well and like to have the odd massage but I wouldn't say I'm high maintenance!

ANY POINTS IN YOUR LIFE THAT MADE YOU LOOK AFTER YOURSELF MORE?

Yes, my father died prematurely from a heart attack and my brother died aged 27 from type 1 diabetes. These events have profoundly affected me – especially my brother being so young. I was 42 at the time and it was the catalyst to me changing my lifestyle.

DO YOU EXERCISE?

Yes, I try and do something active every day, in particular walking, Pilates, yoga, the odd HIIT class and skiing.

YOUR ATTITUDE TO NUTRITION?

As a health and food writer I'm probably more into it than your average person but I'm not a health fanatic. I believe in everything in moderation – including moderation!

WHAT CHANGES HAVE YOU NOTICED SINCE 40?

My body has improved as I have got to grips with nutrition and exercise. Of course, I have a few wrinkles appearing and slightly heavier eyelids but nothing that keeps me up at night.

HOW DO YOU FEEL EMOTIONALLY ABOUT THE PASSING YEARS?

I don't worry about it physically; I just don't like the feeling that I'm running out of time.

WHAT IS YOUR OPINION ON THE MORE INTERVENTIONAL BEAUTY TREATMENTS?

I've had sclerotherapy on some veins on my legs but I don't think I would ever go under the knife facially. In its own way it's quite ageing as you end up with a certain 'look'.

MIMI

MAIN ROLE MODELS
Mother, sister, grandma.

I loved my grandma's sense of style – she was very 1950's, golden dancing shoes and scarlet lipstick. My mum was a 1970's woman – hair, flares, the lot.

HOW AWARE WERE YOU GROWING UP OF BODY IMAGE AND BEAUTY?

Not so much – I was really into music – Northern soul and Rockabilly – so for me it was more about style and look than how my own body felt. I was happy wearing ski pants and getting on the back of a Lambretta! Media didn't feature much until I was 18 and discovered *Vogue*.

DID YOU HAVE STRONG INFLUENCES ON YOUR EATING PATTERNS GROWING UP?

My mum was a nutritionist and home economist, so I grew up understanding not only things about protein/carbs, but also how to make the perfect béchamel.

WERE YOU HAPPY WITH YOUR IMAGE AS A TEENAGER?

Loved it! I dressed in crazy clothes (made most of them myself), and I really liked causing a bit of a stir. I had a huge blonde quiff at one point and thought I looked the bee's knees!

HOW DO YOU FEEL ABOUT SOCIAL MEDIA TODAY?

My girl really has her feet on the ground – kids are trained from an early age about how to interact online, and what's true, what's fake.

WHAT WOULD YOU TELL YOUR 20-YEAR-OLD SELF AND IS YOUR CONFIDENCE NOW HIGHER?

"You are beautiful. Now. Really."

Lower and higher – lower as I think it's harder to be as confident, harder to 'eat the world', but higher because I am more comfortable in my own skin and don't care so much what people think of me.

DO YOU COMPARE YOURSELF TO OTHER WOMEN?

Not really, I admire women my age who have a great sense of style. I am much less confident than I am perceived to be. I think most people are.

DOES BODY IMAGE AND APPEARANCE MATTER TO YOU NOW?

Not so much. I cared more in my 20s and 30s when I worked in the fashion industry. Now I quite like the look of me.

ANY POINTS IN YOUR LIFE THAT MADE YOU LOOK AFTER YOURSELF MORE?

After having kids, and when I saw 50 on the horizon – which inspired me to write *The Midlife Kitchen* with my great friend Sam.

DO YOU EXERCISE?

Yoga class three times a week, great for flexibility, strength and calming the mind.

YOUR ATTITUDE TO NUTRITION?

I am currently having a year of vegetarianism, and it makes you expand your repertoire of cooking. I know enough about nutrition to generally make the 'right' choices. But I do have a soft spot for cake.

WHAT CHANGES HAVE YOU NOTICED SINCE 40?

I have a few crow's feet, which I actually love. A certain softness creeps in.

HOW DO YOU FEEL EMOTIONALLY ABOUT THE PASSING YEARS?

I want to embrace ageing, not fight it. Fairly happy.

WHAT IS YOUR OPINION ON THE MORE INTERVENTIONAL BEAUTY TREATMENTS?

I think it's up to the individual.

HAVE YOU EVER HAD ANY BEAUTY DISASTERS?

My skin came up in a rash after I used a BB cream.

BEAUTY PRODUCTS

Decleor Hydrating Milk SPF 30, By Terry Baume de Rose lip balm, Pantene 3-minute miracle conditioner

SUPPLEMENTS

Occasional vitamin B-complex, Glucosamine, Omega-3 capsules

RUBY HAMMER MBE, 57

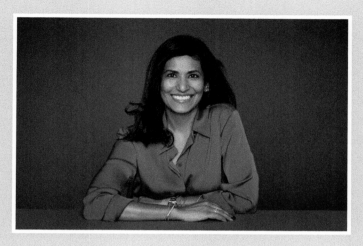

International Makeup Artist, Brand Creator, Consultant and Ambassador. She has done extensive work on photographic shoots around the world, editorial work and also regularly makes speeches and give motivational talks. www.rubyhammer.com including a capsule collection of beauty essentials.

"I did an Economics degree. I thought I would probably go on to work in the UN and work for the diplomatic core. Years later a friend needed an extra pair of hands as a makeup artist and then my career started from there."

MAIN ROLE MODELS

My mum, who died in 2012. My parents were from Bangladesh. We lived in Nigeria until I was 12 then we came to England.

Mum was always fashionable. It was hard to obtain beauty products in Nigeria, and when Dad (a doctor) travelled to England he returned with beauty products for Mum. She was always very glamorous. I remember being fascinated by everything she did. Once I wound her lipstick right up and in the heat it snapped off! Mum was so cross! Years later, I used to give her loads of make-up and products – she said she felt so guilty for having told me off that day!

My father was a very dignified man and my mother very social. If someone was ill, she would cook for them, she could socialise with people of all backgrounds and she had such amazing qualities. My father had such gravitas and they were such a unique couple.

My mum's sister, Aunt Bella, who worked in the United Nations, showed me how exciting entertaining and hospitality could be.

HOW AWARE WERE YOU GROWING UP OF BODY IMAGE AND BEAUTY?

I was skinny but did not understand how advantageous it was to be skinny and wondered if anyone would ever find me attractive. In 1976 we visited America. I received the first positive attention for my appearance. As my confidence grew my personality developed and I realised someone would love me and not just for my looks.

DID YOU HAVE STRONG INFLUENCES ON YOUR EATING PATTERNS GROWING UP?

Mum was curvy, occasionally on diets but never imposed them on us and always cooked fantastic meals. I had two sporty brothers. There was never any negative projection about food.

WERE YOU HAPPY WITH YOUR IMAGE AS A TEENAGER?

Yes, and loved make-up from 14. At 16, I had a Saturday job to get the discount on make-up! I then worked at Harrods in the clothes department to get the clothes discount! I used to do bonkers looks with makeup! If we were going out, my friends would do my hair and I would do our makeup.

WHAT WOULD YOU TELL YOUR 20-YEAR-OLD SELF AND IS YOUR CONFIDENCE NOW HIGHER?

"Prioritise exercise!"

Higher except for my body! Since menopause, 'the belly that I never had before'. I know it would disappear with exercise.

DOES BODY IMAGE AND APPEARANCE MATTER TO YOU NOW?

I see beautiful people at work. I am part of the process that creates the illusion of that image. I have worked with all the supermodels, Victoria's Secret, etc. and when I was younger in a photo next to one I could have been like them. But you make the best of yourself and don't compare. The models know *you will make them feel good being with you and that you are not envious of them.*

I see how hard they work to maintain their figure when we are all going home or going out. They are like mini athletes!

ANY POINTS IN YOUR LIFE THAT MADE YOU LOOK AFTER YOURSELF MORE?

Mum died from lung cancer. I then had a cough for three months and had scans. That was all fine in the end but we have made a pact in our family – if there is *anything* we are worried about we get it checked straight away.

EXERCISE

Our personal trainer often trains my husband who is far more enthusiastic than me; they try to get me to go out with them! I always have excuses.

NUTRITION

As much organic as possible but I am not obsessed, always fresh.

WHAT CHANGES HAVE YOU NOTICED SINCE 40?

Fine lines, loss of volume and firmness, pigmentation, acne on chin.

HAVE YOU EVER HAD ANY BEAUTY DISASTERS?

I plucked my eyebrows down to one hair in a line!

HOW DO YOU FEEL ABOUT AGEING?

Filming *10 Years Younger* I would ask the doctor about treatments available but I would not be interested in actually going under the knife. Work on your face is accessible but consider it carefully; go to qualified doctors and those that you know have a good understanding of the aesthetic and are recommended. I had Botox years ago, not recently. I think they are much more gentle in approach now.

Life is a journey. There are tough bits, parts that are not fair. With the passing years you hope to deal with these without losing your integrity. I always say sleep on it today. Tomorrow is another day.

SUPPLEMENTS

Vitamin D, B12, Turmeric, Lumity, Viviscal, Symprove

WHAT ARE YOUR BEST BEAUTY PRODUCTS OR TIPS?

There are so many fabulous products, Louise, I think it is better to speak in terms of principles rather than products...

NOTHING BEATS PROPER CLEANSING! You should really know your skin and double cleanse the skin with a proper cleansing product for you, whether that is an oil or whatever. Skin wipes are really only for holidays and emergencies – they just don't do the job.

When you are cleansing give your face a good massage – work the products in.

BUY A SET OF PROPER BRUSHES! You can have all the colour palettes and spend a fortune on make-up, but a decent set of brushes is what will make the difference.

RESEARCH THE PRODUCTS FOR YOU. You need to find what is right for you, not your friend. Go to an expert, try a sample from the beauty counter, don't rush and only invest when you know the product is right for you.

YOUR ROUTINE SHOULD BE A REGIME WITH SOME INDULGENCE. Enjoy the smell of the products and the process. You have one life – make sure you live it.

NOURISH AND HYDRATE THE SKIN. I don't just mean moisturise. For example, I use a serum with hyaluronic acid in it which retains the moisture in the skin. You should use products relevant to you and work on the basis of little and often.

SILK PILLOWCASES and a pillow that helps reduce development of wrinkles. I use Illuminage silk pillowcases and a Nurse Jamie shaped pillow. That really helps protect my skin and the pillowcase protects my skin and also my hair. There is less tugging and distortion of the skin at night this way.

FRICTION MIT IN THE SHOWER. Anything to slough off the dead skin and get rid of the dirt. Then you need to *REPLENISH with some kind of multipurpose balm or oil.* Things like Marula Oil from African Botanics. I especially need a thick balm in winter to prevent cracked heels and so on.

DRY BRUSHING. This is always good but I go through phases of doing it religiously then stop for a while.

LUCY BLENKINSOPP, 57

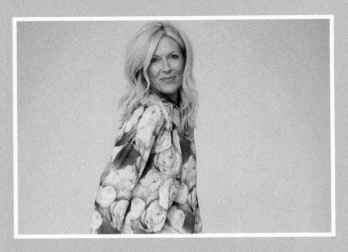

Health, Wellness and Accountability Coach, Yoga Teacher

MAIN ROLE MODELS

My mother was a big influence until I was about 16. She was 40 when she had me, considered pretty old back then. My father owned a couple of hotels and was always busy. Because we had a hotel, my mother never cooked, cleaned or shopped for food, so it was not a traditional childhood. I went to boarding school at 11. There was no health or beauty in our lives, my household was a smoking and drinking environment. I think because Mum served in the war, appearance was not a priority and it was considered quite vain to think about it. I guess I have been the opposite with my children.

HOW AWARE WERE YOU GROWING UP OF BODY IMAGE AND BEAUTY?

I don't remember worrying particularly about my weight or my looks. I have always been confident and self-assured. I loved fashion and always received clothes for Christmas and birthday presents.

DID YOU HAVE STRONG INFLUENCES ON YOUR EATING PATTERNS GROWING UP?

I think my food at school and the hotel was simple and healthy.

WERE YOU HAPPY WITH YOUR IMAGE AS A TEENAGER?

I was secure and pretty popular as a teenager.

HOW DO YOU FEEL ABOUT SOCIAL MEDIA TODAY?

I love it and have so much fun with it. I made many friends and connections, it has certainly changed things up. www.instagram.com/tea.with.lucy.b

WHAT WOULD YOU TELL YOUR 20-YEAR-OLD SELF?

"You don't need someone to complete you. You need to take 100% responsibility for your life and believe in yourself."

DO YOU COMPARE YOURSELF TO OTHER WOMEN?
No.

DOES BODY IMAGE AND APPEARANCE MATTER TO YOU NOW?
It matters enormously that I am fit, healthy, and look and feel good.

ANY POINTS IN YOUR LIFE THAT MADE YOU LOOK AFTER YOURSELF MORE?
When I was 51, I gave up drinking alcohol for six months to learn a 54-page document verbatim, and then after I started drinking again I learned it didn't really suit me so I am teetotal now.

DO YOU EXERCISE?
I am a yoga teacher. I discovered yoga at 49 and went to teachers training at 51 and now, at 57, I teach five or six classes a week and I practise yoga six days a week.

YOUR ATTITUDE TO NUTRITION?
Nutrition is everything. I am a health and wellness coach. I did my training when I was 55 and I believe YOU ARE WHAT YOU EAT!

WHAT CHANGES HAVE YOU NOTICED SINCE 40?
I am still building muscle and flexibility but my skin sags, my neck has changed.

HOW DO YOU FEEL EMOTIONALLY ABOUT THE PASSING YEARS?
My 50s have possibly been my happiest decade. Sometimes I look in the mirror and can't believe how I got here! I am fit and healthy, so I am extremely content about the passing years.

FAVOURITE BEAUTY PRODUCTS
Water, rosehip oil

SUPPLEMENTS
Various algae, Curcumin, Vitamins D & B12, protein powder, Maca powder

EILEEN WILLETT, 53
NANCY ZEFFMAN, 51

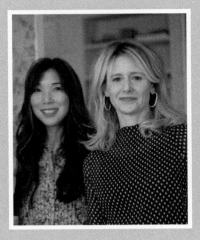

Founders of www.cucumberclothing.com

Eileen trained as a Fashion Illustrator (BFA in Illustration, University of San Francisco) and became Assistant to Head of Menswear Nicole Farhi before having three children. She started accessory brand Wada Bags working as a designer-maker before co-founding **Cucumber Clothing**.

Nancy worked in advertising (Saatchi & Saatchi) before children. She volunteered at Citizen's Advice Bureau and Beanstalk (reading in schools) before co-founding **Cucumber Clothing**.

EILEEN

INTERESTS
Drawing, sewing, writing, beading, crochet, reading, wild swimming, yoga

MAIN ROLE MODELS
My mother always, despite now at 93 her being fairly infirm and suffering from the effects of dementia. Her endless patience, graciousness, sunny personality and desire for honesty and kindness has coloured my view of life in a very positive way. As the child of first-generation Japanese Canadians, she was determined for me to be accomplished and demure so I could become the perfect wife. This may seem bizarre and old-fashioned (and I know

I have fallen short of the mark!), but her emphasis on kindness and graciousness has only ever had a positive effect on me.

My paternal aunt, who was the diametric opposite. Startlingly chic, from an elite Tokyo family, I was fascinated by her gorgeous clothes, her makeup bag full of delicious-looking cosmetics and her air of non-Canadian sophistication. I wanted her wardrobe! At that time every magazine was full of Farrah Fawcett types: tall, tanned, leggy and blonde. To be short and dark strayed far from the then ideal. I still give my hair a bit of a tong to put some Californian wave into it! I began experimenting with punk/ new wave/New Romantics looks in my mid-teens, heavily influenced by the music scene; once I arrived at university I joined a sorority which was all about straight-leg jeans, pleated skirts and Alice bands. Throughout I was obsessed with fashion trends, beauty and style.

HOW AWARE WERE YOU GROWING UP OF BODY IMAGE AND BEAUTY?

Very, in an unfocussed way as a young girl. This became a laser-sharp focus as a teenager.

DID YOU HAVE STRONG INFLUENCES ON YOUR EATING PATTERNS GROWING UP?

My parents. As children of war-era parents, we grew up with the phrase: 'One rice grain could grow a field of rice.' My mother was an early proponent of organic food and healthy balanced diets.

WERE YOU HAPPY WITH YOUR IMAGE AS A TEENAGER?

Absolutely not. Fitting in meant being 'WASPY' and sporty.

WHAT WOULD YOU TELL YOUR 20-YEAR-OLD SELF AND IS YOUR CONFIDENCE NOW HIGHER?

"Stop procrastinating!" My self-confidence is much higher now, mainly because I know myself better.

DOES BODY IMAGE AND APPEARANCE MATTER TO YOU NOW?

In my youth, a lot of emphasis was placed on appearance: looks and manner. I have to confess I find this impossible to shrug off. I reckon to the end of my days I will be applying lipstick and eyeing up dresses!

ANY POINTS IN YOUR LIFE THAT MADE YOU LOOK AFTER YOURSELF MORE?

A family tragedy left me with a large void of time. Hard physical exercise helped fill that space.

DO YOU EXERCISE?

Running, wild swimming, hot yoga or cardio six days a week. I embrace it. I am stronger than I have ever been. Exercise keeps me mentally and physically well.

YOUR ATTITUDE TO NUTRITION?

A bit faddy, hopefully based on sensible knowledge. I still want to lose that last five pounds!

I see a nutritionist, physio and osteopath as and when needed.

WHAT CHANGES HAVE YOU NOTICED SINCE 40?

Ah, too many: gravity taking its toll, hair turning grey, faster weight gain and more difficulty in shaking it, a few wrinkles, bags under the eyes, pigmentation.

HOW DO YOU FEEL EMOTIONALLY ABOUT THE PASSING YEARS?

Reaching the half-century mark does make you think. I embrace the fact I am at a stage in life when after many years of raising a family and juggling work and life, I have more emotional time and space to once again focus on my own hopes and ambitions, both personal and professional.

WHAT IS YOUR OPINION ON THE MORE INTERVENTIONAL BEAUTY TREATMENTS?

As long as this is done safely, with good advice, I'm all for it. At the moment I've had some laser for hyperpigmentation (a real problem for Asian skin) but nothing else – yet. I believe, in the next decade or so, these sorts of interventional 'tweakments' will become as pedestrian as having a manicure or your hair coloured.

TOP FIVE BEAUTY PRODUCTS

111skin serum, Chantecaille China Rose Lip Chic, Origins clay mask, facial oils, Erborian BB cream

SUPPLEMENTS

Probiotics, Evening Primrose oil, fish oil, Vitamin D

NANCY

INTERESTS
Theatre, reading, cooking, dog walking, Netflix.

MAIN ROLE MODELS
My maternal grandmother. She was super stylish, loved travel and cooking, and we had many days out together swimming, shopping and eating out. She taught me to *look for the best*, from choosing a melon in the supermarket (she would spend ages sniffing the end of each one) to appreciating good food and clothing.

HOW AWARE WERE YOU GROWING UP OF BODY IMAGE AND BEAUTY?
Not very. I was a skinny child. My mother made me have short hair until about 12, which meant the greengrocer called me 'sonny'. It really annoyed me. My best friend was a boy who lived up the road – until I decided I hated boys... I do remember, at about 12, going to a friend's birthday party, which was a beauty contest judged by her older brother and sister. I won and all the 'beautiful' girls (who were tall and already developed) thought it was because the judges were being kind. I didn't really think about it. I remember I was wearing an orange T-shirt with 'sunshine girl' written across it. I also remember walking to school at around 15, discussing with a very clever girl that if we had to choose one thing about ourselves, would we choose being 'pretty' or 'clever'. She chose pretty and I thought that was strange. Looks were never really discussed in our house unless to criticise. I don't remember either of my parents ever saying I looked nice. As a teenager, I would do endless makeovers with my friends with cheap make-up and clothes – my mother was not really interested in either. We never really discussed things like that. I would never have dreamt of trying on anything of hers – clothes or makeup.

DID YOU HAVE STRONG INFLUENCES ON YOUR EATING PATTERNS GROWING UP?
We had meat and two veg style suppers every night and never discussed dieting. We occasionally ate out. So a reasonably healthy diet with no off-limits. After school I would often make myself lots of white toast and Marmite. I loved custard cream biscuits and I remember things like Angel Delight. I never understood my friends having treat cupboards as whatever food was in the house was available. I never thought about 'good' and 'bad' food.

WERE YOU HAPPY WITH YOUR IMAGE AS A TEENAGER?
Generally, I don't remember being unhappy about it. I loved *Jackie* magazine, *Top of the Pops*, *Starsky & Hutch*, etc. I was not very worldly – we didn't really discuss issues of the day at home.

WHAT WOULD YOU TELL YOUR 20-YEAR-OLD SELF? IS YOUR CONFIDENCE NOW HIGHER?
"*Be yourself, enjoy life – time moves quickly. Don't try and please everyone, don't worry about everyone liking you. 'Achievement' or 'success' is different to different people. 'Success' is what makes you happy, not what society tells you it is.*"

DOES BODY IMAGE AND APPEARANCE MATTER TO YOU NOW?
I wish it didn't, but I think I have been conditioned that way. I do want to *look and feel good for my age* and I don't want to put on weight and feel dumpy.

ANY POINTS IN YOUR LIFE THAT MADE YOU LOOK AFTER YOURSELF MORE?
After children, I slowly went up a dress size. My PT (also a nutritionist) put me on a special diet with supplements. I lost the extra weight and feel much better now.

DO YOU EXERCISE NOW?
Dog walking, Pilates, PT, gym, basketball

YOUR ATTITUDE TO NUTRITION?

Mainly healthy at home; going out I eat whatever I like.

WHAT CHANGES HAVE YOU NOTICED SINCE 40?

Lines on forehead and around mouth, jaw slightly dropping. Skin less taught, legs a bit veiny. The list goes on...

HOW DO YOU FEEL EMOTIONALLY ABOUT AGEING?

I feel fine about it. Having a daughter makes you realise how quickly time goes. Not that I like wolf whistling, but there is a moment of realisation that time moves on when you notice that the eyes are on your daughter and not you! As I said, I don't want them looking at either of us...

WHAT DO YOU THINK ABOUT MORE INTERVENTIONAL BEAUTY TREATMENTS?

My grandmother had a facelift in her late 60s. I couldn't really see the difference and never understood why. I hope never to do it, but if it makes you feel better, why not? I think the reasons for surgery run deeper than the surgery itself. I don't feel I should judge other people.

TOP BEAUTY PRODUCTS

Alexandra Soveral facial oil, regular facials

SUPPLEMENTS

Omega-3, Vitamin D with K2 in winter, Osteoban in summer, Great Lakes collagen drink

MARIA GRACHVOGEL, 48

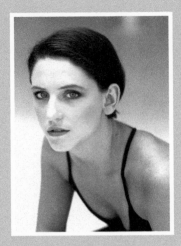

International fashion designer www.mariagrachvogel.com; Instagram @mariagrachvogel

Maria started cutting and sewing clothes aged 10. Her company was established in 1991 and expanded greatly from London Fashion Week 1994 Autumn/Winter.

"I watch a woman try on a garment and see her body language change and she becomes empowered by the clothes. There is a healing process – she is suddenly taller and more elegant. I am very passionate that clothes have a special place in your life and can give you the strength to stand powerful as a woman."

MAIN ROLE MODELS

Mother, aunt, friends. My aunt was immaculately presented, beautifully dressed and gorgeous. I used to stare at her, mesmerised. Our neighbours were Italian and like extended family; we all played board games and they used to let me 'work' in their shop when I was 7! I loved reading about Coco Chanel, *Vogue*, and unlike my friends I already had career aspirations at 12 to have my fashion business. Later on, women like Tracey Woodward and Karen Welman.

HOW AWARE WERE YOU GROWING UP OF BODY IMAGE AND BEAUTY?

In my teens, I was really self-conscious and compared myself to models. I grew extremely fast and was slim. Ironically, now I am heavier but far more comfortable in my own skin. When younger I was really into drawing, painting and climbing trees.

DID YOU HAVE STRONG INFLUENCES ON YOUR EATING PATTERNS GROWING UP?

Mum was always on a diet. Her weight fluctuated and this made me resolve never to diet. I have always had a fast metabolism and do not feel you should deprive yourself of something as you will then crave it. I always listen to my body and its needs.

WERE YOU HAPPY WITH YOUR IMAGE AS A TEENAGER?

My desire to create clothes that flattered me was a great driving force for my career. I do wish I had had more confidence then.

WHAT WOULD YOU TELL YOUR 20-YEAR-OLD SELF AND IS YOUR CONFIDENCE NOW HIGHER?

I do not think I would have listened. My confidence is definitely higher now. I tell my son that life is like a sphere and you have to break through into the 'uncomfortable' to reach the next level.

DO YOU COMPARE YOURSELF TO OTHER WOMEN?

No.

DOES BODY IMAGE AND APPEARANCE MATTER TO YOU NOW?

Not in the same way – I am more into wellbeing than simply external appearance.

DO YOU EXERCISE?

I used to dance, then walking was my main exercise as it fitted neatly into my life. As my studio is so close to home, I have added in a 15-minute HIIT workout three times per week, which has really helped me feel strong as well as fit.

YOUR ATTITUDE TO NUTRITION?

I buy organic and love to eat well but occasionally less healthy – e.g. many croissants in Paris!

WHAT CHANGES HAVE YOU NOTICED SINCE 40?

More wrinkles, grey hair, skin and eyes dryer. My eyes are tired from all the close work!

HOW DO YOU FEEL EMOTIONALLY ABOUT THE PASSING YEARS?

Totally okay with it. I love the wisdom and peace that comes with age.

WHAT IS YOUR OPINION ON THE MORE INTERVENTIONAL BEAUTY TREATMENTS?

Not for me.

HAVE YOU EVER HAD ANY BEAUTY DISASTERS?

At 12 I wanted to look like Prince so had a perm and then my hair fell out leaving a bald patch at the front!

NAME YOUR TOP FIVE BEAUTY PRODUCTS.

Aromatherapy Associates oils, do not use chemicals, a lavender oil containing cleanser, treatment masks at night and most importantly sleep – without it nothing really works!

WHAT DO YOU SEE IN THE FUTURE OF FASHION?

I think it is less designer dictated, now I think the designer's voice resonates with the consumer and this is more a holistic role, not dictatorial. Less is more and we don't need to keep producing. We should become more *conscious* just as with food.

SHAYNE BRODIE, 60

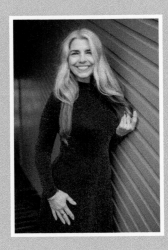

Photo credit Derek Dunlop Photography

Instagram @mssilverlinings; Receptionist for the last 22 years in an advertising agency, and part-time model. Before children, I worked in TV casting for Saatchi & Saatchi.

MAIN ROLE MODELS
My mum was a massive influence, I watched and followed everything she did. She was very clever, funny, beautiful and glamorous. I would thank her for showing me how to be a good parent to my children and a good friend to my friends.

HOW AWARE WERE YOU GROWING UP OF BODY IMAGE AND BEAUTY?
Always very aware.

DID YOU HAVE STRONG INFLUENCES ON YOUR EATING PATTERNS GROWING UP?
When I was 17 my brother became a vegetarian and I decided to try it too, and I haven't eaten meat since.

WERE YOU HAPPY WITH YOUR IMAGE AS A TEENAGER?
Not happy at all.

WHAT WOULD YOU TELL YOUR 20-YEAR-OLD SELF AND IS YOUR CONFIDENCE NOW HIGHER?
"*Don't worry so much, especially don't worry about what other people think.*" In loads of ways it is much higher, and when I look back I wish I had believed in myself more. I still struggle with being a people pleaser.

DO YOU COMPARE YOURSELF TO OTHER WOMEN?
I think I do, but only to women of the same age. I think everyone is more confident than me, but hopefully no one else knows that!

ANY POINTS IN YOUR LIFE THAT MADE YOU LOOK AFTER YOURSELF MORE?
Becoming a single parent – knowing that everything depended on me.

DO YOU EXERCISE?

Zumba – love it – great camaraderie at the class!

YOUR ATTITUDE TO NUTRITION?

I am a vegetarian and really enjoy eating and feeding my children good healthy food. Food is medicine and I try to eat as best I can.

WHAT CHANGES HAVE YOU NOTICED SINCE 40?

Eye bags – wrinkles – and as of a couple of weeks ago those horrid lines around the mouth – argh! I didn't really notice much change until I was about 55 then most days saw something else that wasn't there the day before. "Old age ain't no place for sissies," as Bette Davis once said.

HOW DO YOU FEEL EMOTIONALLY ABOUT THE PASSING YEARS?

I honestly wasn't bothered until recently, but now I am starting to realise that my life is changing and I am not like I always was in some ways. A bit flat, things are changing very quickly. I have just been made redundant after 22 years, and having to go out looking for work at the age of 60 is pretty scary; I am trying to see it as a great opportunity but it's not always easy.

WHAT IS YOUR OPINION ON THE MORE INTERVENTIONAL BEAUTY TREATMENTS?

Don't really have much of an opinion – I've never had anything done, hardly ever had a facial, but never say never... If it makes you happy, why not?

BEAUTY PRODUCTS

Kiehl's Midnight Recovery oil when I can afford it.

SUPPLEMENTS

I have been diagnosed with Vitamin C deficiency and I am often anaemic so take iron.

SUZY READING, 41

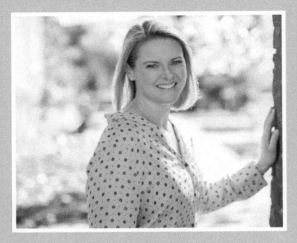

Psychologist and published author. Suzy learned first-hand the transformative power of her now special interest, self-care, when motherhood coincided with the terminal illness of her father. Previously also personal trainer, yoga teacher and health coach. See www.suzyreading.co.uk for more of Suzy's work and links to her books. You can find her on Instagram and Twitter at @suzyreading, and her Facebook page is Suzy Reading: Psychology and Yoga.

MAIN ROLE MODELS

My mother – she lends her calm abiding centre to many and I am grateful to her for her equanimity and for encouraging me to nourish myself. I watched my mum support my father running his psychiatric practice, and loved that so many of his clients would come early for appointments just to have time with her too. In addition to full-time work she drove me to ice skating at 5am six days a week! In retirement I saw her blossom and admired her ability to find a way to make a meaningful contribution. This has shown me how to carve a life imbued with purpose. People often think I have followed my father's career but it's my mum's soothing toolkit that I draw on in my professional life. She has instilled in me the capacity to love and be loved, to care for and facilitate others in their aspirations. One of my favourite mantras is 'I am safe. I am loved. I am held.' I learnt this on a cellular level from my mum.

INTERESTS

Being in nature.

HOW AWARE WERE YOU GROWING UP OF BODY IMAGE AND BEAUTY?

Acutely aware of beauty growing up on the beaches of Australia but at the same time I've always felt a deep appreciation for function over form. As a competitive figure skater, body image was also an integral part of performance.

Dolly magazine and obsessions over Alison Brahe... The image of women in the media definitely created the pressure to be slim.

DID YOU HAVE STRONG INFLUENCES ON YOUR EATING PATTERNS GROWING UP?

My father was a pioneering psychiatrist who advocated for healthy lifestyle choices as an integral part of nourishing mental health. I've always understood that we need to eat for our mood and mental clarity. As an athlete I also appreciated I needed to fuel my body to perform.

WERE YOU HAPPY WITH YOUR IMAGE AS A TEENAGER?

I used to rue my figure skater's thighs... Looking back I had a rocking figure, which now reminds me to check in with what my future grey-haired self would say about my current physical manifestation!

WHAT WOULD YOU TELL YOUR 20-YEAR-OLD SELF AND IS YOUR CONFIDENCE NOW HIGHER?

"Oh darling, throw yourself a bone. Be kind, be tender, be gentle on yourself. You have so much to offer, just get clear on your strengths and unique purpose and things will blossom. Also, there is so much more time than you think!" I'm quite happy with where I am right now. I do wish I had the toolkit I have now when I was 20!

DOES BODY IMAGE AND APPEARANCE MATTER TO YOU NOW?

I am more interested in feeling well nourished. Feeling good is the priority but looking good is part of it. Nothing indulgent about choosing an outfit that fills you with zest. There's no separation between mind and body so when it comes to health, *we need to nurture all layers of our being.*

ANY POINTS IN YOUR LIFE THAT MADE YOU LOOK AFTER YOURSELF MORE?

Motherhood colliding with my father's terminal illness... and my ensuing energetic bankruptcy. I honed my self-care toolkit in clawing my way back to vitality.

DO YOU EXERCISE?

Walking, yoga, gym, running

YOUR ATTITUDE TO NUTRITION?

I eat well to fuel my body, to feed my mind and mental clarity.

WHAT CHANGES HAVE YOU NOTICED SINCE 40?

A little softer around the middle. I've created two people! Hello facial lines... care of sleeplessness and toddler tantrums!

HOW DO YOU FEEL EMOTIONALLY ABOUT THE PASSING YEARS?

I want to preserve my youth with healthy choices but I'm not afraid of ageing. I'm all for savouring the joy of each chapter of life and expressing gratitude for the unique gifts they bring.

HOW DO YOU FEEL ABOUT THE MORE INTERVENTIONAL BEAUTY TREATMENTS?

My friends and I are not having these but if it boosts confidence and is non-harming, why not?

HAVE YOU EVER HAD A BEAUTY DISASTER?

Bruising from an inexperienced waxer... a traumatic experience!

BEAUTY PRODUCTS
Neom facial cleanser balm

SUPPLEMENTS
Magnesium oil spray to promote better sleep.

SALLY BLOOMFIELD, 52

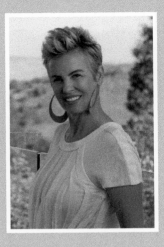

Owner of Bloomfield Hotel in Bali, motivational speaker, soon to be author. Star of *Real Housewives of Melbourne* Season 4. Formerly the Melbourne Editor of *Harper's Bazaar*

MAIN ROLE MODELS

My mum has always been a major role model for me. She always worked and a lot of her friends had really interesting jobs and I aspired to be like them. Women in the workforce was not a foreign thing for me. I admire women all over the world who are juggling families and jobs and just doing what they love to do. I do admire strong women in the public eye; the critics can be harsh, as I know from personal experience being on *Housewives*.

HOW AWARE WERE YOU GROWING UP OF BODY IMAGE AND BEAUTY?

I was lucky that I was slim growing up. I could eat anything, stay up late, party hard and never seemed to suffer. My English mum has the most beautiful skin so I was lucky to inherit this. Life back then was 'fat free' and now we all know that was a huge mistake and false information.

I was always strong and had my own mind. When I was little I loved watching Mum do her hair and makeup; she would let me put on some lipstick and blush. I always knew her and Dad were going out if I could smell her perfume throughout the house. She was and still is an absolute natural beauty.

DID YOU HAVE STRONG INFLUENCES ON YOUR EATING PATTERNS GROWING UP?

My parents were both great cooks and quite ahead of their time. I remember Mum doing cordon bleu and Madame Wivine de Stoop cooking courses, and of course we reaped the benefits in our home. All my friends were having chip rolls at school but Mum would give me pate and lettuce sandwiches – not such a popular choice to swap with anyone! We were never into a lot of processed foods; a big treat to us was lemonade!

WERE YOU HAPPY WITH YOUR IMAGE AS A TEENAGER?

I was pretty confident. I never really had any body issues and never really did much exercise other than school sports. I did have big boobs, which I absolutely hated, but of course was quite popular with all the boys!

WHAT WOULD YOU TELL YOUR 20-YEAR-OLD SELF AND IS YOUR CONFIDENCE NOW HIGHER?

Nothing! That is the whole point of growing up and figuring it out for yourself! Maybe I would have said keep those MC Hammer pants as they will make a huge comeback! There is something to be said for age and wisdom! Confidence is currently at an all-time high!

DO YOU COMPARE YOURSELF TO OTHER WOMEN?

I think I more admire other women of all ages, rather than compare myself. I am confident in some ways and clearly I don't have it all but I do think that people think I am way more confident than I am, which can be good and bad.

DOES BODY IMAGE AND APPEARANCE MATTER TO YOU NOW?

I know that I am happier and more confident when I am taking care of myself. I try not to drink during the week and eat pretty healthily. We all have different ideas about what our ideal is but living an unhealthy lifestyle just doesn't cut it anymore. We have at our fingertips so many choices that it is hard to ignore them anymore.

ANY POINTS IN YOUR LIFE THAT MADE YOU LOOK AFTER YOURSELF MORE?

The diagnosis of my husband and his subsequent death. This would be a huge reason to take better care of myself, not only for me but my boys. It took me on a journey of nutrition and health that changed my life forever.

DO YOU EXERCISE?

I do strength training each week, along with two Pilates classes and try to do two to three walks of about 6 km.

YOUR ATTITUDE TO NUTRITION?

I think after all these years I know how to feed my body for maximum health. I don't believe in crazy dieting, I think it is a way of life that you should strive

to achieve. I am a little up and down in this area, especially due to Ian being sick and opening the hotel in Bali and filming the show; trying to keep a healthy diet and beauty routine has sometimes been a challenge but I feel I'm getting better and better at it.

WHAT CHANGES HAVE YOU NOTICED SINCE 40?

My shape has changed after having kids, things don't seem to bounce back as much as they used to. I have come to terms with the changes though and I understand that I will never be that way again; I am a slightly different me and I am okay with that.

HOW DO YOU FEEL EMOTIONALLY ABOUT THE PASSING YEARS?

I think I now feel at my most confident and self-aware point in life. As you get older you care less about the trivial things in life and focus on everyone just being happy and healthy.

WHAT IS YOUR OPINION ON THE MORE INTERVENTIONAL BEAUTY TREATMENTS?

I have had a little Botox and fillers over the last few years and it makes me feel good and, in my opinion, look a little better... I feel it is each to their own, unless they look like they have re-entered the Earth's atmosphere. Not a big fan!

HAVE YOU EVER HAD ANY BEAUTY DISASTERS?

I once tried to correct my mouth, which turns down when I am concentrating, so had Botox to freeze the muscles but instead it just gave me this odd deranged smile!

NAME YOUR TOP FIVE BEAUTY PRODUCTS.

Lumity Life (capsules and oil), Crème de La Mer if I am spoiling myself, Girl Undiscovered – I love all their natural products, Lacura by Aldi day and night cream and By Terry concealer foundation stick.

SUPPLEMENTS

A company called Organixx for their Bone Broth Protein powder and supplements.

TANYA ROSE, 52

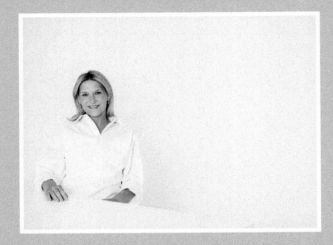

Founder of Mason Rose. Sales, marketing and PR for privately owned 5 star hotels. Established 25 years. www.masonrose.com

"I started my career at the Saint James club in Paris doing everything – chambermaid, restaurant hostess, reservations, and then as a receptionist. After a year the owner of the hotel gave me my opportunity to set up their Paris sales and marketing office. I then came back to the UK and was Head of Sales & Marketing for The Savoy Group for six years."

MAIN ROLE MODELS

My mother. If I can be half as good a mother as she, my life would be complete. My ballet teacher Rosemary Wood who was a taskmaster, but the discipline she installed in us (I danced ballet seriously until I was 14) was invaluable.

My grandmother was an exceptionally strong woman and a great source of love and strength.

INTERESTS

I am on the board of the English National Ballet and I am head of their fundraising campaign. I am also on the board of my old school, Gordonstoun, and The Almeida Theatre .

HOW AWARE WERE YOU GROWING UP OF BODY IMAGE AND BEAUTY?

I was extremely fit and skinny as a teenager as I did gymnastics and ballet for four hours a day. Now that I am going through the menopause this is no longer the case!!

DID YOU HAVE STRONG INFLUENCES ON YOUR EATING PATTERNS GROWING UP?

I ate what I wanted, as I did so much exercise. My mother is a fabulous cook so we always ate very well.

WERE YOU HAPPY WITH YOUR IMAGE AS A TEENAGER?

Very happy. My sister was much more beautiful but it never worried me, as I always had my share of handsome boyfriends and was happy with my own image!

WHAT WOULD YOU TELL YOUR 20-YEAR-OLD SELF AND IS YOUR CONFIDENCE NOW HIGHER?

"If you can dream it you can do it." (Walt Disney)

No, I am delighted that I am the age I am now. I have a wonderful husband, son and family and a thriving business. I am doing everything that I want to be doing and I am extremely grateful to the universe for this.

DO YOU COMPARE YOURSELF TO OTHER WOMEN?

I love all strong women, young and old. I have many mentors that I look up to. I try to mentor younger interns that we have at my company.

ANY POINTS IN YOUR LIFE THAT MADE YOU LOOK AFTER YOURSELF MORE?

Menopause was a trigger to look at how to combat the symptoms.

DO YOU EXERCISE?

10,000 steps every day and train once a week with Jenni Rivett. I should do more but it is hard to fit it all in.

YOUR ATTITUDE TO NUTRITION?

I know I should not eat white carbs! Not always easy when you have a busy day and are lacking energy!

WHAT CHANGES HAVE YOU NOTICED SINCE 40?

Lines on forehead, but my mother and grandmother have great skin so I am hoping that is genetic. I have put on three stone since going through the menopause but am on my way back down again.

HOW DO YOU FEEL EMOTIONALLY ABOUT THE PASSING YEARS?

Happy; I am a secure and emotionally sound person.

WHAT IS YOUR OPINION ON THE MORE INTERVENTIONAL BEAUTY TREATMENTS?

Whatever people are comfortable doing.

HAVE YOU EVER HAD ANY BEAUTY DISASTERS?

I permed and peroxided my hair at 18. I looked like an Afghan hound dog!

BEAUTY PRODUCTS

Creme de la Mer, Eve Lom, Aromatherapy Associates oils, Ila bath salts and body oil.

SUPPLEMENTS

Multivitamin, Vitamin D, Magnesium, DHEA

DR HOLLY WHELAN, 49

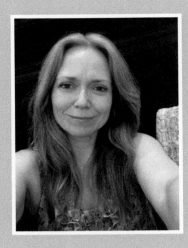

Co-founder www.youngerlives.com, BSc in Biology and PhD in Neuroscience. Holly has worked extensively in consumer health and wellness. Honorary Lecturer at Imperial College.

MAIN ROLE MODELS

I was brought up to believe I could do anything by my father. My self-image was about being an intelligent, independent thinker.

HOW INFLUENCED WERE YOU BY THE MEDIA?

Just probably to become aware of trends, and I remember the fat shaming ethos of the '80s.

HOW AWARE WERE YOU GROWING UP OF BODY IMAGE AND BEAUTY?

As an overweight child my body confidence was affected. I remember my primary school headmaster calling me 'fat' after a weigh-in. I hated clothes shopping as things didn't fit. I wore glasses from 7, and by 13 I wore contact lenses, so clearly I cared enough to want contacts! My best friend and I both had body issues when we were younger, but grew in confidence together trying things out. I have always loved my long hair which I always saw as my crowning glory. As a teenager I grew thinner and gained confidence. My friends influenced me and we tried SunIn spray, metallic lipstick and perms!

DID YOU HAVE STRONG INFLUENCES ON YOUR EATING PATTERNS GROWING UP?

My mother was a great cook but the portions were large. I bought sweets after school and I had a lot of fillings as a child. My mother was constantly dieting. My father was healthy in attitude and weight.

WERE YOU HAPPY WITH YOUR IMAGE AS A TEENAGER?

No, but it didn't hold me back in friendships or achievements. Self-confidence in my academic work and music helped.

WHAT WOULD YOU TELL YOUR 20-YEAR-OLD SELF AND IS YOUR CONFIDENCE NOW HIGHER?

"Self-confidence is sexy. Try things out and be a bit more daring as you have the youth to carry things off and make mistakes." In your 20s the ambitious treadmill to achieve the next goal – promotion, marriage – can make you lose sight of who you are. My confidence is higher now.

DO YOU COMPARE YOURSELF TO OTHER WOMEN?

I compare myself to all sorts of people and find older vibrant women extremely inspirational – Julia Dreyfus, Helen Mirren.

DOES BODY IMAGE AND APPEARANCE MATTER TO YOU NOW?

In my work I need to be a bit of a poster child for a healthy and happy lifestyle. I believe a lot of how you look and are perceived is about your personal energy and approach. I think just aesthetics do not cut it unless you are a model. Attractiveness is the entire package – look, energy, approach.

ANY POINTS IN YOUR LIFE THAT MADE YOU LOOK AFTER YOURSELF MORE?

Leaving home, travel, having children made me start to really realise the importance of self-care whilst caring for others. My marriage breakdown made me embrace positive thinking as the way to cope.

DO YOU EXERCISE?

Exercise videos (HIIT, Rebounding) three times a week. I live in London and don't own a car so aim for 10,000 steps daily. I love walking with my partner and children.

YOUR ATTITUDE TO NUTRITION?

The Mediterranean diet – so delicious and perfect for sharing. My issue is avoiding binge eating with stress (chocolate and cheese)!

WHAT CHANGES HAVE YOU NOTICED SINCE 40?

Sagging of jawline. A few lines. Cellulite. Having to colour my hair regularly. I had early onset cataracts but had surgery to replace my lenses. I need reading glasses which makes me feel old.

HOW DO YOU FEEL EMOTIONALLY ABOUT THE PASSING YEARS?

Happy in some ways but with awareness of the physical impacts, and I try to counter that. I am a strong believer in mental state and, as my father says, you start to seem old when you lose sharpness, get frightened of life and lose curiosity. I see lots of really inspirational older people around me. Old age can be joyful and full of discovery.

WHAT IS YOUR OPINION ON THE MORE INTERVENTIONAL BEAUTY TREATMENTS?

I am frightened, I would not want to look unnatural. If there were a treatment to discreetly sort my jawline I probably would do it!

HAVE YOU EVER HAD ANY BEAUTY DISASTERS?

As a teenager I permed and bleached my hair which made it break off at the roots!

BEAUTY PRODUCTS

Micellar water, moisturiser with sunscreen – tinted and untinted (No7 Protect & Perfect)

SUPPLEMENTS

No, I really have issues with the supplement market as it is so unregulated.

LINDA SULLIVAN, 63

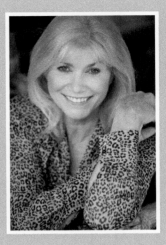

Model and make-up artist www.lindasullivanmakeupartist.com. Previously in a senior role in telecom sales, Linda quit this job to train to be a makeup artist in her mid-50s in a class of 20-year-olds. She regularly appears in TV and editorial work.

MAIN ROLE MODELS
Mum used to put on her makeup with powder and rouge. I used to see the transformation with her lipstick.

HOW AWARE WERE YOU GROWING UP OF BODY IMAGE AND BEAUTY?
I was very aware. I loved fashion and was aware of what could be achieved with makeup. I remember the green eyebrow!

I loved Penelope Tree, Twiggy, Faye Dunaway, Olivia Newton-John.

DID YOU HAVE STRONG INFLUENCES ON YOUR EATING PATTERNS GROWING UP?
Mother was an appalling cook but made the best pastry in the land. Food was not too much of a thing but we had a good Sunday roast. I was skinny as a child naturally and only started putting on weight in my late 30s.

WERE YOU HAPPY WITH YOUR IMAGE AS A TEENAGER?
I was happy once I left school. I did not feel pretty at school.

WHAT WOULD YOU TELL YOUR 20-YEAR-OLD SELF AND IS YOUR CONFIDENCE HIGHER NOW?
"Say yes to opportunities." NO. I would like to be 45 again!

DO YOU COMPARE YOURSELF TO OTHER WOMEN?
No, although when modelling I did not think of myself as a proper model. I don't compare but I do appreciate beauty in other women.

I don't think anyone is truly confident about everything – at work I think women think there is always someone prettier, thinner, etc.

DOES BODY IMAGE AND APPEARANCE MATTER TO YOU NOW?

Appearance matters a lot to me. I am still coming to terms with being a stone over where I want to be in weight. I wish I had protected my hands more.

DO YOU EXERCISE?

Gym three times a week, weightbearing exercise to prevent osteoporosis.

YOUR ATTITUDE TO NUTRITION?

Don't exclude carbs at breakfast, occasional sweet things, no pasta or rice, lots of vegetables.

WHAT CHANGES HAVE YOU NOTICED SINCE 40?

Not much until 55 – lines on face. Suddenly!

HOW DO YOU FEEL EMOTIONALLY ABOUT THE PASSING YEARS?

I'm not keen on the physical manifestations of age, but I'm enjoying the peace of mind and confidence it brings.

WHAT IS YOUR OPINION ON THE MORE INTERVENTIONAL BEAUTY TREATMENTS?

Any surgery that isn't clinically necessary is out of the question for me. For needles, if you iron out one area of the face there is a knock-on effect elsewhere. I've tried and had mixed feelings about it. Many of the mature models I work with have it and on screen it looks great but not always in real life.

BEAUTY PRODUCTS

Elemis skincare, Look Fabulous Forever primer and eye primer, Armani Luminous silk foundation, powder by Terry, LVL eyelash treatment, Elemis Gentle Rose Exfoliator

LINDA SULLIVAN, 63

MELANIE CANTOR, 62

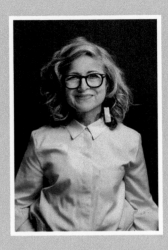

Melanie's first novel *Death and Other Happy Endings* was published June 2019. Prior to this she was an agent to several celebrities, including Melanie Sykes and Ulrika Jonsson.

MAIN ROLE MODELS

My mother was definitely my primary role model although I'm much more open-minded. She was classic war generation: very strong, not overtly emotional yet loving. Her own mother had MS from the age of 30. My mother was eight by the time her mother was crippled from the waist down so became a carer when she was very young. I think that made her stiff upper lip. She didn't like public shows of emotion but became much warmer in her old age! She was a very bright, engaging woman, always elegantly dressed, a great hostess who loved holding dinner parties. She had a wonderful circle of friends but didn't take any prisoners. She loved girly things without being girly and she loved interiors. Every five years she would redecorate our house hence I love the smell of fresh paint. One of the things we enjoyed together was the House & Garden exhibition which we went to over a period of 12 years. The last couple, I

had to push her round in a wheelchair but she wouldn't have missed it for the world. I can't go there anymore because it's too associated with her. My mother died on holiday with me in Cyprus. She was stoical until the end. I think she made me the strong, resilient person I am but I hope I've softened quicker than she did. She was very proud. I think that was something that war generation claimed.

HOW AWARE WERE YOU GROWING UP OF BODY IMAGE AND BEAUTY? DID YOU HAVE STRONG INFLUENCES ON EATING PATTERNS GROWING UP?

I was very aware of body image but somehow feel that was inbuilt. I was aware my mother was very pretty. When I think back to myself as a child, I'm amazed I was so aware when I had good and bad days. I'm lucky in that for most of my life I've been slim. My mother on the other hand was always on a diet. She was a curvy woman, a different shape from me, but she was never satisfied even if you told her she looked great. She always thought she was overweight despite the extra pounds suiting her. She certainly wasn't what I would describe as fat. Maybe her constant dieting made me hate the notion. I've learned to eat in moderation although I'm no saint and have binge days. I'm very aware of the hazards of being overweight so it makes me vigilant with my sons.

WERE YOU HAPPY WITH YOUR IMAGE AS A TEENAGER?

Not unhappy but probably not happy enough. I think we all look back at our younger selves and say, why didn't I realise I was fine?

WHAT WOULD YOU TELL YOUR 20-YEAR-OLD SELF AND IS YOUR CONFIDENCE NOW HIGHER?

I would tell that 20-year-old there would be good and bad moments and I would get through them and not allow either to affect my sense of self-belief or confidence. That I should listen to my intuition and my mother was not always right! That being single is empowering and I should never allow myself to be defined by a relationship, job or another person's perception. My confidence has improved with age and wisdom!

DOES BODY IMAGE AND APPEARANCE MATTER TO YOU NOW?

I care very much about all those things but not for the sake of other people but because it matters *to me*. I am my only judge.

ANY POINTS IN YOUR LIFE THAT MADE YOU LOOK AFTER YOURSELF MORE?

I slipped a disc in my back six years ago. I realised I needed to keep up muscle strength and not get complacent just because I'm slim.

DO YOU EXERCISE?

I used to swim regularly. I wish I still did. Sometimes I get in the habit of doing the seven-minute workout app every morning. I've started yoga but am not committed. Unfortunately, I find exercise boring, but I have a dog in my life now so I walk a lot. Without doubt Mabel has improved my mental and physical states!

YOUR ATTITUDE TO NUTRITION?

I'm a natural healthy eater who has the occasional chocolate/biscuit/pastry binge. I believe in moderation, which sometimes I don't quite manage!

WHAT CHANGES HAVE YOU NOTICED SINCE 40?

At 40 you still look good even if you don't realise it. I'm lucky, my face has aged well, but as soon as I turned 60 my body skin changed due to loss of collagen. Rather a good face though. Clothes hide multiple sins but that's fine by me. I love clothes! Internal atrophying was the worst thing; apparently a classic menopausal symptom. Who knew? I do now so I've started taking HRT.

HOW DO YOU FEEL EMOTIONALLY ABOUT THE PASSING YEARS?

I feel like I'm having my best life now so no complaints.

WHAT IS YOUR OPINION ON THE MORE INTERVENTIONAL BEAUTY TREATMENTS?

I once had filler for the sides of my mouth because friends were doing stuff. Never again! It was a good lesson. I ended up with a massive bruise like I'd been punched in the chin. Plenty of my friends have treatments. Whatever works for you. That said, I'm not keen when it goes too far and you're looking at a clone.

RAE FEATHER, 54

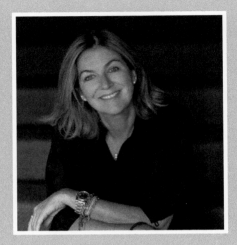

www.raefeather.com. Previously I worked in hospitality and marketing. The Rae Feather online retail lifestyle brand features 'simple things made beautifully' – luxury, monogrammed accessories now recognisable worldwide by the fashion cognoscenti.

MAIN ROLE MODELS

Mother. She was one of 13 children, 9 of them girls. All acted as role models in some shape or form, all naturally beautiful and, as a result, natural in their outlook. They all took great care of themselves but not in any extreme ways. They all wore face cream and some makeup but nothing too extreme. They had a profound effect upon me, especially Mum who continues to keep it real...

HOW AWARE WERE YOU GROWING UP OF BODY IMAGE AND BEAUTY?

When I was young, beauty was not perceived as it is today. I don't believe we were in any way as 'beauty' conscious. My friends and I liked to look good but I don't recall this being a big deal. Makeup consisted of mascara and some lip gloss.

DID YOU HAVE STRONG INFLUENCES ON YOUR EATING PATTERNS GROWING UP?

We ate simply and well. The emphasis of food and health was not nearly as prolific then as it is today... It was more about calories than goodness.

WERE YOU HAPPY WITH YOUR IMAGE AS A TEENAGER?

I was shy and perhaps lacked confidence but overall yes.

WHAT WOULD YOU TELL YOUR 20-YEAR-OLD SELF AND IS YOUR CONFIDENCE NOW HIGHER?

"You are enough."

I am far more comfortable in my skin today. My mind is different. I see the world with more mature eyes and I see that beauty really is in the eye of the beholder.

DO YOU COMPARE YOURSELF TO OTHER WOMEN?

A little. I think this is very natural. I think people perceive me to be more confident than I really am. I think we all have our insecurities and some work harder at hiding them than others.

DOES BODY IMAGE AND APPEARANCE MATTER TO YOU NOW?

It is important; I want to feel good about myself, for me.

DO YOU EXERCISE?

I swim, I walk most days, I spin and I do Pilates religiously once a week.

YOUR ATTITUDE TO NUTRITION?

I like to get my five a day. I like to eat well.

WHAT CHANGES HAVE YOU NOTICED SINCE 40?

My face is more mature! I look after my hair so well, to make allowances for my face! Whereas before a little work went a long way, today a lot of work doesn't go as far!

HOW DO YOU FEEL EMOTIONALLY ABOUT THE PASSING YEARS?

I have questioned my mortality for the first time recently. Want to ensure I leave this world fulfilling all I want to. Be the best mum I can be, a good friend and a good person.

WHAT IS YOUR OPINION ON THE MORE INTERVENTIONAL BEAUTY TREATMENTS?

Totally encourage anyone to do anything that makes them feel better about themselves. I would if I thought it would make me feel better about myself. That is the beauty of age – we should have the confidence to do what is right for us.

BEAUTY PRODUCTS

Guinot Hydrazone Cream, Guinot serum, Kiehl's hand cream

SUPPLEMENTS

MenoSerene, Black Cohosh, Cod Liver oil

URSA CURATOLO, 48

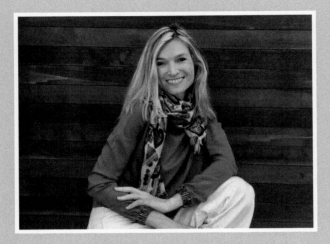

Founder of neweyeonstyle.com. Online personal stylist WISHI.ME www.wishi.me/app/stylist/3fec79cd-0222-11e8-b/profile. Ursa was a Law Graduate from Slovenia, completed a Masters in Austria, moved to Switzerland with her husband and became a private banker. In Seattle she then started as a personal stylist and organised trunk shows while preparing her online store.

MAIN ROLE MODELS

My mother, a textile designer, was my teacher. She taught me appreciation of fashion, which she saw as an art and inspiration to create your own style. She was meticulous about a neat hairdo and outfit. With my mother I learned to appreciate all the charming details I could perceive with the senses. Later I learned from a friend, who was like an older sister. I still only use a dash of pink lipstick or a bit of make-up, just like she showed me, but never leave the house without perfume!

INTERESTS

I redesigned our home interior with inspiration from the Italian style.

HOW AWARE WERE YOU GROWING UP OF BODY IMAGE AND BEAUTY?

I was pretty round as a girl. I didn't really care about my body. In high school, I started being aware of my body as a woman and I became overly sensitive about it.

DID YOU HAVE STRONG INFLUENCES ON YOUR EATING PATTERNS GROWING UP?

When I started high school, I moved in with my father and his wife. I started having problems with my eating habits and eventually developed an eating disorder. My parents never dieted but they took care of their weight. My mother always prepared warm meals, and my aunt cooked for me during college. I had no reason other than insecurity that brought me to have that irrational relationship with food.

WERE YOU HAPPY WITH YOUR IMAGE AS A TEENAGER?

No.

HOW DO YOU FEEL ABOUT SOCIAL MEDIA TODAY?

There is an absurdity of the pressure that comes from those ideal images as they aren't real. Fashion is wrongly judged as a hobby of the rich and labelled as 'superficial'. Young people enjoy taking pride in their appearance. Education in how to dress for confidence is invaluable.

WHAT WOULD YOU TELL YOUR 20-YEAR-OLD SELF AND IS YOUR CONFIDENCE NOW HIGHER?

"Embrace your body and focus on how to highlight your unique self and make it work best for you. It is such a waste of energy trying to be like others."

My confidence is higher. Achievements that come from your own efforts and activities make you confident. *Anything you receive for free does not liberate you of your insecurity.*

DO YOU COMPARE YOURSELF TO OTHER WOMEN?

They are often younger, which is unfair on myself.

DOES BODY IMAGE AND APPEARANCE MATTER TO YOU NOW?

I am an aesthetic with my whole soul, thus stating 'it doesn't matter' would be false, but not for any price.

ANY POINTS IN YOUR LIFE THAT MADE YOU LOOK AFTER YOURSELF MORE?

When I learned about the autoimmune disease I had (CREST syndrome). It took me some time to start living *with it not against it.*

DO YOU EXERCISE?

Dancing, step, weights at the gym.

YOUR ATTITUDE TO NUTRITION?

Too many sweets and carbs. It requires determination to eat healthier.

WHAT CHANGES HAVE YOU NOTICED SINCE 40?

Saggy skin, wrinkles around eyes.

HOW DO YOU FEEL EMOTIONALLY ABOUT THE PASSING YEARS?

I am not indifferent. Being creative can help a lot to keep my mood up and make me FEEL beautiful.

WHAT IS YOUR OPINION ON THE MORE INTERVENTIONAL BEAUTY TREATMENTS?

I tried Botox three times but the results were not as expected, it created circles around my eyes, so I stopped. I never tried fillers. I don't have anything against people doing it; it is a personal decision.

BEAUTY PRODUCTS

Clarins, Dior, Avene, Vichy

NATALIE BANKS, 47

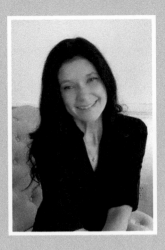

Best-selling novelist. Author of *The Water is Wide*, *The Dark Room*, *The Canary's Song*
www.nataliebanks.net; Instagram @officialnataliebanks; Facebook @NatalieBanksNovels
*"I have been writing since I was 12 years old but was not published until my 40s. I am living
proof that is never too late to pursue your dreams!"*

MAIN ROLE MODELS
My mother, my stepmother Diana, and a friend of
my mother, Mary Lou. My mother influenced me
with how she laughed, cooked, and cared for her
skin. My stepmom was the picture of grace and
unconditional love. Mary Lou taught me how to
look upon others with eyes of love.

INTERESTS
Writing, painting, singing, kayaking, running
and hiking.

HOW AWARE WERE YOU GROWING UP
OF BODY IMAGE AND BEAUTY?
When I was very young, everyone was beautiful
to me. As a teenager, I became more influenced
by television and magazines. These influences
changed the way I looked at others and myself.
In my 30s I realised this was wrong. I heard
about the photo editing and the models starving
themselves. I was able to look and see the beauty
in every woman again.

DID YOU HAVE STRONG INFLUENCES
ON YOUR EATING PATTERNS
GROWING UP?
A close family member was bulimic and self-
critical even though she was thin. I learned to
feel guilty about eating; as I grew older I began
to see the flaw in that way of thinking. Now I eat
whatever I want, within reason.

WERE YOU HAPPY WITH YOUR IMAGE
AS A TEENAGER?
Unhappy and insecure. I never felt good enough
because I held myself to a standard that didn't
exist.

WHAT WOULD YOU TELL YOUR 20-YEAR-OLD SELF AND IS YOUR CONFIDENCE NOW HIGHER?

"Laugh more and don't take life so seriously. MORE moisturiser! MORE sunscreen! Love yourself unconditionally and give yourself a break. Don't stop writing; your passions don't have to come last."

Much higher. I have learned to love myself and be my own best friend.

DO YOU COMPARE YOURSELF TO OTHER WOMEN?

I have in the past when I was worried about ageing but now I have the mindset that my spirit is as young as I choose. I think every single one of us struggles with our self-confidence, no matter the age. I think this time in our life is a difficult one because our roles are changing. The way we see ourselves begins to change and there is a mourning period for our youth. I didn't want this to become my identity, so now I dance more, laugh more, and do everything I can to be beautiful *in my own way*.

DOES BODY IMAGE AND APPEARANCE MATTER TO YOU?

Yes, but differently. I care about how I FEEL about me, rather than what others think about me. If I make changes, they are for me and me only.

ANY POINTS IN YOUR LIFE THAT MADE YOU LOOK AFTER YOURSELF MORE?

Turning 40 got my attention. I got rid of the toxic people, starting saying 'no' more.

DO YOU EXERCISE?

I run, go to the gym and bike, occasional yoga. I blast the music in the living room and dance almost every single day.

YOUR ATTITUDE TO NUTRITION?

I am very health conscious. I try to eat fresh and as healthy as possible. I believe in the 90% rule. As long as I am doing the best I can for my body, there's nothing wrong with a giant order of cheesy fries... or a chocolate bar...

WHAT CHANGES HAVE YOU NOTICED SINCE 40?

I am a fanatic about skincare and water intake, so I don't think I am showing as much in my face as I might have. Muscle tone is looser. Body not quite as flexible.

HOW DO YOU FEEL EMOTIONALLY ABOUT THE PASSING YEARS?

My spirit is still in my 20s. I wish time didn't go so fast. Be as kind as possible (to ourselves and others), live, laugh, learn, and most of all love!

WHAT IS YOUR OPINION ON THE MORE INTERVENTIONAL BEAUTY TREATMENTS?

I wish the younger girls didn't do it because they are comparing themselves to facial tone and lips that just don't exist in the real world.

HAVE YOU EVER HAD ANY BEAUTY DISASTERS?

I had my hair bleached blonde and my hair was breaking off in chunks. I had to get a pixie cut and it didn't grow for years!

BEAUTY PRODUCTS

Eucerin Hyaluron Filler (European version), many products by Dr. Brandt, Atomy Eye Cream, ROC Resurfacing pads weekly, StriVectin Glycolic Peel (once a month)

SUPPLEMENTS

Calcium, Folic Acid, Red Clover, Magnesium, Vitamins E and C

DR JANINE GRAHAM, 46

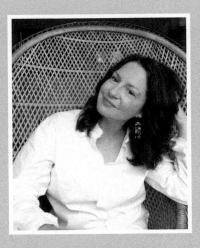

Consultant Medical Oncologist with special interest in melanoma, renal and breast cancer. Clinical Research Lead and Supervisor for trainees.

"I left school at 15 with no qualifications. I trained to be a horse riding instructor and managed a riding school. In my 20s I wanted to become a nurse. After A levels at night school, I did a BSc in Biological Sciences and then trained to be a doctor. I treat patients in both the curative and palliative settings. I have a keen interest in teaching and clinical research."

INTERESTS
Walking, reading, cooking, baking, digital content creation.

MAIN ROLE MODELS
My mother and late grandmother.

My mother taught me to cleanse, tone and moisturise daily. She always had beautiful bottles of perfume on her dressing table, and to this day I remain in love with perfume and the way it can make you feel and the memories it can evoke.

I also worked for a lady (I shall call her LM) when younger who had achieved great things both personally and professionally. I observed her amazing work ethic and achievements; she certainly motivated me to strive for the best and push myself beyond my comfort zone. She was

an amazing cook using organic food grown in her garden, and her love of cooking and creating recipes rubbed off on me.

HOW AWARE WERE YOU GROWING UP OF BODY IMAGE AND BEAUTY?
I was bullied as a child for being small for my age and I was also very thin. I remember wearing lots of layers of tights to make my legs look a bit fatter. I definitely cared about beauty growing up and was keen to maintain a certain image that was groomed and stylish.

HOW INFLUENCED WERE YOU BY THE POPULAR PRESS/TELEVISION/MEDIA?
I was very into music, watching *Top of the Pops* religiously, and followed every fashion trend of

the time and certain people such as Madonna. I remember pop videos being very influential.

DID YOU HAVE STRONG INFLUENCES ON YOUR EATING PATTERNS GROWING UP?

I grew up in a working class family. My parents got divorced when I was little, we didn't have a lot of money, but my mum would make a lot of one-pot meals and soups – potatoes featured a lot! When I was 14 my mother remarried and I went to live with my father. I remember the deep-fat fryer being on most nights. So I wasn't really given examples of healthy eating during my childhood.

WERE YOU HAPPY WITH YOUR IMAGE AS A TEENAGER?

Very self-conscious – always felt I was too thin. I felt top heavy when my breasts began to develop – I remember wearing minimiser bras. On reflection, of course, I wasn't.

WHAT WOULD YOU TELL YOUR 20-YEAR-OLD SELF AND IS YOUR CONFIDENCE NOW HIGHER?

"It's okay to make mistakes because this is how we learn. Don't waste too much time trying to perfect weaknesses. Work on them but work much harder on your strengths and surround yourself with positive people".

DO YOU COMPARE YOURSELF TO OTHER WOMEN?

Yes, usually to women of a similar age.

DOES BODY IMAGE AND APPEARANCE MATTER TO YOU NOW?

I gained a lot of weight after my son's birth. As I began to lose weight I rediscovered my love of fashion and styling. It's important to be happy within yourself. I'm happy in my body and it's just about finding the right styles for your age and body shape.

ANY POINTS IN YOUR LIFE THAT MADE YOU LOOK AFTER YOURSELF MORE?

No, but in work I'm constantly reminded about the results of an unhealthy lifestyle.

DO YOU EXERCISE?

Walking, running at the weekend, gym when on holiday.

YOUR ATTITUDE TO NUTRITION?

I try but at times due to getting busy at work I forget to drink enough water or five portions of fruit and veg. I'm trying very hard to reduce meat consumption and move towards a plant-based diet mainly for the health benefits but also for the planet and the impact on climate change.

WHAT CHANGES HAVE YOU NOTICED SINCE 40?

Jaw softer, forehead and eye wrinkles, top lip thinner. Skin more sensitive. Centripetal weight.

HOW DO YOU FEEL EMOTIONALLY ABOUT THE PASSING YEARS?

I'm not scared of ageing gracefully, it is natural. I have a very stressful job and recently I have been exploring mindfulness as a way of keeping my mind healthy and dealing with stress.

WHAT IS YOUR OPINION ON THE MORE INTERVENTIONAL BEAUTY TREATMENTS?

I'm not judgmental about it, for some people it is the right thing for them. I think if people want to explore these options then I would recommend they do their research first and seek reputable opinions. Being a doctor means that every day I see people with a diagnosis of incurable cancer and this puts things into perspective and makes me remember how important it is to try and live in the moment and be thankful.

JENNI RIVETT, 50s

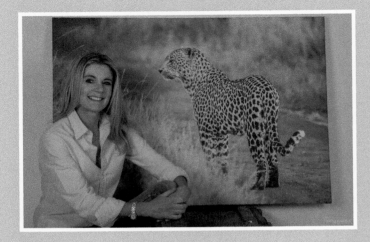

www.jennirivett.com; www.jennirivett-blog.com. Fitness and Nutrition Consultant, specialising in women's health. Former personal trainer to HRH Princess Diana.

"My real passion is strength training and helping women get leaner through correct exercise form. Technique is the number-one factor for me in changing your body shape. I have formulated a dictionary of exercises which are quick, very effective, fun and really get to those 'Mummy bits' us women tend to worry about. I don't believe in heavy weights for women and teach them how to 'switch' their muscles on with very little to no weight at all. My method also includes a very credible HIIT programme and stretching. I advise women on nutrition too and am very into helping them understand how eating healthy and exercising can balance their hormones."

MAIN ROLE MODELS

My mother was the first woman in South Africa to release an exercise 'LP'. She was an absolute inspiration and had the most incredible figure despite having six children. My mum was a great role model but she had her own personal struggles and at times as the eldest daughter I became the carer.

HOW AWARE WERE YOU GROWING UP OF BODY IMAGE AND BEAUTY?

I was pretty aware even though we did not have TV in South Africa. I come from a sporty family so we were always water-skiing, and I was a gymnast and long-distance runner. My mum kept us healthy. I developed a very slight eating disorder in my 20s and I believe this was all part of the influence of the worries of my childhood.

DID YOU HAVE STRONG INFLUENCES ON YOUR EATING PATTERNS GROWING UP?

It was all about meat, veg and potatoes. We did not have the information we have today.

WERE YOU HAPPY WITH YOUR IMAGE AS A TEENAGER?

Pretty happy. We have inherited good genes.

HOW DO YOU FEEL ABOUT SOCIAL MEDIA TODAY?

My daughter is grown up. I feel it is immense pressure for young people.

WHAT WOULD YOU TELL YOUR 20-YEAR-OLD SELF AND IS YOUR CONFIDENCE NOW HIGHER?

"The all or nothing scenario DOES NOT WORK. It is all about balance, and when you go off track – learn to press the DELETE button. Guilt is the worst emotion to have. Your health really is your wealth and do not take it for granted. Laugh more!"

I feel fitter *now* than when I was in my 20s so sometimes I find the age thing awful! I am at my most confident when I am up teaching a class, on a water-ski, or snow skiing.

DO YOU COMPARE YOURSELF TO OTHER WOMEN?

I try not to. I do get a lot of compliments about looking young for my age; sometimes it puts pressure on you to keep trying.

DOES BODY IMAGE AND APPEARANCE MATTER TO YOU NOW?

Nowadays it's more important to feel good, balanced and have all hormones in check and usually this is enough to boost self-esteem. I have always been small and in shape so I guess I would hate it if I couldn't zip up my jeans. Being in your 50s is such a wake-up call. You look great one day when you look in the mirror and bloody awful on another day. I would say I am more concerned with trying to get my face to keep up with my body!

DO YOU EXERCISE?

I've fine-tuned my workouts to be quick and effective. So I try and fit in three 45-minute sessions a week, which include my HIIT training, my 'train like a woman' exercises, five minutes of flexibility and mobility training. Lots of walking in between.

YOUR ATTITUDE TO NUTRITION?

80% of the time I keep myself in check. I have become an intuitive eater and so don't eat much junk. I have a very healthy attitude towards food now and eat quite a lot! I also juice four times a week – beetroot, celery, kale, ginger.

WHAT CHANGES HAVE YOU NOTICED SINCE 40?

More difficult keeping the skin tight! I try and do face exercises.

HOW DO YOU FEEL EMOTIONALLY ABOUT THE PASSING YEARS?

I try to come to terms with it and be the best I can and hopefully be an example to other women.

WHAT IS YOUR OPINION ON THE MORE INTERVENTIONAL BEAUTY TREATMENTS?

Rather go the natural route. Eating well, drinking plenty of water and regular exercise keep you youthful.

TOP BEAUTY PRODUCTS

Tropic range, La Roche-Posay SPF50, Dermalogica Daily Microfoliant, organic virgin cold-pressed coconut oil as make-up remover

SUPPLEMENTS

Multivitamin, Ester C, Pure Arctic Omega-3 Oil, liquid B-complex, Magnesium citrate, Astaxanthin, Vitamin D

KATE TOJEIRO, 48

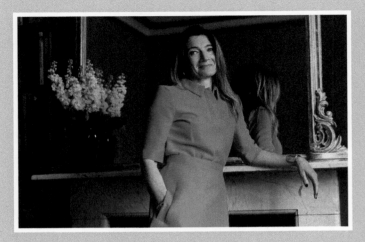

Author of *The Art of Possible – new habits, neuroscience and the power of deliberate action.*
Executive Performance Coach, MD of X fusion, executive coaching and leadership development
consultancy. Trustee for The National Association for Children of Alcoholics (NACOA).
www.katetojeiro.com; Instagram@katetoj #theartofpossible; Twitter @katetoj
*"My passion is enabling others to discover what is possible for them, through encouraging
them to get comfortable with discomfort and take the new, deliberate, different actions that could
change their lives."*

MAIN ROLE MODELS

I admired Joy Adamson, Anne Frank, Karen
Blixen, Angela Rippon and Valerie Singleton. My
English teacher was fantastic and she told us girls
that we could achieve anything and I always read a
lot. We had a babysitter called Aunty Wendy and I
thought she was Wendy from *Peter Pan*! She was
fabulous, the kindest, funniest woman I knew. My
grandmother was very beautiful, introducing me to
moisturiser and the importance of drinking water.
She had amazing skin and always dressed well.
It's definitely down to her that I have a nail polish
obsession! She was a superb cook, she taught us
about the value of fruit and veg in one's diet; she
had a magnificent garden with fruit, vegetables and
flowers which she tended entirely herself.

My childhood was dominated by living with an
alcoholic parent. I believe that some of the difficulties
that played out in my childhood enable me to now use
my voice when others can't. The feeling that you are
somehow lacking as the child of an alcoholic is hard
to shake off. As someone said to me recently, you
hope that you will 'grow out of it'; sadly you don't, but
you can learn how to live with the experiences, for the
better. Hence my work with NACOA.

HOW AWARE WERE YOU GROWING UP OF BODY IMAGE AND BEAUTY?

I always thought I was overweight which I certainly
wasn't. As a young girl, I was blissfully unaware I
think, though I did get bullied because I spoke well.
I was always very particular about how I looked –

perhaps it was part of the façade covering home life. *Girl* magazine every week felt like a friend.

DID YOU HAVE STRONG INFLUENCES ON YOUR EATING PATTERNS GROWING UP?

There was evidence of overeating and undereating in my family. As children we ate well and had no junk food. We were forced to eat some healthy foods that we hated! I still detest marrows and broad beans.

WERE YOU HAPPY WITH YOUR IMAGE AS A TEENAGER?

Happy enough.

WHAT WOULD YOU TELL YOUR 20-YEAR-OLD SELF AND IS YOUR CONFIDENCE NOW HIGHER?

"You are a kind, amazing and unique person and you will be loved for who you are." My confidence is way higher. I think there's something deeply life-changing about being comfortable in your own skin; it can be hard, especially if you have had a difficult experience as a child or indeed an adult. I am confident most days and if I'm not I act 'as if'.

DO YOU COMPARE YOURSELF TO OTHER WOMEN?

I try not to, but yes I'm human. However, I'm inspired by many women and feel honoured to have many friends and clients who are incredible, strong, wonderful women. I look for inspiration in others and always try to be a better person.

DOES BODY IMAGE AND APPEARANCE MATTER TO YOU NOW?

I always make an effort and take pride in how I look, and I know that what I'm wearing impacts on how I'm feeling. I think making an effort for others is important too.

DO YOU EXERCISE?

Dog walking, water skiing, yoga, meditation, occasional blast on an off-road motorbike.

YOUR ATTITUDE TO NUTRITION?

We eat well, drink sensibly. Lots of organic fruit, meat and veg – mostly locally sourced. We have the sweet stuff too but it's a balance.

WHAT CHANGES HAVE YOU NOTICED SINCE 40?

Some things have gone a bit south or east, my eyesight is definitely worse and I have had a couple of basal cell carcinomas removed. I definitely have to exercise more to stay toned and fit.

HOW DO YOU FEEL EMOTIONALLY ABOUT THE PASSING YEARS?

I have two beautiful daughters who inspire, delight and make us immensely proud. I have a general 'don't give a f***' attitude that comes with age. My emotional reaction to physical ageing fluctuates daily, however I feel privileged to be the age that I am, as too many have been denied it.

WHAT IS YOUR OPINION ON THE MORE INTERVENTIONAL BEAUTY TREATMENTS?

It's not for me, mostly because I'm a bit of a wuss about that sort of thing. One acquaintance had a little work done and sadly looked a little like she'd been ironed, which didn't warm one to the idea either.

HAVE YOU EVER HAD ANY BEAUTY DISASTERS?

Going into Oxford Street after filming and forgetting to remove the 'camera' makeup – that wasn't a good look! And of course, being pale, the odd bad fake tan drama.

BEAUTY PRODUCTS

Spiezia face balm, cleanser and exfoliator, water, luxurious scented hand creams, Aromatherapy Associates body oils mixed with a plain moisturiser – my skin is a bit sensitive. I love Australian Gold Botanical Sunscreen for face and body. I'm a bit rubbish at makeup so when I have an event to go to my daughter works her magic.

SUPPLEMENTS

Omega-3 and Wild Nutrition Daily multivitamins and sometimes an iron supplement as I'm occasionally borderline anaemic. Probiotics and Rhythm Life Shots.

CHRISTINA HOWELLS, 52

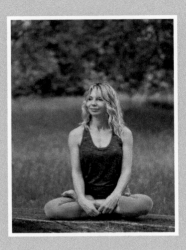

Well-known and highly sought after personal trainer. www.thatgirllondon.com. Worked in film and fashion arenas, lifestyle coach to VIP clients internationally. Sport and Exercise Science Degree MSc Sports and Exercise Psychology Diploma Ed. Nutritional Therapy Yoga Alliance qualified teacher.

WHAT EXERCISE DO YOU DO?

Mobility, bodyweight and strength, walking, hiking, climbing, dancing, Electrical Muscle Stimulation (EMS)

YOUR ATTITUDE TO NUTRITION?

I need to stay in tune with my body and I need to feel alive, not tired and bloated. I eat for nourishment, a fresh lunch and green juices, fish with green veg, cauliflower and couscous for supper. I have breakfast when ready – often after training and maybe only a smaller amount. I feel lighter without it and I feel you are keeping your body in more of a 'fat-burning state' if you eat *after* your morning workout.

WHAT CHANGES HAVE YOU NOTICED SINCE 40?

Not so much then – all at 49 years! More lines, more neck lines. I look mature now and I find

that harder to accept. I need more recovery after exercise, and if I don't keep up mobility training I lock up. I focus on quality over quantity; I don't care for the hardcore circuit-style classes as form is so important to avoid injury and to actually get any benefit.

WHAT DO YOU THINK THE MIDDLE-AGED AND OLDER WOMAN CAN GAIN FROM EXERCISE?

As we age and with the changes in hormones, it's easy to settle and make excuses, believing change is too hard or our efforts won't bring results. Primary ageing is inevitable but the rate at which this happens has *more to do with how we live our lives.*

Physical activity is one of the best forms of preventive medicine you can invest in. In midlife it's not about going hard and fast; this usually ends up being counter-productive, resulting in fatigue, potential injury and eventually demotivating. It's about choosing the right kind of exercise for you. *Quality over quantity* as there is little benefit to be had from poor form. Having fun is essential for adherence, and building in rest aids recovery and reduces injury. Stop the comparisons with others!

You can't out train a bad diet. It's about moderation, not starving yourself or over eating foods with no nutritional value.

Mobility exercises promote a better range of movement by taking the muscles, tendons and joints through their full range of motion with the intent to increase efficiency and quality of motion. This helps you to maintain your posture by decreasing restrictions in the body such as tight hips and upper back. It also allows you to move better and perform tasks such as doing up your dress or getting up off the floor.

Strength training is essential. Muscle is the secret to anti-ageing. We lose muscle from our 30s and this will continue with natural hormone decline. Less muscle means a slightly slower metabolism due to the loss of lean tissue, but more importantly muscle is key to maintaining independence in later life.

To preserve and potentially gain muscle and strength you need to apply the principle of overload whereby you place a stress upon the body beyond what it is accustomed to in order to have a training effect. Gym-based resistance classes incorporating resistance are an obvious choice but remember you can train anywhere using resistance bands, home weights or your body weight.

The maintenance of bone density with ageing is highly dependent on maintaining muscle mass and function. Mechanical forces such as resistance training are essential for the remodelling processes that maintain bone mass. Hormonal and dietary factors are also significant.

Cardiovascular fitness for our heart and lungs should be incorporated into our week. However, endless cardio will do little for your muscle tone, mobility and strength. Furthermore, if you fall, cardio fitness is not going to help you pick yourself up.

BEAUTY PRODUCTS

ILA aromatherapy beauty oil, ULTRASUN SPF 30 tinted moisturiser, Neal's Yard Rose Balm, Pureology shampoo, The Ordinary range

SUPPLEMENTS

Spirulina, Magnesium powder, Osteocare

DIANE KENWOOD, 59

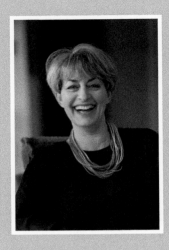

Founder of www.thesearetheheydays.com. A career in TV, Radio, PR, Marketing and Journalism. Editor of the *Marks & Spencer Magazine* and, for 10 years, *Woman's Weekly*.

MAIN ROLE MODELS

My mother has always been my greatest inspiration. She qualified as a lawyer at a time when only 26 women a year did. She only fully retired at the age of 85 and replaced the two days a week work with volunteer roles. She has also set up a number of charities. She's a powerhouse and an amazing example of determination and dedication. She never wore much makeup, but has always loved clothes. Zara is one of her favourite places to shop, and she tries to buy trousers in France as they suit her tiny size.

My parents were both devoted to family. When my girls were growing up I replicated their focus on family meals and spending family time together at the weekends.

HOBBIES

Exercise, travel, singing in a choir, theatre and the arts.

HOW AWARE WERE YOU GROWING UP OF BODY IMAGE AND BEAUTY?

I never felt particularly pretty and was always comparing myself unfavourably to other girls (I'm disappointed to say that's a habit that continues to this day). But I was a swimmer all through my teenage years (I competed for Britain), so my relationship with my body was healthy.

DID YOU HAVE STRONG INFLUENCES ON YOUR EATING PATTERNS GROWING UP?

There was never any talk of dieting or restrictive eating. I was a fussy eater when I was young and in retrospect possibly suffered from some sort of IBS because I would often have spasms of stomach ache and bloating. My eating became more varied as I got older.

WERE YOU HAPPY WITH YOUR IMAGE AS A TEENAGER?

I always felt slightly awkward, gawky and not pretty enough.

WHAT WOULD YOU TELL YOUR 20-YEAR-OLD SELF AND IS YOUR CONFIDENCE NOW HIGHER?

"Stop comparing yourself to other people. You are not only enough, you're bloody marvellous! Say what you're feeling instead of bottling it all up inside." Incomparably higher now.

DOES BODY IMAGE AND APPEARANCE MATTER TO YOU NOW?

Not as much. I've stayed a size 10/12 and always exercised. I'm trying to make peace more with my changing body as it ages and be grateful for the fact that it works as well as it does.

ANY POINTS IN YOUR LIFE THAT MADE YOU LOOK AFTER YOURSELF MORE?

My husband's sudden collapse and death when he was just 60 has had a huge impact on me.

DO YOU EXERCISE?

Pilates, walking, gym, swimming. I also used to dance (Ceroc) twice a week.

YOUR ATTITUDE TO NUTRITION?

I'm less good about food than exercise. I know what I should be eating, but since I've lived alone I am less consistent about preparing fresh meals and eating my five-a-day. When my girls were growing up I always cooked from scratch.

WHAT CHANGES HAVE YOU NOTICED SINCE 40?

There were relatively few in my 40s, but they have definitely accelerated since my mid-50s. My face, which is pretty unlined, has started to sag and become more jowly. I've noticed significant changes in my body. Some of that may be from my husband's death (I firmly believe the body is a repository for stress and trauma). My general suppleness, muscle strength and cardio fitness are noticeably reduced.

HOW DO YOU FEEL EMOTIONALLY ABOUT THE PASSING YEARS?

I do absolutely recognise that it beats the alternative and I remind myself of that when I'm bemoaning the things that make me feel gloomy.

HAVE YOU EVER HAD A BEAUTY DISASTER?

Over-plucking my eyebrows in my teens!

WHAT IS YOUR OPINION ON THE MORE INTERVENTIONAL BEAUTY TREATMENTS?

My only needle treatment was facial acupuncture in my 30s. I have no objections to anyone doing whatever they choose but I do think you can go too far. I wouldn't have fillers or Botox, but I do toy with having an eye and jaw lift. I have friends who have had the eye treatment and they do look better for it. I've just never quite had the courage to have it done – yet...

BEAUTY PRODUCTS

No7 Radiant Results cleanser, Argan oil 5-in-one eye cream, Mac Studio Face and Body Foundation, Code London FFL pre-mascara lash plumper, Maybelline Lash Sensational mascara

SUPPLEMENT

Multivitamin

NICKY HAMBLETON JONES, 47

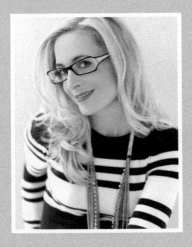

www.nhjstyle.com; Instagram@nhjstyle; Twitter @NHJStyle

Personal Stylist, Fashion Consultant and Founder of NHJ Style Consultancy. Works with individuals, retailers and corporates. Previously TV presenter, Management Consultant and Dietitian.

MAIN ROLE MODELS
My mother, Oprah, Zola Budd. My mum always took a lot of care over her appearance and loved wearing colour, which rubbed off on me. As a 20-something I was fascinated by successful women but found it hard to find those successful in career, love and life. It is difficult to find successful, inspirational women with balance.

INTERESTS
Fashion, fitness, nutrition, interiors

HOW AWARE WERE YOU GROWING UP OF BODY IMAGE AND BEAUTY?
I was aware of keeping slim when I gave up ballet and gained a bit of weight. I don't think I was ever obsessive about body image. Growing up in South Africa, media wasn't a big part of life. The most I had to look at was the local magazines.

DID YOU HAVE STRONG INFLUENCES ON YOUR EATING PATTERNS GROWING UP?
My mum was very conscious of what we ate and encouraged healthy eating. She would also make suggestions as to things I should avoid if she felt I was gaining weight. I think we did Weight Watchers together once when I gained a bit of weight post ballet and at university. It was never negative though, just supportive.

WERE YOU HAPPY WITH YOUR IMAGE AS A TEENAGER?
I don't remember being overly stressed by it.

WHAT WOULD YOU TELL YOUR 20-YEAR-OLD SELF AND IS YOUR CONFIDENCE NOW HIGHER?
"Enjoy your flawless complexion, enjoy the freedom of being young, play the field, follow

your dreams and don't worry about the future." Definitely higher; I am far more in tune with who I am as a person than I was then. Worrying about the future is a work in progress though.

DO YOU COMPARE YOURSELF TO OTHER WOMEN?

I compare myself to others in terms of success all the time. I'm definitely less confident than others probably perceive. I try to stay centred and just focus on me; but it's easier said than done, especially on a PMT day.

DOES BODY IMAGE AND APPEARANCE MATTER TO YOU NOW?

It's everything I am and represent. I have to look and be the best version of myself each and every day. There is a fine balance between nurture and obsession though; it is important not to have unrealistic goals.

DO YOU EXERCISE?

Three to four HIIT classes at the gym, walk my kids to school each day and have recently completed my first triathlon.

YOUR ATTITUDE TO NUTRITION?

As a qualified dietitian, nutrition has always been something close to my heart.

WHAT CHANGES HAVE YOU NOTICED SINCE 40?

Loss of volume around mouth and cheeks. Harder to maintain a flat stomach, and skin elasticity not as good. I also feel more tired after exercise, but these are small things – as long as you have your health you have everything.

HOW DO YOU FEEL EMOTIONALLY ABOUT THE PASSING YEARS?

I feel proud to be 47 and feel I look reasonably good for my age, but it only takes one bad photo to make you feel a bit vulnerable. I'm all over a little cosmetic help here and there though, but have no interest in looking completely fake and plastic. My motto in life is 'little and often', *look after yourself from the inside*. It is about looking your best for the age that you *are*.

WHAT IS YOUR OPINION ON THE MORE INTERVENTIONAL BEAUTY TREATMENTS?

I think used in the right way they can work wonders. Personally I would always choose non-surgical but, hey, if it all falls apart I'll be first in line for a facelift! But right now, a bit of Botox and a spot of fillers is all I need. Everyone must do what they feel works for them. I personally have no issue with intervention as long as you still look normal and like yourself.

HAVE YOU EVER HAD ANY BEAUTY DISASTERS?

I tried to dye my hair red when I was a teenager and it came out black! No idea how that happened!

BEAUTY PRODUCTS

SunSense Daily Face SPF50, Trilogy Rosehip Oil, Bobbi Brown red lipstick, Eyelash curlers, Laura Mercier Secret Camouflage concealer.

SUPPLEMENTS

CurraNZ

DO YOU THINK CLOTHES CAN ELEVATE OUR MOOD IN THE YEARS OVER 40?

Absolutely! Clothes can fundamentally change the way you feel about yourself and the way you see yourself in the mirror. This is particularly powerful for women over 40 who are struggling to juggle the demands of life, adapt to changes in their body shape post-children as well as to life in general if they've left a career to focus on their family. Clothes help you reshape your identity and help you feel confident from the inside out.

WHAT WOULD YOU TELL SOMEONE WHO THINKS THEY HAVE LOST THEIR SENSE OF STYLE IN LATER LIFE? CAN ONE REGAIN IT?

You are never too old to reinvigorate your style, in fact it's something everyone should do at least every 5 to 10 years. It's less about regaining and more about reshaping your style to suit the person you are now and the lifestyle you currently lead. The great thing about clothes is that it's not about you having to adapt yourself to fit the clothes but rather using a style expert to help you find the clothes to fit and flatter the shape you are.

WHAT SKILLS DO YOU AIM TO LEAVE WOMEN WITH AFTER THE STYLING PACKAGE FROM NHJ STYLE?

For starters I strive to open my client's eyes to their untapped potential; once a client sees just how good they can look they want to emulate that feeling every day. Then it's about educating clients around size and fit; so many women are wearing clothes that just don't fit them properly, which reduces the impact of an outfit. Lastly, I show them how to wear colour, nudging them out of their bland, neutral wardrobes into outfits that give you the glow-factor.

TRACEY WOODWARD, 52

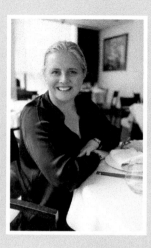

Director of New Products and Partnerships Clean Beauty at Holland and Barrett and Executive Board Member Cosmetic Executive Women. *Previous roles include* CEO Aromatherapy Associates, Head of Business Development of Beauty Marks and Spencer, Director of Sales Aveda, Donna Karan UK Beauty Manager, Kalmar Brand Advisor, mentor to many.

INTERESTS
Dog walking and gardening.

MAIN ROLE MODELS
Mother, sister, cousins and many female mentors on my career journey. Mum told me: "If you want to succeed you have to look like you belong." I always remember this, and she said people will always look at your shoes if they can't decide whether they like you, so make sure your shoes are clean! Everything I am today is because of her. Tracey May, Tracey Jadaa, Hilary Dart, Eileen Border are all role models and now friends. Mary Power taught me to read at 14. I owe her so much; she taught me kindness, humility and gratitude.

HOW AWARE WERE YOU GROWING UP OF BODY IMAGE AND BEAUTY?
I was always so skinny being a premature baby (born at 26 weeks weighing 1lb 13oz) so for many years I looked like a boy. I remember my mum telling me I would get better looking as I got older. I think she was right.

DID YOU HAVE STRONG INFLUENCES ON YOUR EATING PATTERNS GROWING UP?
We went without food growing up – I know how it feels to be hungry. We were poor. I was always grateful to have food, even if it was a bag of chips.

WERE YOU HAPPY WITH YOUR IMAGE AS A TEENAGER?
I had lots of issues with my image as a teenager. I wanted to be like the ladies of *Dynasty* in terms of make-up, shoes, clothes, beauty and success.

WHAT WOULD YOU TELL YOUR 20-YEAR-OLD SELF AND IS YOUR CONFIDENCE NOW HIGHER?
"Nothing ever stays the same, you were so right to

set goals and thank you for not giving up. "Higher now; I know where I belong and where I am going – I have a proven model for success.

DOES BODY IMAGE AND APPEARANCE MATTER TO YOU NOW?

Only because health and wellness are important to me... equally being energised is important too. I have been fat and thin – somewhere in between is ideal. I don't compare myself to other women, I draw inspiration from them. I love to encourage empowerment – my mum always said: "If you think you can, you can, and if you think you can't, you won't."

ANY POINTS IN YOUR LIFE THAT MADE YOU LOOK AFTER YOURSELF MORE?

10 years ago, I had thyroid failure and type 2 diabetes. I refused to take anything apart from thyroxine and *ownership of my health*. I want to be well rested, less stressed and have energy. I am mindful that how I look after myself now will reflect on my next decade of health.

DO YOU EXERCISE?

I walk up to 40 km a week (often carrying weights) with my super-fit dog Stanley!

YOUR ATTITUDE TO NUTRITION AND SELF-CARE?

Balance is key, fruit and veg. I love meat and fish but try to limit it. I also feel the benefits of intermittent fasting. I body brush every day and I have a massage fortnightly.

HAVE YOU EVER HAD A BEAUTY DISASTER?

My body turned green through an evening event with a self-tan product after a magnesium bath! Glad it was not on my face!

WHAT CHANGES HAVE YOU NOTICED SINCE 40?

Less elasticity and tone in body.

HOW DO YOU FEEL EMOTIONALLY ABOUT THE PASSING YEARS?

I am happy with the ageing process because we discover who we are, where we're going and why we are here. I just want to age gracefully. I always compare life to going on holiday. In my 20s I was packing and preparing for the life's journey, now at 52 I feel like I am at the check-in point. I just want to enjoy the next steps and make sure the departure is as smooth as possible.

BEAUTY PRODUCTS

Aromatherapy Associates Inner Strength cleanser and facial oils, Dr. Levy Décolleté crème, QMS tinted moisturiser, Delbove Botanicals, Lebon toothpaste

SUPPLEMENTS

Vitamin D in winter only

YVONNE WAKE, 67

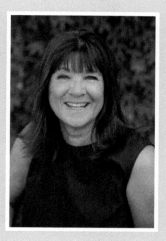

wellbeingandlifestyle.co.uk. Registered Public Health Nutritionist, Fitness Expert, Life Coach, University Lecturer and 'Wellbeing and Lifestyle Consultant' with over 30 years of experience.

"Originally a fitness instructor, I owned the Gym at The Sanctuary in Covent Garden. It was the first 'ladies-only health club' in the world in the 1980s. It wasn't until I was 50 years old that I went to university! My first degree was in Nutrition and Health and then an MSc in Public Health Nutrition at The London School of Hygiene and Tropical Medicine. I then moved on to four years of a PhD studying Childhood Obesity and I had many published works during my academic life. I studied to become a life coach as I was often trying to convey advice about nutrition and exercise and I felt I needed to learn a more psychological approach to doing that. I now have clients all over the world and often work into the night and also run regular retreats in France and elsewhere."

MAIN ROLE MODELS

My mum, now a magnificent 89 years old. Always happy, everyone's friend, an all-encompassing fantastic personality. She started her working life when we were all young as an office cleaner, and many years later became Head of Dispatch (post room) at CBS Music. It was then bought by Sony and Mum became quite a legend. She controlled who came in and out, so she knew everyone! She would talk about meeting Johnny Mathis, Sacha Distel, Meatloaf... I was more interested in fitness than my mother.

The Pankhurst Ladies, Coco Chanel, Maya Angelou, Ella Fitzgerald, Anne Frank, Rosa Parks, Rosalind Franklin and the Queen of England.

One of my great real-life role models later on in my 50s was Carol Nobel, my first lecturer at Surrey University. She taught me to look far deeper into the scientific world; she pushed me academically!

HOW AWARE WERE YOU GROWING UP OF BODY IMAGE AND BEAUTY?

I had zero awareness. I had no vanity. I look at the pictures now from when I was younger and think I was so pretty but did not realise! My father was always telling us that we were beautiful and my mother was never critical. So many people do not have that love acknowledged and that is probably why life coaching is so in demand these days.

DID YOU HAVE STRONG INFLUENCES ON YOUR EATING PATTERNS GROWING UP?

We always ate healthily. Simple meals, there were no sweets or chocolate. There were no diets, there was no fridge, so food was often kept on the windowsill. In the garden we grew our own vegetables. Mum was still working a full-time job with three children. We used to meet her at the King's Cross bus stop from work and carry her shopping home – she cooked every day from scratch.

HOW INFLUENCED WERE YOU BY THE POPULAR PRESS, TELEVISION AND MEDIA?

Not really and not now. I am still a scientist and want real proof and evidence. When I was studying my PhD I was studying secondary school children to see if changing the environment around them – school snacks, home food – would change their behaviour and thus reduce obesity. Thus I am used to looking for precise facts.

HOW HAPPY DID YOU FEEL WITH YOUR IMAGE AS A TEENAGER?

Very happy – I thought I was the bee's knees!

WHAT WOULD YOU TELL YOUR 20-YEAR-OLD SELF AND IS YOUR CONFIDENCE NOW HIGHER?

"Don't be too concerned about what others say, realise that criticism is really coming from the one who said it and is really in essence reflecting how they feel about themselves.

Don't try and impress friends – be more interested in school work. Don't be so worried about having boyfriends!" I wish I had studied more when I was young but then I had three wonderful children and lived in different countries and had wonderful experiences!

Yes, my confidence is higher naturally with age.

DO YOU EXERCISE?

Yoga, I have a personal trainer, walking, I have a pool and swim daily.

I teach stretch classes on my retreats.

YOUR ATTITUDE TO NUTRITION?

Because of my knowledge I could not go off my healthy eating path. No processed food. I might have chips in a restaurant once a year. I cook everything from scratch. I believe in organic food. I have read lots of papers on organic farming. I feel that it is like an insurance policy in your future not an expense. Not all organically labelled food is accurately labelled. If it is seasonal it is more likely to be correctly sourced. Talk to the farmers in the market – it may not need to be labelled organic if not sprayed with pesticides and so on. Get to know the farmers.

BEAUTY PRODUCTS

Antipollution facials, anti-ageing hydrating facial mask with clay, say every five months, I use a moisturiser with SPF 50 in it – so I am a new convert (I went to a facialist and they did one of those photos of sun spots on your face!).

DO YOU CONSULT WITH ALTERNATIVE HEALTH PRACTITIONERS?

I have a GP who is also an alternative practitioner. She is called Dr Tatiana Bosch. She is a conventional GP who then trained in Reflexology, Acupuncture, Chinese medicine, Reiki, Functional and Integrated Medicine. She gives me a lot of advice about healing naturally. I follow some Gerson principals, coffee enemas, homeopathy.

My father died of liver cancer (but was a non-drinker) and I first saw Tatiana presenting with puffy eyes and an itchy neck. That was the first time I met her. She diagnosed liver problems and taught me a detox which I perform regularly and all the symptoms disappeared.

SUPPLEMENTS

Vitamin D. I take a homeopathic detox (Heel from Germany) twice a year in January and October for six weeks and notice the difference within two weeks.

WHAT DO YOU THINK ABOUT EATING PATTERNS THAT ADVOCATE TREAT DAYS?

You should not need this if you are eating well normally. It suggests you are craving something. It is also never a good idea with children or adults to ever reward with food. I think food needs to be completely separate from any reward/ punishment ideas.

DO YOU THINK THERE ARE ANTI-AGEING FOODS?

I think that if you are feeding your gut the correct food you will see a massive impact on health in the skin. Just the same as smoking and drinking cause detrimental effects on the skin. If the foundations are good in your diet and gut, you will see the benefits on the outside.

CINDY ROBINS, 54

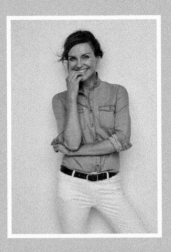

Photo copyright of Cindy Robins, not to be reproduced
without permission, provided courtesy of Bruno Juminer

Model with Models One and Yoga Teacher www.cindyrobinsyoga.com; Instagram @cindyrobins
   Cindy has modelled for many brands including Max Factor, Marks and Spencer, Avon, Phase
Eight, Aquascutum, Hotter Shoes, J D Williams, plus editorials and shows. She is a Scaravelli-
inspired yoga teacher who teaches group classes and one-to-one and also teaches at Lovelong
House Residential Rehabilitation Centre.

MAIN ROLE MODELS
My mum was very stylish and used to make clothes
herself. She sadly died when I was 18.

Aunt Buffy. She always looks fabulous and
stylish. She has such an attitude of freedom – she
doesn't care what others think!

My grandmother was head of the YWCA
(Young Women's Christian Association in the
south) and within that she ran a Saturday club
for mentally handicapped adults. That was an
inspiration to me and I would go along and help
my grandparents. She also influenced me to love
the idea of great family dinners.

My Scottish grandmother was incredibly elegant
in her tweed suits, blue rinse and sensible shoes.

HOW AWARE WERE YOU GROWING UP OF BODY IMAGE AND BEAUTY?
I was aware of body shape and at 14 was happy
with my body. At 16, I was told to lose weight by
my first modelling agency, despite being slender!

I loved fashion magazines, Bananarama,
Madonna! I have always loved fashion and used to
transform my friends for discos!

DID YOU HAVE STRONG INFLUENCES ON YOUR EATING PATTERNS GROWING UP?
My mother was always on a diet and made me a
bit obsessed. I do remember my teacher being
shocked that I had only taken a flask full of hot
bouillon and some Ryvitas once for a school

lunch! That was normal in our house but we were also a 'three meals a day' family.

WERE YOU HAPPY WITH YOUR IMAGE AS A TEENAGER?

I did ballet and was always active. At 16 I left school and we had to travel to Singapore. I was recommended for a modelling interview through a friend. I did not receive compliments about my appearance from my parents, simply because it wasn't valued in that way. I was shy with modelling to start with and didn't think I was good enough.

WHAT WOULD YOU TELL YOUR 20-YEAR-OLD SELF AND IS YOUR CONFIDENCE HIGHER NOW?

"Do yoga, eat clean, trust in yourself and have confidence." Higher now.

DO YOU COMPARE YOURSELF TO OTHER WOMEN?

Sometimes for work it is inevitable. I don't really compare to other women in daily life.

DOES BODY IMAGE AND APPEARANCE MATTER TO YOU NOW?

I feel more comfortable in my body now than when I was 20 years old. I was in Mauritius last month for a swimsuit shoot, modelling with a lovely girl who was 25 years old. She was in the bikinis and I was in the swimsuits!

DO YOU EXERCISE?

Yoga daily, teach six classes a week, a power walk.

YOUR ATTITUDE TO NUTRITION?

I love cooking and always cook fresh. I eat well – no meat/dairy or gluten. I suffer from eczema and avoid any food that can cause inflammation. I do eat fish, as it is so nutritious. I use coconut milk.

HOW OFTEN DO YOU USE SUN PROTECTION ON YOUR FACE?

I use Heliocare factor 50 every day.

DO YOU CONSULT WITH OTHER HEALTH PRACTITIONERS?

I have acupuncture, homeopathy, Indian facial massage, reiki and foot massage. I see a naturopath for a broader view.

SUPPLEMENTS

Nettle and Quercetin, Vitamin C, Vitamin D, Acidophilus.

TELL ME ABOUT YOUR SKINCARE REGIME AS EVERYONE WILL WANT TO KNOW!

I cleanse with Emma Hardie balm and give my face a good massage, usually in the evening or when I feel my skin needs it. Alternatively, I use Ren Gentle Cleansing wash along with my Magnitone (electrical brush) depending upon how my skin is feeling.

I use SKYN eye mask gels and Dr. Organic Rose Mask.

I use ENVIRON products every day which have greatly improved my skin and got rid of pigmentation. At night I use a super moisturiser and Arbonne Aloe Vera Eye Gel which is light and moisturises without puffiness. I like Calendula Baby Body Lotion and Weleda Skin Food for my hands. CACI facials and facial acupuncture.

WHAT TIPS HAVE YOU PICKED UP FROM MAKE-UP ARTISTS AT WORK?

Less is more with foundation. I use a Laura Mercier tinted moisturiser – it makes your skin look good and has good coverage. Burberry Face Contour.

Use a brow pencil slightly lighter than your natural colour and use small thread strokes.

HOW DO YOU HONESTLY FEEL ABOUT AGEING?

I can look at Daphne Selfe or my aunt and see that women can still look amazing as they age. I am embracing life at 50 plus.

HOW DO YOU FEEL ABOUT MORE INTERVENTIONAL BEAUTY TREATMENTS?

I think it is a personal decision and if you are desperately unhappy it might be the right thing. I can only say how I *feel today* and that I don't want to do it and I will embrace what I have – who knows in a few years' time? My agent supports me in being natural.

DR LOUISE PENDRY, 52

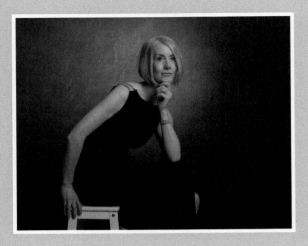

Senior Lecturer in Psychology at Exeter University. After optician and bank jobs, I studied Psychology then worked as an account manager in a marketing firm. I returned to academia for research then a PhD. I specialise in Social Psychology and Stereotyping. Currently my research includes ageism and gendered ageism and I am commissioned to write features for national press, radio and magazines.

INTERESTS
@silverserenity4 on Instagram. Country walks with family.

MAIN ROLE MODELS
My mum and two sisters started modelling when I was about 10. It was hard to not be swept along with the make-up and hair fascination. Mum emphasised we had to make the best of ourselves; my parents were so proud of us. I wore make-up in my teens and grew my hair. I recall Mum giving me Oil of Ulay and obsessing about wrinkles.

HOW AWARE WERE YOU GROWING UP OF BODY IMAGE AND BEAUTY?
I learned that appearance was all. I recall pretty women on magazines, Miss World beauty contests, little else.

DID YOU HAVE STRONG INFLUENCES ON YOUR EATING PATTERNS GROWING UP?
One of my sister's boyfriends would tease her about her weight, and tease me (despite me being slim) that I was getting a 'big bum'. She was getting married and went on a diet and I joined her, learning about calories. Bad mistake. This gave me a complex I really didn't need. My relationship with food from 16-25 was not great. I went from enjoying food to seeing it as the enemy, coincidentally growing larger across these years (I now know the psychology – why thought suppression can lead to rebound effects, making us *do the very thing we are trying not to do* even more). That comment about my bum set me on a path of diet and self-loathing. I recovered, I returned to eating when hungry, stopping when full, *enjoying*

food. My weight reverted to my set point and has not budged, pregnancies aside, for 30 years.

WERE YOU HAPPY WITH YOUR IMAGE AS A TEENAGER?

I was tall and skinny and not remotely attractive (I thought). My dad was head of our Catholic secondary school and I was really not encouraged to experiment image-wise.

WHAT WOULD YOU TELL YOUR 20-YEAR-OLD SELF AND IS YOUR CONFIDENCE NOW HIGHER?

"Don't believe ageing is all bad, don't spend decades fighting it. Eat well, exercise, be kind to yourself. Try not to be influenced by what others think of you. Be bold. Take risks. Dive in."

Much higher. Accepting my age has been a game changer. I stopped dyeing my hair a few years ago and that was a turning point. As my hair grew out my confidence grew in.

DOES BODY IMAGE AND APPEARANCE MATTER TO YOU NOW?

Yes. I'm learning to love my wrinkles, and exercise *not to lose weight* but to get fitter and stronger – I'm investing in my future and my body needs to be up to it!

ANY POINTS IN YOUR LIFE THAT MADE YOU LOOK AFTER YOURSELF MORE?

Turning 50 brought things into sharp focus. I'd traded on being fairly slim my whole life, but my inner health was a mystery.

DO YOU EXERCISE?

Gym classes and workouts. I look for opportunities to exercise as part of my day (lunchtime walks).

YOUR ATTITUDE TO NUTRITION?

Most days we cook from scratch. Rarely eat meat, lots of pulses and veggies.

WHAT CHANGES HAVE YOU NOTICED SINCE 40?

More wrinkles, boobs are a bit lower, though to be honest I am in pretty good shape, no cellulite. Wrinkles especially around my eyes. The odd blemish.

HOW DO YOU FEEL EMOTIONALLY ABOUT THE PASSING YEARS?

I'm way more chilled about it, with brief moments of doubt! A sense of calm has settled over me in recent years.

WHAT IS YOUR OPINION ON THE MORE INTERVENTIONAL BEAUTY TREATMENTS?

I don't think I'd do it. I have considered eyelid surgery but I'm okay as I am.

BEAUTY PRODUCTS

Liz Earle Hot Cloth Cleanser and Polish, homemade scrub – coconut oil, olive oil, sugar, Veil under-eye concealer, Daniel Sandler Watercolour blusher

VANESSA COWAN, 42

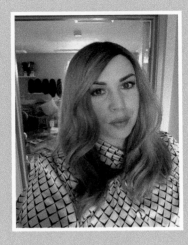

Wig specialist. Vanessa's own diagnosis with Alopecia Totalis led her to create www. glamorousbutterfly.co.uk. Instagram @glamorousbutterfly76. Previously Avon lady, Arts Liaison Officer, Civil Service Admin Officer, Garage Receptionist, Optical Advisor.

MAIN ROLE MODELS

My beautiful late mum, a style icon to me. I inherited my love of fashion, make-up, hair, shoes, life and all things beauty from her. Without much money she always looked glamorous, on trend, in a classy kind of way. She took pride in her appearance, wore make-up every day, changing hairstyles and always smelling lovely and exotic. I thank my mum every day as she has helped to mould and shape the person I am, not just with my style but also how I am emotionally, spiritually and my personality.

HOW AWARE WERE YOU GROWING UP OF BODY IMAGE AND BEAUTY?

I was overweight from about 9 to 15 so I was always very self-conscious. It didn't help that I had short hair too. Once I hit 16 (after a terrible few months when I was ill) I lost a lot of weight and grew my hair long. I used to look at Mum and think *'Yep, that's how I want to look when I'm older'.*

DID YOU HAVE STRONG INFLUENCES ON YOUR EATING PATTERNS GROWING UP?

My uncle who used to give me cakes and sweets as a way of showing his love! At home I was never allowed sweet things. Mum and Dad always seemed to be on some sort of 'fad diet'. My gran used to grow all her own veg and cook from scratch... vegetable soup and stewed rhubarb.

WERE YOU HAPPY WITH YOUR IMAGE AS A TEENAGER?

TV and magazines were a big influence. Image-wise 13 to 15 were the worst years. Then at 16, although still painfully shy, I got an older, cooler boyfriend and I really began to love the way I looked. I swam for the county from 11 to 13. Then I used a gym, hill and fell walked, spinning, boxercise and yoga.

HOW DO YOU FEEL ABOUT SOCIAL MEDIA?

Children, especially girls, grow up far too fast, a lot of it influenced by social media. I am thankful we did not have it in childhood.

IS YOUR CONFIDENCE NOW HIGHER THAN AT 20?

Much higher. Although still, in a social situation, I have little confidence deep down. I was a painfully shy child. I used to make Mum do everything! Phone calls, letters. When I was 16, Mum was diagnosed with breast cancer and during the next four years it spread to her bones. When she passed away, as the eldest child I had to practically grow up overnight.

DOES BODY IMAGE AND APPEARANCE MATTER TO YOU NOW?

More than it should really. I struggle with my weight. Through many different illnesses and injuries my weight has fluctuated since the age of 17. There isn't really a day goes by when I don't think '*I wish I was slimmer*'. I think people think I am more confident than I am.

ANY POINTS IN YOUR LIFE THAT MADE YOU LOOK AFTER YOURSELF MORE?

My mum and aunt dying young of cancer.

Also, at 38 when you suddenly lose your hair, eyebrows, lashes and body hair it really shakes your confidence.

DO YOU EXERCISE?

Walking, yoga.

YOUR ATTITUDE TO NUTRITION?

I always eat my five (usually seven) a day, cook from scratch, drink green tea, take vitamin D, drink little alcohol, try to avoid gluten. My downfall is sugar. I have a sweet tooth.

WHAT CHANGES HAVE YOU NOTICED SINCE TURNING 40?

A couple of fine lines, particularly around one eye! Facial hair arrgghhh!

HOW DO YOU FEEL ABOUT AGEING?

I look after my skin and wear make-up and generally don't look my age (so I'm told) so I feel okay about it. Plus, you can't stop time! A lot has happened in my life – sad, heart-breaking events. I'm learning to accept these things and am thankful every day that I am here and on the whole healthy.

HOW DO YOU FEEL ABOUT MORE INTERVENTIONAL BEAUTY TREATMENTS?

I've never personally had these treatments. The closest is having my eyebrows tattooed (lost due to alopecia). I am not opposed to it if there is a genuine obvious need. I do not like young people having procedures and tweaks. I just want to shout *"You have no lines, you are flawless, you are beautiful, please don't change!"*

BEAUTY PRODUCTS

Myroo range, coconut oil, Liz Earle Cleanse and Polish, Weleda Calendula Weather Protection Cream, La Roche-Posay SPF30 face cream.

SUPPLEMENTS

Vitamin D3

SALLY BEATON, 40

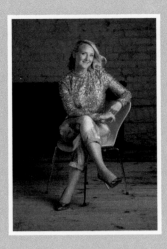

Founder of www.womenwithsparkle.com. Women's Holistic Nutritionist + Life Coach. Previously Choreographer, PR and Marketing Manager

MAIN ROLE MODELS

I used to watch my mum put her makeup on thinking she was beautiful but she was always scrutinising herself. My peers at school always seemed effortlessly glamorous and I felt like their short, 'funny' friend. Growing up, I felt inadequate no matter how much I tried to improve my appearance. Breaking away from the constant scrutinising and feelings of inferiority in regards to other women set me on my path to being the woman I am today though – one who sparkles!

INTERESTS

Dogs, roller-skating, hip-hop dancing.

HOW AWARE WERE YOU GROWING UP OF BODY IMAGE AND BEAUTY?

I was OBSESSED! I adored playing with hair and make-up as a young girl and was mesmerised by the '90s supermodels – Cindy, Naomi, Helena – they just seemed to *glow with health*.

MAGAZINES

Growing up I read *Just17*, *Cosmopolitan*, *More*.

DID YOU HAVE STRONG INFLUENCES ON YOUR EATING PATTERNS GROWING UP?

My mum and my friends always seemed to be on a diet! Food seemed to be the *enemy* of women around me.

WERE YOU HAPPY WITH YOUR IMAGE AS A TEENAGER?

No. I felt like the one the boys never fancied. How sad this was the barometer of my worth then.

HOW DO YOU FEEL ABOUT SOCIAL MEDIA TODAY?

I can't bear to think of the pressure for young girls, with the competition for likes/followers/ risqué pics, etc.

WHAT WOULD YOU TELL YOUR 20-YEAR-OLD SELF AND IS YOUR CONFIDENCE NOW HIGHER?

"You're beautiful. You're unique. You have a path and a purpose that no one else has. Follow your passions and set the world alight." My confidence is sky high compared to my teens and 20s. I feel like in my 40s I shook off the idea I need to look/act like someone else and I enjoy being me!

DO YOU COMPARE YOURSELF TO OTHER WOMEN?

Women fascinate me. The mistake is we've looked to a narrow group of women for how we're *meant to look*, we haven't realised that variety is gorgeous. I long for us to all be on a beach, admiring ourselves and women of *all* shapes – the same way we do trees, flowers or dogs.

DOES BODY IMAGE AND APPEARANCE MATTER TO YOU NOW?

Yes. I want to be in *total partnership with my body* and cherish it. Loving and looking after myself are what I aim to do daily and teach other women how to do the same.

ANY POINTS IN YOUR LIFE THAT MADE YOU LOOK AFTER YOURSELF MORE?

A breast tumour at the age of 30 turned my life around. I started looking at food as medicine and stopped drinking alcohol.

DO YOU EXERCISE?

Yes, in accordance with my cycle. Women are not designed to exercise the same way every day. I rotate walking, Rebounding, dancing and rest.

YOUR ATTITUDE TO NUTRITION?

Nutrition has to be personalised as no two people are the same. I stay away from foods/drinks that contribute to excess oestrogen and inflammation and avoid dairy 90% of the time (cream tea with friends or pizza with loved ones is always allowed though!). I fast 12-16 hours overnight as this balances my energy and keeps my weight stable (I never weigh myself though). I listen to my body instead of ignoring it like I used to.

WHAT CHANGES HAVE YOU NOTICED SINCE 40?

Softer jawline, lines around my eyes, stomach more rounded, nipples changed position, but I have more passion, purpose and confidence so I'm happy for the trade.

HOW DO YOU FEEL EMOTIONALLY ABOUT THE PASSING YEARS?

I embrace it. I don't want to waste the next 20 years wishing I was something/someone else. Who cares if my boobs aren't perky or my eyes have lines, as long as they sparkle (my eyes not my boobs – although maybe my boobs too – ha ha!).

WHAT IS YOUR OPINION ON THE MORE INTERVENTIONAL BEAUTY TREATMENTS?

I don't know enough about the procedures out there to know how damaging/poisonous they are to women's precious bodies. A friend has something called 'fire and ice' and looks wonderful. As long as the treatment is for you and not to fit a narrow, male-led standard of beauty, then why not?

HAVE YOU EVER HAD ANY BEAUTY DISASTERS?

Patchy fake tan! An ex's mum once said, "I'd love to pay for you to have your tan done professionally" – I stopped after that!

BEAUTY PRODUCTS

Dr. Bronner's Castile soap, Neal's Yard Wild Rose Beauty Balm (cleanser/moisturiser), Origins Vitazing tinted moisturiser with SPF.

SUPPLEMENTS

A variety depending upon my current needs, but remember the quality of the supplement is key (I use food-based ones), and flaxseed oil.

GRACE FODOR, 53

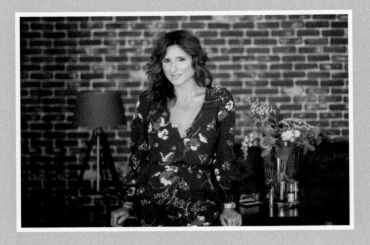

Founder of www.studio10beauty.com. *"My instincts were telling me that there was a huge gap in the market for a high-performing capsule collection of quick-fixes that target and are designed specifically for maturing and mature skins. I am passionate about not only redefining beauty for women as they age, but redefining age. Challenging the many outdated misconceptions of middle-age that leave many women feeling invisible, undervalued and unattractive."*

MAIN ROLE MODELS
Audrey Hepburn and Grace Kelly always made me sigh with joy at their elegance. My mother, beautiful inside and out, was my biggest influence. One of those women who always made an effort, always elegant. Her lessons have stayed with me. She passed away two years ago. From her, I learned compassion and empathy and how to forgive. Dad taught me to be fearless and unafraid, Mum showed me vulnerability is not a sign of weakness.

HOW AWARE WERE YOU GROWING UP OF BODY IMAGE AND BEAUTY?
I felt no awareness of how I looked until a sense of boys when I was 14 made me aware of body image. Interestingly, in comparison to my daughters, this happens much younger because of sexuality driven music, film and social media – also peers with 'selfie culture'.

DID YOU HAVE STRONG INFLUENCES ON YOUR EATING PATTERNS GROWING UP?
My parents' culture was that food sits at the heart of the family. No diets. They were great gardeners, growing most of their vegetables and fruits and we ate healthy, freshly cooked meals.

WERE YOU HAPPY WITH YOUR IMAGE AS A TEENAGER?
Up and down.

WHAT WOULD YOU TELL YOUR 20-YEAR-OLD SELF AND IS YOUR CONFIDENCE NOW HIGHER?
"Right now, you're full of ambition – eager

to make your mark on the world and start building the empires planned in your head. You've worked hard, you've got great business instincts and are going to go far. I know you feel insecurities you often don't show in public – around being alone, being liked and needing to fill your days to escape a brain that often feels far too busy. You will get to see wonderful places and explore parts of the planet that you don't yet have the confidence to do. Trust me, you should – you won't discover until you are 50 how much you enjoy your own company."

Far higher. I have such a better understanding of who I am and am aware of my own priorities and boundaries.

DO YOU COMPARE YOURSELF TO OTHER WOMEN?

No, I want to look the best I can look, no point comparing that with anyone else. I do look at the careers of women I admire and think 'I want to get there'.

DOES BODY IMAGE AND APPEARANCE MATTER TO YOU NOW?

I won't lie and say it doesn't matter. I work out most days, I love clothes and I run a makeup brand, so clearly I care about it. I will say that I care about it for myself not others.

ANY POINTS IN YOUR LIFE THAT MADE YOU LOOK AFTER YOURSELF MORE?

My mother's death made me realise I really needed to make time for my emotional needs and wellbeing. I reassessed how to protect my mental and emotional resilience.

DO YOU EXERCISE?

Yes, yoga, Pilates and weights. I do weights to restore the natural loss of muscle mass that occurs with age and to help rebuild it and maintain my bone density.

YOUR ATTITUDE TO NUTRITION?

Food is about pleasure and nourishment. I'm very aware of the importance of diet on my mood, hormones and overall wellbeing so I try to be really careful.

WHAT CHANGES HAVE YOU NOTICED SINCE 40?

Fine lines and a loss of definition but I learned great skin and make-up tips to help me work with that! I have to work harder to stay in shape.

HOW DO YOU FEEL EMOTIONALLY ABOUT THE PASSING YEARS?

I love getting older and I want everyone else to – there's still such stigma in society about it. I remember, when I turned 50, feeling anxious as if it was the beginning of the end for me. Now I'm all about a positive mindset and embracing the shift with as much energy as I can.

WHAT IS YOUR OPINION ON THE MORE INTERVENTIONAL BEAUTY TREATMENTS?

Absolutely down to the individual. I advocate inclusive ageing which means ageing however you want to. I always say though, to have a good friend be honest with you as it's easy to lose sight of how you really look.

HAVE YOU EVER HAD ANY BEAUTY DISASTERS?

The thing is they weren't really disasters, it's just that time moves on and we learn more. I wouldn't go with a perm again though!

TOP BEAUTY PRODUCTS

Sarah Chapman Skinesis Overnight Facial, Heliocare 360 sunscreen, Cult 51 Day Cream, Studio 10 Miracle Effect Priming Serum, Tatcha's at-home spa kits.

SUPPLEMENTS

Rejuvenated collagen shots

HILARY DART, 62

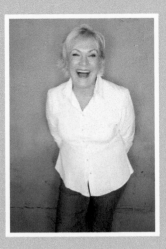

Owner of Hilary Dart Associates (since 2003). Hilary works with beauty brands as a Consultant. She is highly respected within the beauty industry and is currently Company Secretary for Cosmetic Executive Women UK having cofounded the organisation. Previously fashion retail – trained at House of Fraser, junior fashion buyer at Selfridges, Head of Beauty at Selfridges, UK Managing Director of Beauty at Calvin Klein, Global President of Beauty at Calvin Klein in New York.

MAIN ROLE MODELS
My mother and four sisters were a great influence on me. My father died when I was young. We were brought up with a stoical influence, great humour and an irreverent outlook. We were always told you CAN do...

HOW AWARE WERE YOU GROWING UP OF BODY IMAGE AND BEAUTY?
I was really aware.

I used to use my pocket money for *Petticoat* magazine, then get my sisters to pay to read it! I caught the bus to St Albans to admire the clothes.

DID YOU HAVE STRONG INFLUENCES ON YOUR EATING PATTERNS GROWING UP?
We knew we weren't allowed to be fat. We had home-cooked meals. We might have a treat like a sugared doughnut on a Friday. We were constantly playing outside and running around, active.

WERE YOU HAPPY WITH YOUR IMAGE AS A TEENAGER?
Yes.

HOW DO YOU FEEL ABOUT SOCIAL MEDIA TODAY?
It can be a blessing and curse. My daughter can keep in contact with all of her extended family easily. There is a large amount of damage potentially from it, though. It takes away the emotion of conversing. I totally ban phones from mealtime or even in the sitting room. I was in a large company recently and a young employee was having problems but it was all communicated

via email. When I said why don't you pick up the phone she looked at me astonished. But of course it worked!

WHAT WOULD YOU TELL YOUR 20-YEAR-OLD SELF AND IS YOUR CONFIDENCE NOW HIGHER?

"It will all come right in the end. Make sure you live the moment, grasp every opportunity and don't overthink it!"

Higher – I am more philosophical now; my confidence then was the enthusiasm of youth.

DO YOU COMPARE YOURSELF TO OTHER WOMEN?

Yes. Then I also realise there is photoshopping. I think that there are great influences out there like Helen Mirren that show you can have confidence and lead vibrant lives as you age. I think the Queen is a great role model for positive ageing.

DOES BODY IMAGE AND APPEARANCE MATTER TO YOU NOW?

Really important. We are very influenced by first impressions and I think if you have let yourself get very unhealthy from lifestyle not disease, it suggests that you have a lack of self-respect and self-care. I think when we go through menopause we can easily feel we lose our sex appeal and we have to work to keep that.

DO YOU EXERCISE?

Gym (cardio/weights/stretching), horse ride, walking, Pilates with Reformer

YOUR ATTITUDE TO NUTRITION?

We both cook at home, a lot of pulses and fish. We do not have readymade meals. Frozen sweetcorn and peas is about the limit on that! I am allergic to pork and beef (very *unusual*) so we have a lot of fruit, vegetables, eggs, smoked salmon. I don't buy organic – I get fruit and veg from Tesco or Waitrose. We used to have our own chickens!

HOW DO YOU FEEL EMOTIONALLY ABOUT THE PASSING YEARS?

It is the journey we are on. We cannot turn back; with age comes wisdom. It is a privilege denied to others, don't ever forget.

HAVE YOU EVER HAD ANY BEAUTY DISASTERS?

I used self-tan instead of sun protection and the next day had to go to work and important meetings – my hands looked so awful!

BEAUTY PRODUCTS

Aurelia night rose jasmine sandalwood face oil, Aurelia eye cream and morning gel, Elemis cleansing balm, MIO Boob Tube, MIO Shrink to Fit.

SUPPLEMENTS

Glucosamine, Chondroitin, Krill, used MenoHerbs in menopause

WHAT DO YOU THINK ABOUT THE FUTURE OF THE BEAUTY INDUSTRY?

The east and west coast USA is very dynamic, as well as emerging markets such as South Korea. I remember years ago at Avon NY there was an eyebrow director! That was never here then. They are pushing the boundaries and the way we adopt them here is important.

WHAT WOULD SURPRISE OUTSIDERS ABOUT THE INDUSTRY?

That it is really friendly and the barrier between the consumer and the staff on the shop floor should not really be there, yet women still find it intimidating. They are truly friendly.

WENDY EULER, 51

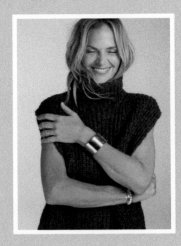

Founder of www.goodbyecroptop.com. *"Goodbye Crop Top is a place where women can come and understand how beautiful it is just to be... to be your age but do it with gumption, with strength, and to look damn good in the process."* Wendy lives in Bozeman, Montana.

"I sold radio ads in San Francisco in the '90s, living on commission. As I stood one night in a grocery store spending my last dollars on a tin of tuna and a bottle of wine, a woman walked by and said to the cashier, 'Hey, we need to get on that radio advertising programme tomorrow.' I knew in that moment a guardian angel was with me. I approached her explaining my work... and she bought an entire programme from me the next day! My career moved on to digital ad sales. I became Director of International Ad Sales for the largest recipe site in the world. I then moved on from my marriage and went on to meet the love of my life. He inherited my little girls and we had a baby together. After a few years off, I decided to pursue my love of style and writing so started the website."

MAIN ROLE MODELS

There were not many women in my real life that I emulated as far as fashion. One of the sales girls at my high school job was really cool. I even remember her scent which was almost foreign! I loved Paulina, Cindy, Christy, the supermodels of the '80s in magazines. That whole look – healthy, beautiful. As you can deduce I sort of lived in a fantasy! Lauren Hutton, Diane Keaton.

HOBBIES

Gardening, decorating (need to make more time for those!), love helping friends with wardrobes and outfits for occasions.

HOW AWARE WERE YOU GROWING UP OF BODY IMAGE AND BEAUTY?

I was quite a 'dork' with a mullet and braces in high school. I started comparing myself when I hit college and felt pretty insecure then. I eventually grew out of it. I've always had good, long-term friends who have loved me as I am. I was very influenced by MTV and was always aspiring to leave home for a big city.

DID YOU HAVE STRONG INFLUENCES ON YOUR EATING PATTERNS GROWING UP?

I am a Kansas girl. My father was a physician but we lived on a cattle ranch. I grew up eating meat and potatoes for the most part alongside junk food. I thought we were eating healthy, but in hindsight not so much.

WERE YOU HAPPY WITH YOUR IMAGE AS A TEENAGER?

I did not know any different and was pretty content in my own skin. I always had kind, good friends and their families around me. So I felt okay about myself... until college.

HOW DO YOU FEEL ABOUT SOCIAL MEDIA TODAY?

It is the bane of my existence with my children (ironic as I have to be on Instagram at least four hours daily). My hope and wish is they learn how to use it in good ways. There is a lot of positive if you are following along with healthy and happy people; there is a lot of negative if kids are comparing themselves. I remind my daughters often that comparison is the thief of joy. I have fairly strict rules around phone use, no phones in the bedroom and so on.

WHAT WOULD YOU TELL YOUR 20-YEAR-OLD SELF AND IS YOUR CONFIDENCE NOW HIGHER?

"Start 'not caring what others think' NOW. Stop worrying so much about things that never actually happen. Understand empathetic people are the ones you want to hold close." The cliché is true: 'youth is wasted on the young!' My confidence is high. I attribute this to a lot of hard knocks, choosing happiness over misery, which

involved making some very tough choices. I'm really taking care of myself now more than ever... health, exercise, meditation.

DOES BODY IMAGE AND APPEARANCE MATTER TO YOU NOW?

I believe if one is doing all they can to be healthy, making good choices about the company they keep, moving, learning every day, body image follows. If you feel good on the inside, you are most likely going to like your reflection.

DO YOU EXERCISE?

Weights and running twice a week, HIIT and yoga once a week plus occasional cardio.

YOUR ATTITUDE TO NUTRITION?

I try to live the 80-20 rule. I love juicing, the way healthy food makes me feel. But I'll also eat a cheeseburger and drink a beer with the best of them. For me, I need the balance. When in Rome... I'll always eat pasta in Italy!

WHAT CHANGES HAVE YOU NOTICED SINCE 40?

Oh Lord, where do I start? Sallow... a few more wrinkles around the eyes. Looking tired... but eating well, eating good fats, moving, and HAPPINESS reflects in a healthy looking face.

HOW DO YOU FEEL EMOTIONALLY ABOUT THE PASSING YEARS?

I feel lucky. Every bit of sadness, happiness has led me to where I am today. I'm so grateful and blessed. I'm loved, I love, I have a family and a husband I adore and respect who feels the same about me.

WHAT IS YOUR OPINION ON THE MORE INTERVENTIONAL BEAUTY TREATMENTS?

I believe it is an individual choice. If people look at you and think or say 'wow you look really rested, good, healthy' you are doing something right. You can have secrets if you so choose. But when you walk in a room and the reaction is 'what the hell have you done, you look like another person or an alien' maybe it's gone too far! Saying that, if looking like another person or an alien makes YOU happy, go for it! Just make sure it's done for the right reasons.

HAVE YOU EVER HAD A BEAUTY DISASTER?

In my 20s my hair caught fire on a candle (in a bar) and burned off! I had to cut the other side the next day and of course it grew out eventually.

BEAUTY PRODUCTS

Always trying new things.

SUPPLEMENTS

Vitamin D, Turmeric, Fish oil, B Vitamins, C, PQQ, Antioxidant, Ubiquinol

TRACY ACOCK, 58

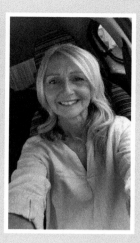

Instagram @returnofthecornishbird. Now retired, Tracy worked in Cancer Services in the NHS for over 20 years as a Nurse Specialist working with patients with secondary (incurable) breast cancer. She only started nursing training in her 30s after bringing up her sons. She now lives in Cornwall and has started her blog and website www.returnofthecornishbird.com *"encouraging other women to empower, inspire and encourage with healthy lifestyle changes – from menopause to muscles!"*

MAIN ROLE MODELS
My mother... she was very glamorous and definitely set the bar high for looking after myself. I would never describe it as a negative influence, but it wasn't encouraged or expected to work towards a career and I'm so glad this has changed today.

HOW AWARE WERE YOU GROWING UP OF BODY IMAGE AND BEAUTY?
I have suffered with my own dieting pressures since aged 13 after a chance remark made me think I was 'fat'. I wasn't but it has stayed with me all these years.

DID YOU HAVE STRONG INFLUENCES ON YOUR EATING PATTERNS GROWING UP?
Different times back then I'm afraid; the eating disorders weren't recognised or the awareness highlighted.

WERE YOU HAPPY WITH YOUR IMAGE AS A TEENAGER?
I was popular but very dependent on approval I'd say.

HOW DO YOU FEEL ABOUT SOCIAL MEDIA TODAY?
It's hard even as a grounded adult not to get sucked into 'likes' and approval that we know is not real life... such a potential challenge for teens who may have low self-esteem.

WHAT WOULD YOU TELL YOUR 20-YEAR-OLD SELF AND IS YOUR CONFIDENCE NOW HIGHER?
"Work hard at school, sun cream at all times, learn how to meditate."

Higher, as I am in such a good place with fitness and nutrition it has given me a new spark about life generally (who knew?!).

DO YOU COMPARE YOURSELF TO OTHER WOMEN

I do... doesn't everyone?!

DOES BODY IMAGE AND APPEARANCE MATTER TO YOU NOW?

This does make me feel a bit shallow but my fitness lifestyle has given me a whole new mindset, in a totally positive way... 'It's not too late' is my message and I am so passionate about that. Working with all the fabulous and brave patients in my life just made me so grateful for health, to be honest.

ANY POINTS IN YOUR LIFE THAT MADE YOU LOOK AFTER YOURSELF MORE?

I think my job definitely never allows me to take things for granted, and I want to take responsibility for my health as I age.

DO YOU EXERCISE?

Joined a gym three years ago, tried classes, but once I had a personal training session I got hooked. Instagram became part of my 'journey', as people described me as an inspiration, and I wanted to learn even more.

YOUR ATTITUDE TO NUTRITION?

I am quite disciplined and eat healthily, with balance. I have a good knowledge in nutrition and my mindset changed since starting lifting weights and resistance training, knowing that food is fuel. I then started to think what I could do to empower other women with this knowledge and passion and the website was born!

WHAT CHANGES HAVE YOU NOTICED SINCE 40?

Things going downwards! Joints ache but training has helped.

HOW DO YOU FEEL EMOTIONALLY ABOUT THE PASSING YEARS?

Just lucky to be here, health is everything!

BEAUTY PRODUCTS

Lumity skincare, No Wrinkles night moisturiser by This Works, BB cream SportFX cosmetics, Benefit Clarifying Gel

SUPPLEMENTS

Probiotics, Fish Oils, Magnesium

GILLIAN THOMSON, 40

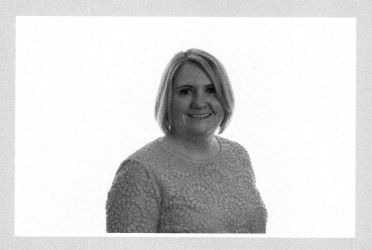

Director of www.act-clean.com supplying cleaning to the world's top hotels. Twitter @act_clean. Degree in Hotel and Hospitality Management. Worked in operations for Gordon Ramsay Holdings previously. *"I cleaned holiday chalets and played the bagpipes for the tourists in my home town as my first job!"*

MAIN ROLE MODELS

Mum. She was in the local Young Wives Club, PTA, Brownies and supported my dad in his business clubs. I remember her with sheer black tights, patent high heels, blue eyeshadow, with the scent of Dior on nights out! We loved this, as those evenings we had cake before bed! Everything she ever did was for her family.

Grandma was simply the kindest person I've ever met and I still think of her daily. A glamorous Northern Irish lady of brilliant humour, musical with old-fashioned values and never judged anyone.

They taught me honesty, integrity and to never underestimate the value of the likeability factor. They nurtured my strong moral compass.

HOW AWARE WERE YOU GROWING UP OF BODY IMAGE AND BEAUTY?

Not aware. I remember experimenting with SunIn, fake tan, makeup but not in a negative way. I loved Kylie in *Neighbours*, *Juliet Bravo*, *The A-Team* but really I preferred reading to TV.

DID YOU HAVE STRONG INFLUENCES ON YOUR EATING PATTERNS GROWING UP?

My aunt was on the Rosemary Conley Hip & Thigh diet, never smoked, obsessive about aerobics – got breast cancer and then a brain tumour and died at 53. My mum drinks and smokes and is in generally great health heading towards 70. I don't remember her dieting. We had no fizzy drinks, processed meals or chocolate, but lots of white bread, chips, crisps.

WERE YOU HAPPY WITH YOUR IMAGE AS A TEENAGER?

Reasonably. I was badly bullied but not because of how I looked or talked.

HOW DO YOU FEEL ABOUT SOCIAL MEDIA TODAY?

It is frightening and I am determined to learn more before my daughter reaches that age.

WHAT WOULD YOU TELL YOUR 20-YEAR-OLD SELF AND IS YOUR CONFIDENCE NOW HIGHER?

"Care less what others think. Be here for a good time, not everyone makes it to a long time. Learn empathy. Don't try to behave like a man. No one ever wished they had worked more and had less fun!"

Much higher. At 20 I was deputy department head in a hotel with 100 younger, longer-serving colleagues. Now I'm the leader of a business, I'm surrounded with smart people who care about me. I don't have to compete.

DO YOU COMPARE YOURSELF TO OTHER WOMEN?

I probably compare myself to my peers and sometimes find myself lacking as they all seem so successful. Then they say the same thing.

DOES BODY IMAGE AND APPEARANCE MATTER TO YOU NOW?

As I get older I realise I like the nice things in life and have no discipline at all. I'm in danger of becoming mutton dressed as lamb if I don't sort it out.

ANY POINTS IN YOUR LIFE THAT MADE YOU LOOK AFTER YOURSELF MORE?

Turning 40!

DO YOU EXERCISE?

I walk, but still not enough. It's on the list of things to sort out this year.

YOUR ATTITUDE TO NUTRITION?

I have a very positive attitude to eating everything I want, which is probably nutritionally a disaster.

HOW DO YOU FEEL EMOTIONALLY ABOUT THE PASSING YEARS?

There is nothing I can do about it as it comes to us all. All you can do is to embrace every stage of life and have a good time. Find fun and joy in as much as you can.

WHAT IS YOUR OPINION ON THE MORE INTERVENTIONAL BEAUTY TREATMENTS?

Never done it, don't think I will, but no judgement on anyone who does.

BEAUTY PRODUCTS

Urban Veda Facial Wash (rose), Toner, Crème de la Mer

SUPPLEMENTS

Vitamin C

DR JULIET MCGRATTAN, 47

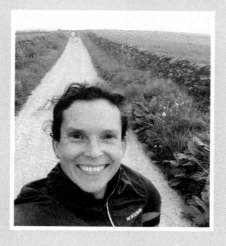

www.julietmcgrattan.com. **Author of** *Sorted: The Active Woman's Guide to Health.* **Women's Health Lead and Master Coach for 261 Fearless.** *"I graduated from the University of Dundee in 1996 and immediately began working as a junior doctor. I passed diplomas in Child Health, Obstetrics and Gynaecology and Family Planning and qualified as a GP in 2002. I have worked in a variety of locations including New Zealand and Shetland but settled in Lancaster where I became a salaried GP in a busy town-centre practice in 2003. I officially relinquished clinical work in 2019."*

HOBBIES & INTERESTS

I love to run, for myself and for others, and I volunteer every week as a coach in my local 261 Fearless club. I enjoy being outside, walking my dog, baking, and hanging out with my husband and kids.

WHO WERE YOUR MAIN FEMALE ROLE MODELS GROWING UP IN TERMS OF EXERCISE, NUTRITION AND BEAUTY?

I was a keen dancer and singer as a child so my main role models were my dance teachers or on *Top of the Pops*! My parents weren't big on exercise and I grew up in the era of chicken kievs and Findus Crispy Pancakes. In terms of beauty, my information came from *Girl* and *Just Seventeen* magazines and from my friends.

WHAT WOULD YOU TELL YOUR 20-YEAR-OLD SELF AND IS YOUR CONFIDENCE NOW HIGHER?

I was always confident as a child and a young woman. In fact, I think I'm possibly less confident now than I was then. I was a high achiever and had a lot of success in my studies and hobbies. I embraced opportunities and wasn't afraid to try things. I'm certainly wiser now but repeatedly suffer imposter syndrome and generally worry more than I used to. I would tell that confident 20-year-old that she was amazing, to keep going and just be herself. I would warn her that the junior doctor years would be harder than she thought and that she needed to take care of herself but she would get through it and her life ahead would bring her all she dreamed of. I'd also ask to have a quick word with her 47-year-old self to give her a confidence boost!

DOES BODY IMAGE AND APPEARANCE MATTER TO YOU NOW?

Yes, it does. I don't spend hours looking in the mirror, I'm not keen on shopping and I don't have a complicated beauty routine but looking good is still important to me. Being a runner helps because it maintains my weight and figure without me having to give it much thought. It does mean I spend a lot of my days in running kit, but I still enjoy nice clothes and dressing up to go out. I know I'm terribly lacking in makeup skills because I don't wear it much! I don't relish ageing but I'm reasonably happy with myself when I stand naked in front of the mirror. I don't spend a lot of time worrying about what others think of me, I'm happy in my own skin.

ANY POINTS IN YOUR LIFE THAT MADE YOU LOOK AFTER YOURSELF MORE?

I haven't always been good at making myself a priority. Being a busy mum and a doctor I've gone whole days without going for a wee, skipped more meals than I've eaten and generally not been terribly good to myself. It's only recently that I've really become aware of how I suffer when I don't take time to look after myself. I feel much more in tune with my body than I ever did, and I notice the effect on me when I've not slept enough, drunk too much or am overworked. Previously in life I've just cracked on and got away with it but I can't now. I've assumed this is because of my age and am finding it fascinating to see how delicate the balance is and how even small changes can have a positive effect on my feelings and behaviours.

TELL ME ABOUT YOUR AVERAGE WEEK IN TERMS OF EXERCISE.

I do some form of exercise every day. I have a dog so I have to either walk or run with her. On average I run three times a week, sometimes it's four – anything from two to ten miles. Every now and then I'll go for a swim and I'll do a few core exercises at home when I suddenly realise I haven't done any for ages. I try to minimise my sedentary time and work standing up sometimes or at least get up and move around a bit. That's something I've had to consciously work on since becoming a writer.

YOUR ATTITUDE TO NUTRITION?

I love food! There's nothing I enjoy more than a really good meal out with my husband. I cook a lot and I bake too. I have a sweet tooth and eat plenty of treats. To me, food is a pleasure and I enjoy it. I'm aware also that it's a fuel, and to maintain my running hobby I need to eat well so I do eat lots of fruit, vegetables and healthy fats. We eat as a family whenever we can, we chat and we usually have pudding. I hope that my kids are growing up with a sensible attitude to food and nutrition and see mealtimes as an enjoyable part of their day – even if they do have to put their plates in the dishwasher!

WHAT CHANGES HAVE YOU NOTICED SINCE 40?

Obviously there are some wrinkles and grey hairs but I expected those. My skin is a bit drier and so is my hair; it seems to need cutting every six weeks when previously I'd have got away with at least six months! I've got a few annoying little skin tags appearing on my neck. I don't think my breasts have changed and as long as I'm keeping a check on my exercise and diet then I haven't noticed any weight gain yet. I am aware that this body gets more tired more easily, takes longer to recover after a long run and I can't tolerate sleep deprivation like I used to.

NAME YOUR TOP FIVE BEAUTY PRODUCTS.

Clarins Foaming facial wash, Clinique Dramatically Different Moisturiser, Burt's Bees lip balm, Clarins hand cream, My amazing bed!

MELISSA POE, 52

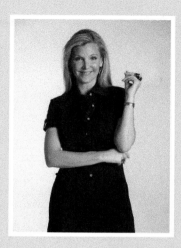

Runway model and pageant queen in her early years, Melissa became a reality show star on *Big Rich Texas,* which is now syndicated worldwide. She is also a swimsuit/cover-up designer. She has worked as a Human Resources Manager/Director of Administration in the oil and gas exploration industry for the last 26 years and lives in Dallas, Texas.

INTERESTS
Cooking, gardening, travel, wine, being active (Pilates Megaformer or Barre), and I'm happiest when I'm entertaining family/friends.

FEMALE ROLE MODELS
Ingrid Bergman and Grace Kelly (my early teens to about 40). From the age of 40 to now, I've become my own role model.

HOW AWARE WERE YOU GROWING UP OF BODY IMAGE AND BEAUTY?
Because I was tall and skinny growing up, I often felt awkward, gawky and so uncomfortable with my body. I was 10 years old when a stranger told me I should be a model, and from that moment on I'd save every penny I could to spend on fashion magazines and get lost in them.

DID YOU HAVE STRONG INFLUENCES ON YOUR EATING PATTERNS GROWING UP?
No, because I grew up poor and sometimes food was scarce, so my sisters and brothers and I had very little choice but to eat what was put on the table... mostly fried potatoes, chicken, catfish, deer meat. Vegetables and fruits were rare. I changed from that way of eating when I started my first job as a grocery store cashier at the age of 15, by eating fruit on my breaks instead of junk food and buying fruits and vegetables to contribute to our family's nightly dinners.

WERE YOU HAPPY WITH YOUR IMAGE AS A TEENAGER?
Not really. Took me until I was 15 to start embracing my height and angular face and not seeing those features as oddities.

WHAT WOULD YOU TELL YOUR 20-YEAR-OLD SELF AND IS YOUR CONFIDENCE NOW HIGHER?

I would actually prefer to go back to my five-year-old self and tell her that she will survive and that she is valued and loved and ultimately will have the best life ever. By the time I was 20 I knew my life was going to be good... just didn't know what that really looked like yet.

DO YOU COMPARE YOURSELF TO OTHER WOMEN?

I used to compare myself all the time. Took me until I was about 50 to stop the comparisons. There is always going to be someone prettier, smarter and who seems to have it more together than you. Comparisons stop when you realise your own unique talents, identity, value and beauty. There is no one like you or me... We are all powerful, cherished, unique, precious, BELOVED daughters of Abba Father!

DOES BODY IMAGE AND APPEARANCE MATTER TO YOU NOW?

Only in the aspect that in order to be your best self you have to take care of yourself, and that only comes from honouring and truly loving yourself.

ANY POINTS IN YOUR LIFE THAT MADE YOU LOOK AFTER YOURSELF MORE?

I encountered high blood pressure last year due to stress in dealing with family issues, along with health issues that led up to a hysterectomy. I had to learn to destress by learning to meditate and take up yoga... and I'm not a big fan of yoga. HA!

DO YOU EXERCISE?

Yes, but not as much as I should these days. I work out maybe two to three days a week with the Pilates Megaformer. It's the best cardio/core training for my body, and it's the only exercise that has truly changed the shape of my body.

YOUR ATTITUDE TO NUTRITION?

Eat to Live is my motto! Nutrition is everything. I truly believe the body can heal itself with nutrient-rich food. I really don't believe in diets except for eating 'clean' like the 'Whole30' way of eating. I do my best to eat clean most days but when the weekend rolls around I allow myself to have cheese and a few bad carbs (bread, chips and so on).

WHAT CHANGES HAVE YOU NOTICED SINCE 40?

Fine lines and wrinkles started taking up residence on my face at about age 42, my metabolism started slowing down, AND the big one... menopause at age 47! That was shocking to me.

HOW DO YOU FEEL EMOTIONALLY ABOUT THE PASSING YEARS?

Time passing by doesn't really bother me because I feel like every passing year I'm much wiser and smarter. What does bother me is that as I get older my parents are getting up there in age as well... Saddens me that I may not have my parents around in 15-20 years.

WHAT IS YOUR OPINION ON THE MORE INTERVENTIONAL BEAUTY TREATMENTS?

My opinion is "You do you, girl!" If an invasive beauty procedure/treatment makes you feel good about yourself, then by all means do it for you.

HAVE YOU EVER HAD ANY BEAUTY DISASTERS?

No, thank goodness!

NAME YOUR TOP FIVE BEAUTY PRODUCTS.

1) Aveeno Absolutely Ageless Blueberry Nourishing Cleanser
2) Josie Maran's Argan Milk Intensive and Argan Face Oil
3) EltaMD UV Clear SPF 46 moisturising Facial Sunscreen
4) Organic virgin coconut oil
5) Forever Young BBL laser face treatments twice a year (best non-invasive treatment you can ever do for your face)!

TELL ME ANY SUPPLEMENTS YOU TAKE.

Activated B-Complex, Ubiquinol (Co-Q10), vitamins D3 and K, DIM Estro, Niacin and Krill oil

MAGGIE MCMILLAN, 66

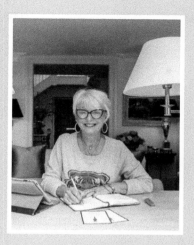

Originally trained as a speech therapist specialising in special needs, and became the first female salaried director of a national charity THE DOWN SYNDROME ASSOCIATION. After having her first child, Maggie set up a small fundraising consultancy for small charities, then in 10 years off, alongside being a mummy, qualified in Nutrition, Historic Garden Design and learned to cook international cuisines. In France she trained as an image consultant and worked seriously on it after her husband's death in 2006. Her consultancy includes personal branding, impact and wardrobe, and works across most corporate sectors with men and women, often senior. She runs workshops for individuals and groups, and clients include popstars, politicians, CEOs, sixth-formers and grannies! She trains other consultants and is on the board of the SMARTWORKS charity.

MAIN ROLE MODELS
Mum, teachers and contemporaries. I was brought up to expect the 'banana skin', that you should never think too much of yourself and that it was inappropriate to brag (my mum). I was taught to consider the cost of any purchases I wanted. My teachers embraced my work ethic and, as I was clever, boosted my confidence. My peers regarded me as a swot! My German teacher encouraged my linguistic aptitude and my maths teacher was endlessly patient. My mum showed me love and understanding even though we were so different emotionally and intellectually.

HOBBIES
Gardening, cooking, baking and decorating.

HOW AWARE WERE YOU GROWING UP OF BODY IMAGE AND BEAUTY?
I was always aware that I had no boobs when my friends had developed, and I was desperate to have a bra. I always wanted to be prettier, especially after my first boyfriend at 16.

DID YOU HAVE STRONG INFLUENCES ON YOUR EATING PATTERNS GROWING UP?
We always ate healthily with plenty of fruit and veg; Mum was an amazing baker. I don't

remember craving sweet things then as they were readily available but I certainly crave them now. Mum used to refer to my father being overweight but carried on baking for all of us!

WERE YOU HAPPY WITH YOUR IMAGE AS A TEENAGER?

No – I was thin and thought myself 'pokey' looking! I had some terrible perms which I hated – I never had long hair though I am not sure why, I always wanted it! I loved *Petticoat* magazine but the looks seemed unattainable.

HOW DO YOU FEEL ABOUT SOCIAL MEDIA TODAY?

The huge pressure concerns me. I see in my daughters the evolution of 'Everyone else's life is perfect' syndrome and their blind acceptance of total lack of privacy.

WHAT WOULD YOU TELL YOUR 20-YEAR-OLD SELF AND IS YOUR CONFIDENCE NOW HIGHER?

You cannot control the behaviour of others but you can control your reaction to it. Worrying about the future and the past is exhausting and futile. My confidence is higher now.

DOES BODY IMAGE AND APPEARANCE MATTER TO YOU NOW?

Because of my work it is very important to me. I worry constantly about the way I look. I HATE ageing and looking in the mirror. I am terrified of death and want to turn the clock back.

ANY POINTS IN YOUR LIFE THAT MADE YOU LOOK AFTER YOURSELF MORE?

The death of my first husband in 2006 from bowel cancer and the sudden death of my second husband in 2017 from total organ failure/sepsis. Since both deaths I have been desperate not to leave my girls alone.

DO YOU EXERCISE?

Dog walking, Pilates, about to join a gym!

YOUR ATTITUDE TO NUTRITION?

Meals are healthy but too many chocolate items in between! I struggle to make breakfast if working then crave something sweet. I would rather give up alcohol than chocolate.

WHAT CHANGES HAVE YOU NOTICED SINCE 40?

Bags under eyes, wrinkles, latterly around mouth and neck and décolletage. Increasingly dry skin. Middle-aged spread. Ageing hands. Bingo wings.

HOW DO YOU FEEL EMOTIONALLY ABOUT THE PASSING YEARS?

Would love to have the resources to have surgical intervention and just want to turn back the clock and look young and attractive.

HAVE YOU EVER HAD A BEAUTY DISASTER?

Dyed my white hair blonde and it emerged with a ginger tint – my children called me the ginger whinger!

WHAT IS YOUR OPINION ON THE MORE INTERVENTIONAL BEAUTY TREATMENTS?

Whatever works for you and makes you feel confident. I had an eyelift but wish I had researched more as I have wonky eyebrows. Would love some cryotherapy too!

BEAUTY PRODUCTS

PIXI Double Cleanse, Tata Harper eye cream, Beauty Pie retinol moisturiser, Sarah Chapman face mask, SkinLab products.

SUPPLEMENTS

D3 for memory

TRACEY MCALPINE, 59

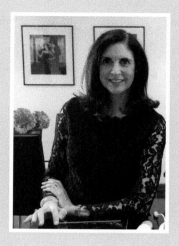

Founder of www.fightingfifty.co.uk

"Following a successful career in advertising, working at some of the top London agencies including Saatchi & Saatchi, I took a long career break to bring up my two children. It was only when I hit 50 that I realised how much negativity there was surrounding older women. Not only that, there was also a marketing misconception surrounding ageing. Companies were targeting me with details of a walk-in bath, funeral plans and chair lifts. Supposedly, I had become frail, infirm and approaching death. I didn't relate to this in the least and nor did my peer group. We were running companies, climbing mountains and caring for families. We were not about to give up!

I felt I had to do something to challenge these stereotypes and perceptions of ageing. We all want to look good and feel well regardless of age. I created the website 'Fighting Fifty' as a platform to share knowledge and information from leading experts. And to speak to women as they are now, in the prime of their lives.

Fighting Fifty has given me a creative outlet where I can use my marketing skills combined with my love of photography, cooking, health, beauty and fitness. Best of all, it has enabled me to meet some wonderful and inspirational women."

MAIN ROLE MODELS

My mother was, and still is, a huge influence in my life. Healthy living has always been a part of our lives, and during my teens and early 20s there wasn't a diet we didn't try or an exercise video we didn't own. We tried everything, from the Cabbage Soup Diet to the Cambridge Diet. We even did circuit training together which was quite unusual in the '70s, unless you were an athlete. I was very aware of body image and appearance when I was growing up but having children completely changed my focus. I was far more concerned about giving them a healthy diet, and taking care of them, than I was worrying about my weight or appearance.

WHAT WOULD YOU TELL YOUR 20-YEAR-OLD SELF AND IS YOUR CONFIDENCE NOW HIGHER?

I would definitely tell my younger self that every age is amazing; it's a gift to be cherished. I would also mention just how quickly it goes. One minute you're 25 and the next you're 50, literally in a blink of an eye. So, enjoy every moment and try to keep learning. We are never too old to learn a new skill. I have a different type of confidence now I'm older. One that only comes with age and life experiences.

DO YOU COMPARE YOURSELF TO OTHER WOMEN?

I don't directly compare myself to other women, but I do admire so many and sometimes wish I could be more like them.

DOES BODY IMAGE AND APPEARANCE MATTER TO YOU NOW?

Yes, very much so. I feel I owe it to myself to keep well, control my weight and to exercise. I feel better when I look better, it's that simple.

DO YOU EXERCISE?

I'm a fair-weather runner. I started running at 47 to take part in the Race for Life, supporting a friend going through cancer treatment, and have kept it up. I like to work out at home using a Whole Body Vibration FlexxiCore Challenger and hand weights, HIIT, walking.

YOUR ATTITUDE TO NUTRITION?

I love healthy food and don't follow diets, but I'm very aware of what I eat and when. Understanding that food is for fuel and not just for pleasure helps to change your mindset and make healthy choices.

WHAT CHANGES HAVE YOU NOTICED SINCE 40?

Changes to my skin, hair and body are part of the natural ageing process and I have accepted them. Eating sensibly and only drinking the occasional glass of wine has helped me keep my weight down, and exercise has helped keep my body reasonably well toned.

HOW DO YOU FEEL ABOUT THE PASSING YEARS?

I am hugely grateful to have lived as long as I have and look forward to many more years ahead. My only concern is not being able to look after myself in my later years. I believe that functional fitness is the key to independent living. If I can carry my shopping home, change a light bulb and dress myself I should be fine.

WHAT IS YOUR OPINION ON THE MORE INTERVENTIONAL BEAUTY TREATMENTS?

Everyone has a choice how they look and how they age. I am not in any way against interventional beauty treatments, but they aren't for me. I am perfectly happy to laser my own face, use red light therapy and radio frequency devices at home, but at present I don't want any invasive treatments. Of course, I might change my mind in the future!

BEAUTY PRODUCTS

SPF daily, e.g. Ark Skincare Skin Protector SPF 30 Primer, Skin Alchemists The Humble Warrior cleanser, Temple Spa Eye Truffle, Bodhi & Birch Super25 Botanical Serum, Kiss The Moon Love Night Cream for Hands

SUPPLEMENTS

Omegas, Lutein eye supplement, Magnesium, Collagen shots

MELANIE SYKES, 49

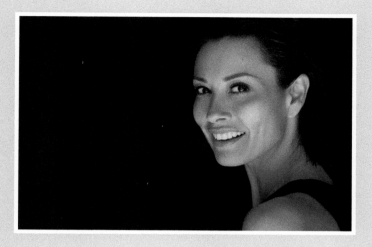

TV and Radio Presenter, Model and Editor-in-Chief of online magazine www.thefrankmagazine.com

MAIN ROLE MODELS

My mum always worked, so I learned my work ethic from both her and Dad. When I was modelling the supermodels were aspirational in terms of giving me something to aspire to be, within my industry. They were commanding high fees and getting them and were not being taken for a ride. I love any women, especially women who have power who support other women, it's really that simple.

HOW AWARE WERE YOU GROWING UP OF BODY IMAGE AND BEAUTY?

I was a very skinny and flat-chested teenager. I was the youngest in my year, so very immature mentally and physically. I was self-conscious and quite shy. I never felt beautiful and I was never told I was. I blossomed when I hit 17 and somebody suggested I be a model. I was not very comfortable in front of the cameras but managed to wing it and after all this time I still feel the same. Being a model didn't make me feel beautiful, it was just a job I did.

DID YOU HAVE STRONG INFLUENCES ON YOUR EATING PATTERNS GROWING UP?

I have always had a huge appetite – Dad and I would hoover up any leftovers! I can eat a lot but just try not to. I'm healthier now than I have ever been though. Mum was always on a diet, but I didn't feel swayed either way by it growing up, I was just naturally thin. During my modelling days I tried all sorts of different eating plans. In the modelling world I had to stay skinny, which I struggled with. I would fluctuate weight-wise quite a lot.

WERE YOU HAPPY WITH YOUR IMAGE AS A TEENAGER?

I was embarrassed of my skinny, tall body, I used to round my shoulders to disguise how flat-chested I was. I just wasn't comfortable in my own skin as a teenager and was so self-conscious.

HOW DO YOU FEEL ABOUT SOCIAL MEDIA TODAY?

I'm lucky my boys have absolutely no interest in social media which is just brilliant. But I can see how it could affect young minds. Adults fall foul of it too. I have to be involved in it for my work. If it wasn't for that I probably would not really get involved. It can be a very toxic place.

WHAT WOULD YOU TELL YOUR 20-YEAR-OLD SELF AND IS YOUR CONFIDENCE NOW HIGHER?

"Always speak your truth and don't let any man tell you what to do!" I am very confident in myself and sometimes the complete opposite. I am a walking contradiction. I absolutely know my worth in my personal life and at work but can feel insecure at times also.

DO YOU COMPARE YOURSELF TO OTHER WOMEN?

I feel *inspired* by women older than me. They show me where I would like to get to. Confidence isn't a constant state of play, it's something to be nurtured and worked on. We should support each other in that.

DOES BODY IMAGE AND APPEARANCE MATTER TO YOU NOW?

My physique is very important to me because if I am in shape, I feel good. Yoga keeps me mentally strong and my body flexible. I would never describe myself as a fanatic when it comes to fitness. It is woven into my life because it's part of my being, as important as food and water. It affects my parenting skills, my stamina for long days at work, my mental health and hopefully my longevity.

ANY POINTS IN YOUR LIFE THAT MADE YOU LOOK AFTER YOURSELF MORE?

I stopped drinking when I hit 45 and then every now and again I would have a blowout. Now I am sober two and a half years and I will never drink again. It's poison to me physically and mentally.

DO YOU EXERCISE?

I do about three hours of hot yoga, one hour of gym every week. I love exercise, and even if I am not in the mood I will still go because I know I will feel better afterwards. If my body is tired though I don't go. It's a 12-year habit that has paid me back in spades!

YOUR ATTITUDE TO NUTRITION?

Not drinking, I have developed a sweet tooth! I like dark raw chocolate. I have to make an effort to eat fruit, but thankfully I do like vegetables. I am very aware now of what I put into my body. I try to eat less meat than I naturally crave and really try to get as many nutrients into my diet as possible.

WHAT CHANGES HAVE YOU NOTICED SINCE 40?

Actually more specifically it's been since turning 45 that I have noticed my face change. The skin is thinner and I have lines around my eyes. My nose is longer too! Skin on my neck has gone crepey, hands veiny, my knees and elbows look different LOL but it's a process I embrace, but it can be a little scary.

HOW DO YOU FEEL EMOTIONALLY ABOUT THE PASSING YEARS?

I'm embracing it! My personality and work life are developing in amazing ways, along with parenting becoming more interesting as the kids get older. So to those ends it's fantastic. The aesthetics however are a different dynamic, but I keep healthy and that's all I can do.

WHAT IS YOUR OPINION ON THE MORE INTERVENTIONAL BEAUTY TREATMENTS?

I have nothing against plastic surgery. I will never say never to a little facelift, LOL; if Jane Fonda can live with it so can I!

SUPPLEMENTS

B12, Omega 3-6-9, Shatavari, Ashwagandha, Bio-Biloba

JULES WILLCOCKS, 57

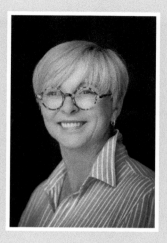

www.bodyballancer.co.uk. *"After 35 years as a business consultant I co-founded Body Ballancer Systems UK. This arose out of a chance encounter with an utterly miraculous piece of kit – the Ballancer lymphatic massage system – at a spa in Spain. As soon as I tried it, I decided to buy one once back in the UK. I was so impressed that the distributor Naomi and I joined forces and ended up creating our company three months after meeting."*

MAIN ROLE MODELS

My aunts. The elder one in terms of behaviour – very calm, level-headed and open-minded; the younger in terms of lifestyle, beauty and fashion as she was outgoing and vivacious with lots of friends and a hectic social life. I became a 'mini-me' of my younger aunt, copying her clothing, make-up and love of jewellery – this was the 1980s, so flamboyance was pretty much obligatory; the older aunt taught me to always try to see the other person's point of view, no matter how at variance it was with your own, and to be unfailingly polite and respectful of whoever you came into contact with irrespective of age, gender or social status.

HOW AWARE WERE YOU GROWING UP OF BODY IMAGE AND BEAUTY?

Unlike today, there simply was not the pressure to look any particular way; you were allowed to be a 'normal' teenager and for that I am eternally grateful. I was neurotic about the odd spot and spent about a week obsessing about the size of my thighs at 15, but I can honestly say that was it.

We were the first on our street to get a TV, but there was simply not the content that exists today. The only newspapers in the house were the tabloids – none of which held any interest for me. I was kept supplied with 'age-appropriate' magazines but even then I don't recall taking anything in them to heart (though any mention of Donny Osmond possibly having a girlfriend would make me sick with grief!).

DID YOU HAVE STRONG INFLUENCES ON YOUR EATING PATTERNS GROWING UP?

My great-grandmother (Nanna) lived with us and was almost exclusively responsible for the diet of the entire family. Three no-nonsense delicious home-cooked meals a day, and the occasional treat of homemade cakes and pastries. The only takeaway was the sacred Friday night fish and chips. There was never any obsessing over food in any way.

WHAT WOULD YOU TELL YOUR 20-YEAR-OLD SELF AND IS YOUR CONFIDENCE NOW HIGHER?

"Everything you are aspiring to right now, you will achieve, and more." Yes, because I have everything I need to lead a happy, healthy and productive life. On the whole, I think I appear to be more confident than a lot of women, but note the operative word 'appear'. I may be very nervous inside but outwardly come across as super self-assured, and I think that is likely to be the same for a lot of women. I am the archetypal 'extroverted introvert' as indeed most of the women in my family are.

DO YOU COMPARE YOURSELF TO OTHER WOMEN?

Only with women of my own age and I think I'm doing pretty damn well! Even those of a similar vintage who look spectacular – Elle Macpherson, Jennifer Aniston et al. – don't bother me terribly as that is almost their full-time job. And they are bloody good at it, so all power to them!

DOES BODY IMAGE AND APPEARANCE MATTER TO YOU NOW?

It matters to me that I look good for my age, not younger. My husband is extraordinary for his age and I really believe I owe it to him to look my best. That may be seen by some as 'anti-feminist' but to me it's about respect for him and for me. I look after my skin, and hair really IS everything. Enough said.

ANY POINTS IN YOUR LIFE THAT MADE YOU LOOK AFTER YOURSELF MORE?

At 55 I found I couldn't even fit into my 'big clothes'. This made me take stock of my lifestyle. I embarked on a year of spa/clinic holidays, shed 10 kilos and became much more vigilant in terms of any 'creeping' gains. This was not just for sheer vanity and wanting to be skinny – being the size I was, was making me miserable and I didn't want to become one of those middle-aged ladies blaming *everything but themselves* for poor physical shape.

DO YOU EXERCISE?

Light workout twice a week with a PT, Hypoxi training (a form of low-impact cycling designed to burn fat), Pilates Reformer classes to improve my core strength. I regularly use my beloved Ballancer.

YOUR ATTITUDE TO NUTRITION?

I have recently found intermittent fasting and the PROLON fasting Mimicking Diet (which I do every quarter) work for me.

I consider myself to be very well informed on nutrition and know precisely what works best for me. I cook from scratch every day.

WHAT CHANGES HAVE YOU NOTICED SINCE 40?

Most of the bits that should be pert have decidedly lost the fight with gravity. Skin quality on legs and arms reducing, losing elasticity since 55.

WHAT IS YOUR OPINION ON THE MORE INTERVENTIONAL BEAUTY TREATMENTS?

I invest regularly.

Botox (three times a year); fillers (once a year on average); RadioFrequency/Ultrasound skin tightening every 18 months, laser resurfacing (three a year), thread lifting every 18 months, upper eyelid surgery – done about 10 years ago and probably will redo in the next year or so.

HAVE YOU EVER HAD ANY BEAUTY DISASTERS?

I only ever had professional, full-face make-up applied once for a posh evening 'do' 30 years ago and I looked like a circus clown. Never again!

NAME YOUR TOP FIVE BEAUTY PRODUCTS.

Clarisonic cleansing brush, Dr Dennis Gross LED light mask three mins per day, Ginza moisturising sheet mask (astonishing but indulgent), Cicalfate Repair Cream (calming), any Retinol product

SUPPLEMENTS

Vitamin D3, Iron (monitored by doctor), Omega-3

ALICE HART-DAVIS, 57

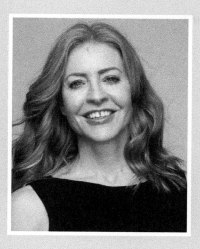

"After a Modern History degree at Oxford, I worked as a journalist at *Vogue*, then *The Telegraph*, writing, commissioning and editing. Freelance since 1997, I now specialise in beauty and non-surgical cosmetic treatments – writing, commissioning and editing – for the *Daily Mail*, *The Times* and *The Telegraph*. In 2019, I launched **Tweakments Guide Ltd** and self-published a book – *The Tweakments Guide: fresher face*, and I now run the business and website www. thetweakmentsguide.com. This aims to demystify the world of non-surgical cosmetic procedures."

HOW AWARE WERE YOU GROWING UP OF BODY IMAGE AND BEAUTY?

I grew up in the countryside and was happily unaware of body image until I was found to be overweight by the doctor and put on a diet age 11. It worked but I have been self-conscious of my body shape since.

At school, we experimented with mascara and blue eyeshadow and obsessed over Debbie Harry, Olivia Newton-John and Chrissie Hynde but were largely unaware of 'beauty'.

WERE YOU HAPPY WITH YOUR IMAGE AS A TEENAGER?

No. I disliked my heavy face and body shape and believed 'thinner would be better' so ate as little as possible. The food at boarding school wasn't great, so that wasn't hard, but eating normally in the holidays stopping me tipping into anorexia.

WHAT WOULD YOU TELL YOUR 20-YEAR-OLD SELF AND IS YOUR CONFIDENCE NOW HIGHER?

"Be brave and find your voice. Get better at setting boundaries. Find mentors. Don't keep things for best. Stay kind, and be kinder to yourself. Stop worrying about how you look and what other people think. People-pleasing and constant dieting are a waste of energy. Dance more. Know that you are enough. Wear sunscreen. Find ways to give back."

My confidence is a million times higher now.

DO YOU COMPARE YOURSELF TO OTHER WOMEN?

No, we can't be anyone but ourselves. I prefer to celebrate other women in all their forms and finery, and admire their different qualities. I try to learn from other women.

DOES BODY IMAGE AND APPEARANCE MATTER TO YOU NOW?

Yes, massively. It shouldn't, but I also know that how we look drives how happy we feel about ourselves. My appearance also matters in that I no longer feel a need to minimise myself.

DO YOU EXERCISE?

Cycling, dog walking, intensive weight training three times a week, interval sprints on treadmill for cardio weekly, plus plenty of yoga.

It took me a long time to realise that yoga and meditation are just about showing up and doing the practice, rather than achieving any particular end.

YOUR ATTITUDE TO NUTRITION?

I try to eat sensibly but have researched and tried just about every fad diet. I read keenly all the latest research so know the value of vegetables, whole grains, beans and pulses and so on, but of course if there's cake on offer I'm not going to say no! We cook well from scratch every night within the family.

WHAT IS YOUR OPINION ON THE MORE INTERVENTIONAL BEAUTY TREATMENTS?

I've been writing about and trying out minor cosmetic medical procedures for 20 years and I'm still an advocate for *good, understated cosmetic work*. I recognise the potential of good tweakments to encourage confidence and this can be a great boost, say, to older women in the workplace, alongside a great haircut and wardrobe.

MY GENERAL TOP FIVE

Botox, done with a light hand, is great for softening frown lines and crow's feet and the muscles that pull an ageing neck into stringy bands.

Fillers, used intelligently, to replace volume and structure where needed.

Intense pulsed light or laser for pigmentation marks and thread veins.

'Injectable moisture' treatments such as Profhilo which help hydrate and recondition the skin from the inside.

Red light therapy, one of the few no-pain-but-lots-of-gain treatments. I have a home-use mask and try to use it daily.

NAME YOUR TOP FIVE BEAUTY PRODUCTS

Sunscreen, antioxidant day serum, prescription retinoid night product, body lotion, a fabulous fragrance.

TELL ME ANY SUPPLEMENTS YOU TAKE REGULARLY

Liposomal vitamin C – that's vitamin C encased in liposomes, which are minute, fatty protective spheres, because that way it a) doesn't upset the stomach (b) makes it through to the gut and is properly absorbed. I was put through a study with this stuff last year, and it made such a measurable difference to my skin elasticity, hydration and collagen production that I've felt obliged to keep taking it.

Collagen supplements – (Totally Derma, Skinade, or Absolute Collagen) with a dose that delivers around 8,000 mg of hydrolysed collagen – that's collagen that has been fragmented into a form that is easily absorbed in the body – and which has studies to show that it works. Like the vitamin C, these allegedly help with joint maintenance and dry scaly shins, as well as the face.

Vitamin D, as my levels are always low, even when I've had a sunny holiday and had my legs and back in the sun.

Vitamin B12, to help with energy levels

Magnesium, for general calming-down

Melatonin, for its hormonal action, as well as to help with sleep.

Thank you for the immense generosity of spirit that allowed these women to share their personal stories.

You will have seen how lives can be changed over 40, before this was maybe just the rehearsal! With courage and a little caution thrown to the wind YOU might now improve your future health and happiness. Take that walk, start a club, design a business, volunteer, eat more greens, meditate, look at the sky and know there is no limit to what can happen now. Do whatever makes you smile and laugh more than ever!

It has been an honour and a delight to share this journey with all contributing to it and now you, dear reader. I wish you all luck, tenacity and passion in creating your own **best life**.

ACKNOWLEDGEMENTS

Never did I imagine what a journey these pages would take me on. Words cannot suffice to thank you all for giving your time, energy, humour and inspiration to this project. Let us hope that many women will be touched and motivated by it in the years to come.

Professional thanks to The British Medical Association and the Royal College of General Practitioners for enabling me to have access to all online medical research reading resources.

Elizabeth of www.ruby-roux.com for all the professional photography in this book; fate brought us together for the book yet we grew up in the same road never knowing each other. You are stuck with me now, lovely.

Matador for allowing me to bring the dream to life exactly as I imagined.

Suzy Reading, Terrence the Teacher, Roja Dove, Jack Cassidy, Dr Louise Pendry, Raman Malhotra, Dr Naji Tabet, Nicky Gough, Dr Alastair Smith, Andrew Yelland, Liz O'Riordan, Professor Janice Rymer, Sophie Dopierala at CoppaFeel!, Stephanie and Hayley at Kegel8, Positive Pause Jo and Ann, Christien Bird, Dr Justine Hextall, Dr Juliet McGrattan, Jenni Rivett, Dr Olga Rutherford, Vanessa Cowan, Shelley Osborne-Shaw, Louise Coyle, Becks Armstrong, Professor Dawn Skelton, Frances Stephens, Dr Suzanne Barr, Jackie Lynch, Dr Holly Whelan, Dr Mark Cobain, Professor Jose Ordovas, Yvonne Wake, Nicky Hambleton-Jones, Professor Carolyn Mair, Dr Peter Venn, Clare Baumhauer, Maxine Laceby, Dr Jenna Macciochi, Shelley Von Strunckel, Athena Lamnisos and Lydia Brain at Eve Appeal, Katie Pande, Willow and Eve, The Burlington Hotel.

Limitless thanks to the incredible women who let me into their lives to ask them personal and pertinent questions and who were just so willing to share their wisdom.

Tracey Woodward, your enthusiasm and interest took the book to a higher echelon.

Dr Roger Duckitt, your Clarithromycin and sense were the keys that saved me. No words suffice.

Gratitude for the friendships created and the old friendships that saw me through this process.

To all my wonderful followers on social media – especially Instagram. You all have a special place in my head as I write, overwhelmed by your kindness and unlimited love, wishing me on to the finishing line. Who knew we would start such a movement of fabulous women all thinking the same?

Melanie Sykes for giving me the platform to write for the fabulous www.thefrankmagazine. com and for showing me that voice messages are a 'thing'. Thank you, darlin', for believing in me, and thank you to Tony Parsons, my writing idol, for connecting us.

Rhalou Allerhand at Hearst Magazines and Juliet for helping me become a working mum again through working for www.netdoctor.co.uk after this book was complete.

Jenni Rivett, I didn't expect to find a dear friend forever; Yvonne Wake, you had me at the word 'lunch' – your intense kindness and support have literally warmed my heart; Terrence the Teacher, shared life experience united us immediately; Juliet McGrattan, just to know another 'writing doctor' helped me not feel alone; Nicky H-J, I can't look at red without seeing your gorgeous face; Tanya Rose, you truly reflect the hashtag 'women empowering women'; Suzie Barr, thank you for patiently answering constant nutrition niggles; Jules Willcocks, thank you for the enforced relaxation at my writing peak with the Body Ballancer; Lou Pendry, not just two 'Dr Louises' but writing and life buddies; Shelley Osborne-Shaw, for resetting my batteries and listening to my relentless ramblings with a smile; Shelley von Strunckel, reading your stars was only surpassed by having your kind words in my inbox.

Emma at Rarebrandmarket, for my first speaking gig; 'Mother of teenagers' Jo, for asking me to write for her; Jackie Lynch, for letting us bounce ideas on her podcast and reach so many women; the Kegel 8 ladies for wonderful support; Grace Fodor for interviewing me; Kate Thornton, what a first podcast; Positive Pause Jo and Ann, thank you for letting me spread the word; Frances Stephens, thank you for letting me chatter to your lovely ladies; The Women's Institute, for loving my ideas and laughing loud.

Vix, you are my rock and sounding board, let's return to simple times of painting cupboards; Caroline, my darling, this is what happens when you meet and think 'it's someone else normal'; Jane, Kati and Andrea, all together we make up the friends forever five, ten children and so many laughs and tears; Mo, your love and calmness centre me; Amy the younger sister I never had; Claire, your laughs and makeup skills kept me smiling; Wendy, your advice stays with me always; Yvette, my book, your shop – dreams do come true; Amanda and Justin showed me real men do listen to podcasts; David and Liz you knew I could do it before I did; Louise, since 15 we have laughed together, Auntie Ellen would be proud.

Roz and Olga, Physiology soulmates with a connection of pure love and laughter; Rey and Mims, for all the laughs, sense and nonsense, always the Nutford trio in my heart; Dr Hazel Adams, for teaching me the Physiology of Obstetric Anaesthetics but more importantly what it was to be a doctor and mummy; Dr Richard Baxter, for your kindness and not thinking I am mad to write; to my work colleagues, I learned something different from each of you; Dave Prince, I still hope for you to bring the tea in; Ronnie and Michelle, we are now on the same train; Justine, thank you for seeing this could be something when I almost didn't believe it myself.

To my darling mother, who brought me up believing I could achieve absolutely anything I put my mind to. To my lovely father, because of you I always wanted to go the extra mile – call me eccentric – and surprise them.

To my dearest, darling, quite remarkable husband, who has loved me as I give everything to these pages, and for the wonderful Daddy that he is. Little did I know that the little boy whose hair was standing on end as he touched the Van der Graaf Generator in science class would become my husband, love of my life and soulmate.

To our beautiful children, you are my heart and my everything – may you always have our love with you and discover your own path and fly.

REFERENCES

Happiness

1. Laura E. Kurtz, Sara B. Algoe, Putting laughter in context: Shared laughter as behavioural indicator of relationship well-being, Journal of The International Association for Relationship Research 24.8.15

2. Berk L.S. et al., Modulation of neuroimmune parameters during the eustress of humor-associated mirthful laughter, Altern Ther Health Med. 2001 Mar;7(2):62-72, 74-6.

3. R. Mora_Ripoli, The therapeutic value of laughter in medicine, Altern Ther Health Med. 2010 Nov-Dec;16(6):56-64.

4. Zeidan F. et al., Mindfulness meditation-based pain relief: a mechanistic account, Ann N Y Acad Sci. 2016 Jun;1373(1):114-27

5. 'Don't overthink it, working a little mindfulness into your day could go a long way toward remedying a whole host of ills' by Ben Kallen, March 11 2013 Los Angeles Magazine

6. 'Doctor struggling with work-life balance experiences positive outcome in mindfulness program for mixed audience' September 18, 2018 www.beaumont.org

7. Meditation may serve as pain-relief alternative to opioids by Denise Dador, April 18, 2019, Circle of Health

8. Chiesa A. and Serretti A., Mindfulness-based stress reduction for stress management in healthy people: a review and meta-analysis, J Altern Complement Med. 2009 May;15(5):593-600.

9. Koszycki D. et al., Randomized trial of a meditation-based stress reduction program and cognitive behavior therapy in generalized social anxiety disorder, Behav Res Ther. 2007 Oct;45(10):2518-26.

10. Levine G.N. et al., Meditation and Cardiovascular Risk Reduction: A Scientific Statement From the American Heart Association, J Am Heart Assoc. 2017 Sep 28;6(10).

11. Barrett B. et al., Meditation or exercise for preventing acute respiratory infection: a randomized controlled trial, The Ann Fam Med. 2012 Jul-Aug;10(4):337-46.

12. Obasi C.N. et al., Advantage of meditation over exercise in reducing cold and flu illness is related to improved function and quality of life, Influenza Other Respir Viruses. 2013 Nov; 7(6): 938–944.12

13. Last N. et al., The Effects of Meditation on Grey Matter Atrophy and Neurodegeneration: A Systematic Review, J Alzheimer's Dis. 2017;56(1):275-286.

14. Sivasankaran S. et al., The effect of a six-week program of yoga and meditation on brachial artery reactivity: do psychosocial interventions affect vascular tone?, Clin Cardiol. 2006 Sep;29(9):393-8.

15. Rao R.M. et al., Effects of a yoga program on mood states, quality of life, and toxicity in breast cancer patients receiving conventional treatment: A Randomized Controlled Trial, Indian Journal of Palliative Care, 23(3): 237-246, 2017 Jul-Sep.

16. Krishnakumar D. et al., Meditation and Yoga can modulate brain mechanisms that affect behaviour and anxiety – A modern scientific perspective, Ancient Science, 2(1):13-19, 2015 Apr.

17. Vanhuffel H. et al., Contribution of mindfulness meditation in cognitive behavioural therapy for insomnia, Encephale, 2017 Feb 14

18. Pascoe M.C. et al., Mindfulness mediates the physiological markers of stress: Systematic review and meta-analysis, Journal of Psychiatric Research 95:156-178, 2017 Aug 23

19. Ball E.F. et al., Does mindfulness meditation improve chronic pain? A systematic review. Current Opinion in Obstetrics and Gynaecology, 2017 Sep 28.

20. Ponte Marquez P.H. et al., Benefits of mindfulness meditation in reducing blood pressure and stress in patients with arterial hypertension, J Hum Hypertens. 2019 Mar;33(3):237-247

21. Kuyken W. et al., The effectiveness and cost-effectiveness of mindfulness-based cognitive therapy compared with maintenance antidepressant treatment in the prevention of depressive relapse/recurrence: results of a randomised controlled trial (the PREVENT study), Lancet 2015; 386: 63-73

22. Sarkar C. et al., Residential greenness and prevalence of major depressive disorders: a cross-sectional, observational, associational study of 94,879 adult UK Biobank participants, Lancet Planet Health. 2018 Apr;2(4):e162-e173

23. Chetelat G et al., Reduced age-associated brain changes in expert meditators: a multimodal neuroimaging pilot study, Nature.com/scientific reports, 31.8.17

24. Black D.S. et al., Mindfulness meditation and the immune system: a systematic review of randomized controlled trials, Ann N Y Acad Sci. 2016 Jun;1373(1):13-24

25. Farias M. et al., Has the science of mindfulness lost its mind?, Br J Psych Bull. 2016 Dec; 40(6): 329–332.

26. Does mindfulness work? BMJ 2015;351:h6919

27. Evidence for mindfulness Mersey NHS study

28. Miller M. et al., The effect of mirthful laughter on the human cardiovascular system, Med Hypotheses. 2009 Nov;73(5):636

29. Tinker Ready, Meditation apparently good for the heart as well as the mind June 7 2000 CNN.com

30. Kegel J., The Power of the Mind. Stress – the Missing Piece, Journal of Lancaster General Hospital Spring 2013 – Vol 8, no.1

31. Bhasin M. K. et al., Specific Transcriptome Changes Associated with Blood Pressure Reduction in Hypertensive Patients After Relaxation Response Training, J Altern Complement Med. 2018 May;24(5):486-504.

32. Meditation in general practice (letter P. Joan Bishop) Br Med J (Clin Res Ed) 1981; 282:528

33. Canter P., The therapeutic effects of meditation, BMJ 2003;326:1049

34. Levin L.S. et al., Self-Care in health, Ann. Rev. Public Health 1983. 4:181-201

35. Ellen Bard, 45 simple self-care practices for a healthy mind, body and soul, Tiny Buddha

36. The self-care continuum, Self Care Forum.

37. The Economic burden of minor ailments on the NHS in the UK, Self Care Journal, 105-116, September 2010

38. Jones R., Self Care, Editorial BMJ 2000;320:596

39. Limb M., Technology must not replace human contact in drive for self care, conference hears, BMJ 2014;348: g4278

40. Parkin S., Has dopamine got us hooked on tech? The Guardian 4.3.18

41. Journaling for mental health, University of Rochester Medical Center

42. Writing about emotions may ease stress and trauma, Harvard Health Publishing Harvard Medical School

43. Power M., Dear Diary... The surprising health benefits of journaling, The Telegraph, 21 July 2017

44. Sample I., Keeping a diary makes you happier, The Guardian, 15 Feb 2009

45. Rajmohan V. et al., The Limbic system, Indian J. Psychiatry. 2007 Apr-Jun; 49(2):132-139

46. Kiecolt-Glaser et al., Olfactory Influences on Mood and Autonomic, Endocrine and Immune Function, Psychoneuroendocrinology, 2008 Apr;33(3):328-339

References: The Psychology of Ageing and The Genetics of Ageing

1. The Telomere Effect, Elizabeth Blackburn PhD and Elissa Epel PhD, Orion Books, 2017

2. Wilkinson P. et al., Depression in older adults, Editorial, BMJ 2018;363: k4922

3. Happy People live longer, Minerva, BMJ 2018;363: k4600

4. www.brainhealthregistry.org/
5. Ward R.A., How Old Am I? Perceived Age in Middle and Later Life, International Journal of Aging and Human Development 71, no.3 (2010):167-84
6. Ersner-Hershfield H. et al., Poignancy: Mixed Emotional Experience in the Face of Meaningful Endings, Journal of Personality and Social Psychology 94, no.1 (Jan 2008): 158-67
7. Levy B.R. et al., Longevity Increased by Positive Self-Perceptions of Aging, Journal of Personal and Social Psychology 83, no.2, (August 2002): 261-70
8. Low C. A. et al., Psychosocial Factors in the Development of Heart Disease in Women: Current Research and Future Directions, Psychosomatic Medicine 72, no.9 (Nov 2010): 842-54
9. Nolen-Hoeksema S., The Role of Rumination in Depressive Disorders and Mixed Anxiety/Depressive Symptoms, Journal of Abnormal Psychology 109, no.3 (Aug 2000): 504-11
10. Understanding Depression, NIMH
11. Wolkowitz O.M. et al., Of sound mind and body: depression, disease and accelerated aging, Dialogues in Clinical Neuroscience Vol 13, no 1, 2011
12. Querstret D. et al., Assessing Treatments Used to Reduce Rumination and/or worry: A systematic Review, Clinical Psychology Review 33, no.8 (December 2013): 996-1009
13. Friedman H.S. et al., Personality, Wellbeing, and Health, Annual Review of Psychology 65 (2014): 719-42
14. Shanahan M.J. et al., Conscientiousness, Health and Ageing: The Life Course of Personality Model, Developmental Psychology 50, no. 5 (May 2014): 1407-25
15. Friedman H.S. et al., Personality, Well-Being, and Health, Annual Review of Psychology, Vol. 65:719-742
16. Conklin Q. et al., Telomere Lengthening After Three Weeks of an Intensive Insight Meditation Retreat, Psychoneuroendocrinology 61 (November 2015): 26-27
17. Welch A.A. et al., Healthier ageing, BMJ 2012;344: e1214
18. Shammas M., Telomeres, cancer and ageing, Curr Opin Clin Nutr Metab Care 2011 Jan; 14(1): 28-34
19. Leung C.W. et al., Soda and Cell aging: Associations between Sugar-Sweetened Beverage Consumption and Leukocyte Telomere Length in Healthy Adults from the National Health and Nutrition Examination Surveys, American Journal of Public Health 104, no. 12 (Dec 2014): 2425-31
20. Richards J.B. et al., Higher Serum Vitamin D Concentrations Are Associated with Longer Leukocyte Telomere Length in Women, American Journal of Clinical Nutrition 86, no. 5 (Nov 2007): 1420-25
21. Healthy Aging: Lessons from the Baltimore Longitudinal Study of Aging, July 2010 (updated 2015)
22. Latifovic L. et al., The influence of alcohol consumption, cigarette smoking, and physical activity on Leukocyte telomere length, Cancer Epidemiology, Biomarkers and Prevention. 25(2):374-80, 2016 Feb.
23. Bansal N. et al., Association between kidney function and telomere length: the heart and soul study, American Journal of Nephrology, 36(5):405-11, 2012
24. Mathur M.B. et al., Perceived stress and telomere length: A systematic review, meta-analysis, and methodologic considerations for advancing the field, Brain, Behavior, & Immunity, 54:158-68, 2016 May
25. Haussmann M.F. et al., Telomere dynamics may link stress exposure and ageing across generations, Biology Letters, 11(11), 2015 Nov.
26. Simons M.J., Questioning causal involvement of telomeres in ageing, Ageing Research Reviews, 24(Pt B):191-6, 2015 Nov.
27. Wojcicki J.M. et al., Cord blood telomere length in Latino infants: relation with maternal education and infant sex, Journal of Perinatology, 36(3):235-41, 2016 Mar.
28. Lin P.Y. et al., Shortened telomere length in patients with depression: A meta-analytic study, Journal of Psychiatric Research, 76:84-93, 2016 May
29. Oliveira B.S. et al., Systematic review of the association between chronic social stress and telomere length: A life course perspective, Ageing Research Reviews, 26:37-52, 2016 Mar.
30. Freitas-Simoes et al., Nutrients, foods, dietary patterns and telomere length: Update of epidemiological studies and randomised trials, Metabolism: Clinical and Experimental, 65(4): 406-15, 2016 Apr.

References: Eye Health
1. https://www.boots.com/sunglasses/uv-protection-myths-busters
2. http://lookafteryoureyes.org/

3. Dart J.K.G., Disease and risks associated with contact lenses, British Journal of Ophthalmology 1993;77:49-53
4. www.rnib.org.uk Understanding Age-related Macular Degeneration
5. National Eye Institute, Facts about Presbyopia
6. RNIB and RC Opth Nov 2010 Cataracts information
7. allaboutvision.com, Jegtvig S.J., Can a healthy diet prevent cataracts?

References: Protecting Mental Health and Memory

1. Pink J. et al., Dementia: assessment, management and support: summary of updated NICE guidance, BMJ 2018;361: k2438
2. Robinson K., Nutrition and Dementia, BDA.org.uk
3. Lourida I et al., Mediterranean diet, cognitive function and dementia: a systematic review, Epidemiology. 2013 Jul;24(4):479-89
4. Golf for older people, Minerva, BMJ 13.10.18
5. Abas B. et al., Letter BMJ Seasonal Affective Disorder: the miseries of long dark nights, Br Med J (Clin Res Ed). 1987 Dec 12;295(6612):1504-5.
6. Lara R.W. et al., The Can-SAD study summarised by BMJ updates 'Light therapy and fluoxetine both work in Seasonal Affective Disorder', BMJ Vol 332 3.6.06
7. Drug and Therapeutics Bulletin Clinical Review, Management of Seasonal Affective Disorder, BMJ 2010;340:c2135
8. McMahon B. et al., Seasonality-resilient individuals downregulate their cerebral 5-HT transporter binding in winter – A longitudinal combined C-DASB and C-SB207145 PET study, European Neuropsychopharmacology, Vol 28, Issue 10, October 2018, Pages 1151-1160
9. Matheson G.J. et al., Diurnal and seasonal variation of the brain serotonin system in healthy male subjects, Neuroimage Vol 112, 15 May 2015, Pages 225-231
10. Menculini G. et al., Depressive mood and circadian rhythm disturbances as outcomes of Seasonal Affective Disorder treatment: a systematic review, Journal of Affective Disorders, Volume 241, 1 December 2018, Pages 608-626
11. Danilenko K.V. et al., Dawn simulation vs bright light in Seasonal Affective Disorder: Treatment effects and subjective preference, Journal of Affective Disorders, Volume 180, 15 July 2015, Pages 87-89.
12. Mind 2019 Seasonal Affective Disorder Guide
13. April 2015 Seasonal Affective Disordered (SAD) Guide Royal College of Psychiatrists
14. Rastad C. et al., Patients' Experience of Winter Depression and Light Room Treatment, Psychiatry J. 2017; 2017: 6867957
15. Symptoms Seasonal Affective Disorder NHS guide.
16. UNSW Sydney, How well will your brain age? Older Australian Twins Study unlocking the secret of ageing, 27.2.18

References: Dental Care and why it can change your life

1. Poklepovic T. et al., Interdental brushing for the prevention and control of periodontal diseases and dental caries in adults, Cochrane Oral Health Group 2013

References: Health Screening and Breast Health

1. www.gov.uk/topic/population-screening-programmes (England)
2. www.nidirect.gov.uk/information-and-services/health-services/health-screening-programmes (Northern Ireland)
3. www.nhsinform.scot/healthy-living/screening/screening-in-scotland (Scotland)
4. gov.wales/topics/health/protection/public-health-screening/?lang=en (Wales)
5. www.breastcancercare.org.uk
6. www.coppafeel.org
7. www.association of breastsurgery.org.uk 'best practice diagnostic guidelines for patients presenting with breast symptoms'.
8. NICE document 'Breast cancer-recognition and referral'
9. NHS.UK 'How should I check my breasts?'
10. NHS.UK Overview breast cancer screening

11. NHS.UK Breast pain cyclical
12. Amit Goyal 'Breast pain' BMJ Clin Evid 2011;2011: 0812
13. Karen Robock 'Breast Practices' Canadian Living October 2018
14. Patient.info health information leaflets
15. Staten A. and Staten P., Practical General Practice: Guidelines for Effective Clinical Management published 2.8.19
16. Lee Y-K. et al., Vaginal pH-balanced gel for the control of atrophic vaginitis among breast cancer survivors: a randomized controlled trial, Obstetrics and Gynaecology, 117(4): 922-927, Apr 2011
17. Hickey M. et al., A randomized, double-blind, crossover trial comparing a silicone-versus water-based lubricant for sexual discomfort after breast cancer.

References: Wisdom in our femininity

1. NICE pathways 2018 Menopause overview
2. NICE pathways 2018 Managing menopausal symptoms
3. Hickey M. et al., 'Non-hormonal treatments for menopausal symptoms', BMJ 2017; 359:j5101
4. Red Whale Course 'Menopause and HRT' from NICE menopause CKS/NG23 (2015), British Menopause Society Guidelines (2017) and BNF (2019) Summary advice for practitioners including 'Menopause and HRT: which HRT?', 'HRT: formulations', 'Menopause: alternative treatments' January 2019
5. Rymer J., Brian K., Regan L., HRT and breast cancer risk, we must prevent another setback in women's health, BMJ 2019;367:I5928
6. Roberts H., Hickey M., Managing the menopause: An update, Maturitas, The European Menopause Journal, April 2016, Volume 86, Pages 53-58
7. Breast Cancer Screening – The Essentials, Royal College of General Practitioners Online Course completed 19.2.18
8. Bloating and other abdominal symptoms: could it be ovarian cancer? Royal College of General Practitioners Online Course completed 31.1.18
9. Leach M.J., Moore V., Black cohosh (Cimicifuga spp.) for menopausal symptoms. Cochrane Database of Systematic Reviews 2012, Issue 9.
10. Lambert M.N.T., 'Combined Red Clover isoflavones and probiotics potently reduce menopausal vasomotor symptoms', PLoS One. 2017 Jun 7;12(6):e0176590. doi: 10.1371/journal.pone.0176590
11. Newton K.M. et al., 'Efficacy of yoga for vasomotor symptoms: a randomized controlled trial', Menopause. 2014 Apr;21(4):339-46. doi: 10.1097/GME.0b013e31829e4baa.
12. Sternfield B. et al., 'Efficacy of exercise for menopausal symptoms: a randomized controlled trial', Menopause. 2014 Apr;21(4):330-8. doi: 10.1097/GME.0b013e31829e4089.
13. J. Woyka, 'Consensus statement for non-hormonal-based treatments for menopausal symptoms', Post Reprod Health. 2017 Jun;23(2):71-75. doi: 10.1177/2053369117711646.
14. M. Hunter and M. Smith in collaboration with the British Menopause Society 'Cognitive Behaviour Therapy (CBT) for menopausal symptoms. Information for women', Post Reproductive Health 2017, Vol. 23(2) 77-82
15. Nick Panay 'Chapter 47:Menopause and the postmenopausal woman' from Dewhurst's Textbook of Obstetrics and Gynaecology, Seventh Edition
16. Patient: Alternatives to HRT authored by J. Payne
17. Amelia Hill 'Menopause experts say compounded HRT is unsafe' The Guardian 26.8.19
18. Meczelekalski B. et al., 'Genetics of premature ovarian failure', Minerva Endocrinol. 2010 Dec;35(4): 195-209
19. Chapman C et al., 'The genetics of premature ovarian failure: current perspectives', Int J Women's Health 2015;7:799-810
20. Labrie F. et al., Effects of intravaginal DHEA on the female sexual function in postmenopausal women, Hormone Molecular Biology and Clinical Investigation, Volume 25, Issue 3
21. Scheffers C.S. et al., Dehydroepiandrosterone for women in the peri- or postmenopausal phase, The Cochrane Library 22.1.15
22. Avis N. E. et al., Longitudinal changes in sexual functioning as women transition through menopause: results from the Study of Women's Health Across the Nation, Menopause. 16(3):442-452, May 2009
23. Politi M.C. et al., Revisiting the Duration of Vasomotor Symptoms of Menopause: A Meta-Analysis, Journal of

General Internal Medicine, September 2008, Volume 23, Issue 9, pp 1507-1513

24. Hickey M. et al., Depressive symptoms across the menopause transition: findings from a large population-based cohort study, Menopause 23(12):1287-1293, Dec 2016

25. Stuenkel C.A. et al., Treatment of Symptoms of the Menopause: An Endocrine Society Clinical Practice Guideline, The Journal of Clinical Endocrinology and Metabolism, Volume 100, Issue 11, 1.11.15, p 3975-4011

26. Perrone G. et al., Menopausal symptoms after the discontinuation of long-term HRT in women under 60: a 3 year follow up, Gynaecol Obstet Invest. 2013;76(1):38-43

27. Elkins G.R. et al., Clinical hypnosis in the treatment of postmenopausal hot flashes: a randomized controlled trial, Menopause 2013 Mar;20(3): 291-8

28. Carmody J.F. et al., Mindfulness training for coping with hot flashes: results of a randomized trial, Menopause 18(6):611-620, Jun 2011

29. Carolyn E., Acupuncture for menopausal hot flashes: clinical evidence update and its relevance to decision making, Menopause 24(8):980-987, Aug 2017

30. Goulis D.G. et al., EMAS position statement: Non-hormonal management of menopausal vasomotor symptoms, Maturitas, July 2015 Volume 81, Issue 3, Pages 410-413

31. Ensrud K.E. et al., Effects of estradiol and venlafaxine on insomnia symptoms and sleep quality in women with hot flashes, Sleep, Volume 38, Issue 1, 1.1.15, p 97-108

32. Drewe J. et al., A systematic review of non-hormonal treatments of vasomotor symptoms in climacteric and cancer patients, Springer Plus 2015, 4:65

33. Drugs and Therapeutics Bulletin. 55(5):57-60, 2017 May, Testosterone Therapy for menopausal women.

34. Milman L.W. et al., Higher serum testosterone levels correlate with increased risk of depressive symptoms in Caucasian women through the entire menopausal transition, Psychoneuroendocrinology, 62:107-123, 2015 December

35. El Khoudary S.R. et al., Cardiovascular Fat, Menopause, and Sex Hormones in Women, The SWAN Cardiovascular Fat Ancillary Study, Journal of Clinical Endocrinology and

36. Metabolism, 100(9):3304-12, 2015 Sep.

37. Alexander J.L. et al., Testosterone and libido on surgically and naturally menopausal women, Women's health, 2(3):459-77, 2006 May.

38. Heather B. Patisaul and Wendy Jefferson, The pros and cons of phytoestrogens, Front Neuroendocrinol. 2010 Oct; 31(4);400-419.

39. Kegel8 Bladder Diary

References: Skin

1. Guyuron B., et al., 'Factors contributing to the facial aging of identical twins', Plast 2009 Apr;123(4):1321-31. doi: 10.1097/PRS.0b013e31819c4d42.

2. Clatici V.G. et al., Perceived age and life style. The specific contributions of seven factors involved in health and beauty, Maedica (Buchar), 2017 Sep, 12(3):191-201

3. Flament F. et al., Effect of the sun on visible clinical signs of aging in Caucasian skin, Clin Cosmet Investig Dermatol. 2013 Sep 27;6:221-32

4. Randhawa M. et al., Daily use of a facial broad spectrum sunscreen over one year significantly improves clinical evaluation of photoaging, Derm Surgery 42(12):1 Oct 2016

5. Fourtanier A. et al., Sunscreens containing the broad-spectrum UVA absorber, Mexoryl SX, prevents the cutaneous detrimental effects of UV exposure: a review of clinical study results, Photodermatology, Photoimmunology and Photomedicine, 24(4): 164-74, 2008 Aug.

6. Gilchrest B.A., Sun exposure and vitamin D deficiency, Am J of Clinical Nutrition, 88(2):5705-5775, 2008 Aug.

7. Seite S. et al., The benefit of daily photoprotection, J of the American Academy of Dermatology, 58(% suppl 2): S160-6, 2008 May

8. Nolan K. et al., Moisturizers: Reality and the skin benefits, Dermatologic Therapy, Vol 25, 2012, 229-233

9. Perper M. et al., Tranexamic acid in the treatment of melasma: a review of the literature, American Journal of Clinical Dermatology, 2017 Mar 10

10. Zhou L.L. et al., Melasma: systematic review of the systemic treatments, International Journal of Dermatology,

2017 Feb. 27

11. Dayal S. et al., Combination of glycolic acid peel and topical 20% azelaic acid cream in melasma patients: efficacy and improvement in quality of life, Journal of Cosmetic Dermatology, 16(1):35-42, 2017 Mar.

12. Becker S. et al, Melasma: An update on the clinical picture, treatment and prevention, Hautarzt, 68(2): 120-126, 2017 Feb

13. Ju Q. et al., Sex hormones and acne, Clin Dermatol. 2017 Mar – Apr;35(2):130-137. doi: 10.1016/j.clindermatol.2016.10.004

14. Dessinioti C., et al., Propionibacterium acnes and antimicrobial resistance in acne, Clin Dermatol. 2017 Mar – Apr;35(2):163-167

15. Kontochristopoulos G. et al., Chemical peels in active acne and acne scars, Clin Dermatol. 2017 Mar – Apr;35(2):179-182. doi: 10.1016/j.clindermatol.2016.10.011.

16. Rai R., et al., Laser and light based treatments of acne, Indian J Dermatol Venereol Leprol. 2013 May-Jun;79(3):300-9. doi: 10.4103/0378-6323.110755.

17. Kosmadaki M. et al., Topical treatments for acne, Clin Dermatol. 2017 Mar – Apr;35(2):173-178. doi: 10.1016/j.clindermatol.2016.10.010.

18. Barros B., et al., Hormonal therapies for acne, Clin Dermatol. 2017 Mar – Apr;35(2):168-172. doi: 10.1016/j.clindermatol.2016.10.009.

19. Kiayani A.J. et al., Association Of Serum Testosterone And Sex Hormone Binding Globulin Levels In Females With Acne Based On Its Severity, J Ayub Med Coll Abbottabad. 2016 Apr-Jun;28(2):357-359.

20. Pavlidis A.I. et al., Therapeutic approaches to reducing atrophic acne scarring, Clin Dermatol. 2017 Mar-Apr;35(2):190-194

21. Aslan I. et al., Decreased eicosapentaenoic acid levels in acne vulgaris reveals the presence of a proinflammatory state, Prostaglandins Other Lipid Mediat. 2017 Jan;128-129:1-7.

22. Samantha Brick 'The adult acne epidemic' by Samantha Brick 1.3.12 Daily Mail

23. India Sturgis 'The rise of adult acne is 'like an epidemic', The Telegraph 18.1.16

24. www.proactiv.co.uk

25. Kerry Potter 'Wrinkles and spots? How to treat midlife acne', by Kerry Potter the Telegraph 30.4.19

26. Goulden V. et al., 'Prevalence of facial acne in adults', J Am Acad Dermatol. 1999 Oct;41(4):577-80.

27. Information presented at American Academy of Dermatology's 70th annual meeting by Professor B.J. Schlosser MD PhD FAAD 'Hormonal factors key to understanding acne in women' March 2012

28. Bowe W.P. et al., Acne vulgaris, probiotics and the gut-brain-skin axis-back to the future? Gut Pathogens 2011, 3:1

29. Santer M. et al., 'Views of oral antibiotics and advice seeking about acne: a qualitative study of online discussion forums', Br J Dermatol. 2017 Sep;177(3):751-757

30. Francis N.A., et al., The management of acne vulgaris in primary care: a cohort study of consulting and prescribing patterns using the Clinical Practice Research Datalink', Br J Dermatol. 2017 Jan;176(1):107-115

31. Abokwidir M. et al., Rosacea Management, Skin Appendage Disord 2016;2:26-34

32. Bissett D.L., et al., 'Niacinamide: a B vitamin that improves aging facial skin appearance', Dermatol Surg. 2005 Jul;31(7 Pt 2):860-5; discussion 865 (The Proctor and Gamble Company).

33. Farris P.K., 'Topical vitamin C: a useful agent for treating photoaging and other dermatologic conditions', Dermatol.Surg.2005 Jul;31(7 Pt 2): 814-7; discussion 818.

34. Pha Mix, Alpha Hydroxy Acids or Retinol: Which is best?, Dec 22, 2008

35. Kornhauser A. et al., Applications of hydroxyl acids: classification, mechanisms, and photoactivity, Clin Cosmet Investig Dermatol., 2010;3:135-142

36. Sorg O. et al., Topical retinoids in skin ageing – a focused update with reference to sun-induced epidermal vitamin A deficiency, Dermatology 2014;228:314-325

37. Handler M.Z. et al., Neocollagenessis, Dermal Fillers, Aesthet Dermatol Basel, Karger, 2018, vol 4, pp27-35

38. Roenigk H.H., Treatment of the aging face, Dermatologic Therapy, Vol 13, 2000, 141-153

39. Rendon M.I. et al., Evidence and considerations in the application of chemical peels in skin disorders and aesthetic resurfacing, J Clin Aesthet Dermatol, 2010 Jul; 3(7): 32-43

40. Fluhr J.W. et al., Tolerance profile of retinol, retinaldehyde and retinoic acid under maximised and long term clinical conditions, Dermatology 1999;199 (suppl 1):57-60

41. Jegasothy S.M. et al., Efficacy of a new topical nano-hyaluronic acid in humans, J Clin Aesthet.Dermatol. 2014 Mar, 7(3):27-29

42. Seite S. et al., Histological evaluation of a topically applied retinol-vitamin C combination, Skin Pharmacology and Physiology, 2005;18:81-87

43. Manela-Azulay M. et al., 'Cosmeceuticals vitamins', Clin Dermatol. 2009 Sep-Oct;27(5)

44. Burke K.E., 'Interaction of vitamins c and E as better cosmeceuticals', Dermatol. Ther. 2007 Sep-Oct;20(5):314-21.

45. Knuutinen A., et al., 'Smoking affects collagen synthesis and extracellular matrix turnover in human skin', Br J Dermatol. 2002 Apr;146(4):588-94.

46. Figueres J.T.et al., 'An overview of the beneficial effects of hydrolysed collagen intake on joint and bone health and on skin ageing', Nutr Hosp. 2015 Jul 18;32 Suppl 1:62-6. doi: 10.3305/nh.2015.32.sup1.9482.

47. Choi F.D., et al., 'Oral Collagen Supplementation: A Systematic Review of Dermatological Applications', J Drugs Dermatol. 2019 Jan 1;18 (1):9-16.

48. Kim D.U., et al., 'Oral intake of low molecular weight collagen peptide improves hydration, elasticity, and wrinkling in human skin: A randomized, double-blind, placebo-controlled study', Nutrients. 2018 Jun 26;10(7).

49. Proksch E. et al., Oral supplementation of specific collagen peptides has beneficial effects on human skin physiology: a double-blind, placebo controlled study, Skin Pharmacology and Physiology 2014;27:47-55

50. Schunck M. et al., Dietary supplementation with specific collagen peptides has a body mass index-dependent beneficial effect on cellulite morphology, J Medicinal Food, 2015 Dec 1; 18(12): 1340-1348

51. Catherine de Lange, Can a drink really make skin look younger, The Guardian, 27.9.15

52. Proksch E. et al., Oral intake of specific bioactive collagen peptides reduces skin wrinkles and increases dermal matrix synthesis, Skin Pharmacology and Physiology, 2014;27:113-119

53. Elizabeth Siegel, 'How to layer your skin-care products in the correct order' Allure April 15, 2019.

54. '"In the know" want the best results from your skincare products', Red Promotion February 2019 Red Magazine.

55. The Dermstore Blog 'Antioxidants in skin care: How do they work and which ones are the best?'

56. EWG's Guide to Sunscreens 'The trouble with ingredients in sunscreens'

57. Chemical Vs. Physical Sunscreens – Art of Skin Care 24.5.17

58. Emma Brancatisano Chemical Versus Physical Sunscreen: What's the difference? Health (Australia) 30.11.16

59. *www.bbcgoodfood.com › howto › guide › eat-your-way-fabulous-skin*

60. www.healthline.com/nutrition/12-foods-for-healthy-skin

61. Sonia Haria, Is this the new skin saviour? The Telegraph

62. Choi F.D. et al., Oral Collagen Supplementation: A Systematic Review of Dermatological Applications, Journal Drugs Dermatol 2019 Jan; 18(1): 9-16

63. Sorg O. et al., Topical Retinoids in Skin Ageing: A focused update with reference to sun-induced epidermal vitamin A deficiency, Dermatology 2014;228:314-325

64. Danby F.W., Nutrition and aging skin: sugar and glycation, Clin Dermatol. 2010 Jul-Aug;28(4):409-11

65. Loader J. et al., Effects of sugar-sweetened beverage consumption on microvascular and macrovascular function in a healthy population, Arterioscler Thromb Vasc Biol 2017 Jun;37(6):1250-1260.

66. Universiteit Leiden, Research – Looking older: the effect of higher blood sugar levels.

67. Reigle K.L. et al., Non-enzymatic glycation of type 1 collagen diminishes collagen-proteoglycan binding and weakens cell adhesion, Journal of Cellular Biochemistry, Vol 104, issue 5, 1.8.08

68. Dr Perricone, Sugar, starch, and Glycation: The not-so-sweet science of ageing

69. Parabens in cosmetics, FDA

70. Foods to help keep your skin healthy, Elaine Magee, Web MD

71. Mary Jo DiLonardo, What's in Your Personal Care Products?, WebMD

72. Kirchhof M.G. et al., The health controversies of parabens, Skin Therapy Lett, 2013 Feb;18(2):5-7

73. Hafeez F. et al, An overview of parabens and allergic contact dermatitis, Skin Therapy Lett. 2013 Jul-Aug; 18(5):5-7

74. Cooper A.J. et al., Modern management of acne, Med J Aust. 2017 Jan 16;206(1):41-45

75. Barbara Casassus, Hormone disrupting chemicals: the slow progress to regulation, BMJ 2018;361:k1876

76. Ferneini E.M. et al., Surgeon's Guide to Facial Soft Tissue Filler Injections: Relevant Anatomy and Safety Considerations, Journal of Oral and Maxillofacial Surgery, 75(12):2667.e1-2667.e5,2017 Dec.

77. Barolet D. et al., Infrared and Skin: Friend or Foe, J Photochem. Photobiol B. 2016 Feb: 155: 78-85

78. Schroeder P. et al., The role of near infrared radiation in photoaging of the skin, Exp Gerontol 2008 Jul;43(7):629-32

References: Hair loss

1. Goluch-Koniuszy Z.S., Nutrition of women with hair loss problem during the period of menopause. *Prz Menopauzalny.* 2016;15(1):56–61. doi:10.5114/pm.2016.58776.
2. https://www.nhs.uk/conditions/hair-loss/coping-tips-for-women/
3. Amr Salam et al., Non-hormonal treatments for menopausal symptoms – letter in response – Hair loss is an important symptom of the menopause BMJ 2017;359:j5101.
4. Cunningham C. et al., Case Report Recurrent episodes of hair loss in a 37 year old woman BMJ 2012;345:e6798.
5. Zuuren E.J. et al., Evidence-based treatments for female pattern hair loss: a summary of a Cochrane systematic review. Br J Dermatol. 2012 Nov;167(5):995-1010
6. Fabbrocini G. et al., Female pattern hair loss: A clinical, pathophysiologic, and therapeutic review, *International journal of women's dermatology* vol. 4,4 203-211. 19 Jun. 2018
7. https://www.health.harvard.edu/staying-healthy/treating-female-pattern-hair-loss
8. Allure The Best Hair Loss Treatments for Every Budget by Jessica Chia October 15, 2018
9. www.bad.org.uk/leaflets Patient information leaflets; Female Pattern Hair Loss, Alopecia Areata, Frontal Fibrosing alopecia
10. Park, Song Youn et al. 'Iron plays a certain role in patterned hair loss', Journal of Korean medical science vol. 28,6 (2013): 934-8
11. Rasheed H. et al., Serum ferritin and vitamin d in female hair loss: do they play a role? Skin Pharmacol Physiol. 2013;26(2):101-7
12. Deloche C. et al., 'Low iron stores: a risk factor for excessive hair loss in non-menopausal women', Eur J Dermatol. 2007 Nov-Dec;17(6):507-12.
13. National Cancer Institute 'Hair Dyes and Cancer Risk'
14. Trust me, I'm a Doctor 'Are my wash products damaging my skin?'
15. Environmental Working Group's Skin Deep Cosmetics Database
16. Panhard S. et al., 'Greying of the human hair: a worldwide survey, revisiting the '50' rule of thumb', Br J Dermatol 2012 Oct; 167(4): 865-73

References: A broader approach

1. Elkins G.R. et al., Clinical hypnosis in the treatment of post-menopausal hot flashes: a randomized controlled trial. Menopause 2013 March; 20 (3):
2. Carpenter J. et al., Non-hormonal management of menopause-associated vasomotor symptoms: 2015 position statement of the North American Menopause Society.
3. Menopause 2015, volume 22, issue 11.
4. Hickey M. et al., Non-hormonal treatments for menopausal symptoms. BMJ 2017; 359.
5. Valentine K.E. et al., The efficacy of hypnosis as a treatment for anxiety: a meta-analysis. International Journal of Clinical and Experimental Hypnosis, 2019; volume 67, issue 3.
6. Acupuncture for you, leaflet provided by the British Acupuncture Council
7. Yun Y. et al., Effect of facial cosmetic acupuncture on facial elasticity: an open-label, single arm pilot study, Evid Based Complement Alternat Med. 2013: 424313
8. Donoyama N. et al., Cosmetic acupuncture to enhance facial skin appearance, a preliminary study, acupmed-2012-010156
9. Doran V., An introduction to facial revitalisation acupuncture, EJOM Vol 5 no. 5
10. Wakefield M.E., The yang and yin of facial acupuncture – Part 4, Acupuncture Today
11. Nora Isaacs, Hold the chemicals, bring on the needles, The New York Times, Fashion and style, 13.12.07

References: Bone Health and Exercising

1. Strong, Steady and Straight: Physical activity and Exercise for Osteoporosis, Royal Osteoporosis Society
2. 15 tips for preventing osteoporosis, Readers' Digest 2013
3. Radojka Bijelic et al., Risk Factors for Osteoporosis in Postmenopausal Women Med Arch. 2017 Feb 71 (1): 25-28
4. Pim Pellikaan et al., Ranking of osteogenic potential of physical exercises in postmenopausal women based on femoral neck strains, PLOS One Journal April 4, 2018

5. Danginh Hu et al., Fruit and vegetable consumption and the risk of postmenopausal osteoporosis: a meta-analysis of observational studies, Food and Function Issue 5,2018

6. www.bda.uk.com Calcium food fact sheet

7. V.H. Stiles et al., A small amount of precisely measured high-intensity habitual physical activity predicts bone health in pre- and post-menopausal women in UK Biobank. International Journal Of Epidemiology 2017 Dec 1;46(6): 1847-1856

8. John J. B. Anderson et al., Calcium intake form diet and supplements and the risk of coronary artery calcification and its progression among older adults: 10-year follow-up of the Multi-Ethnic Study Of Atherosclerosis (MESA) Journal of the American Heart Association, 2016;5

9. Yi-Hsueh Lu et al., Twelve-Minute Daily Yoga Regimen Reverses Osteoporotic Bone Loss Topics in Geriatric Rehabilitation 2016 Apr; 32(2): 81-87

10. Vibration or exercise – which is the best therapy for bone loss? Review of current study at Griffith Menzies Health Institute Queensland

11. Duration of osteoporosis treatment, National Osteoporosis Soceity

12. NHS website 'Healthy Body – Food for strong bones'

13. Fung et al., Soda consumption and risk of hip fractures in postmenopausal women in the Nurses' Health Study Americal Journal Clinical Nutrition 2014 Sep; 100(3):953-8

14. Professor Juliet Compston, Weight change and risk of fracture in postmenopausal women, British Medical Journal 2015; 350

15. Richard L. Prince et al. Prevention of Postmenopausal Osteoporosis – a comparative study of exercise, calcium supplementation, and Hormone-Replacement Therapy, The New England Journal Of Medicine 1991;325:1189-1195

16. Tonya S. Orchard et al., Magnesium Intake, bone mineral density, and fractures: results from the Women's Health Initiative Observational Study American Journal Of Clinical Nutrition 2014 Apr; 99(4)

17. Setor Kwadzo Kunutsor et al., Low serum magnesium levels are associated with increased risk of fractures: a long term prospective cohort study, European Journal of Epidemiology 2017; 32 (7)

18. Bolland M.J. et al., Should adults take vitamin D supplements to prevent disease? BMJ 2016;355: i6201

19. Dawn Skelton, Susie Dinan, Malcolm Campbell, Olga Rutherford, Tailored group exercise (Falls Management Exercise – FaME) reduces falls in community-dwelling older frequent fallers (an RCT), Age and Ageing, Volume 34, Issue 6, 1 November 2005, 636-639

20. Dawn Skelton Effects of physical activity on postural stability, Age and Ageing 2001; 30-S4:33-39

21. R. Hubbard et al. Falls recorded by the general practitioner and the subsequent risk of hip fracture: a case-control study using the UK general practice research database. Age and Ageing, Volume 30, Issue suppl_4, ! November 2001, 4120.

22. Lauren Slayton, What's the deal with oat milk? And all our fave milks, Foodtrainers.com21.

23. 'One minute of running per day associated with better bone health in women', University of Exeter Website

24. Pizzorno L., The Complete Guide to Caffeine and Osteoporosis,

25. Royal Osteoporosis Society (formally National Osteoporosis Society) UK-based www.ros.org.uk

26. National Osteoporosis Foundation USA-based www.nof.org

27. International Osteoporosis Foundation www.iofbonehealth.org

28. Jelleyman C. et al., The effects of high-intensity interval training on glucose regulation and insulin resistance: a meta-analysis.

29. Wippert P. et al., Stress and Alterations in Bones: An Interdisciplinary Perspective, Front Endocrinol (Lausanne) 2017;8:96

30. Edwardson C.L. et al., Reducing sedentary behaviour in the workplace, BMJ 2018; 363:k3870

31. NICE guidelines Osteoporosis: assessing the risk of fragility fracture

32. Peripheral X-ray absorptiometry in the management of osteoporosis, ROS.org.uk

33. Lu Y.H. et al., Twelve-Minute Daily Yoga Regimen Reverses Osteoporotic Bone Loss, Topics in Geriatric Rehabilitation 32, no.2 (April 2016): 81-87

34. Dunn C.A. et al., Midlife women, bone health, vegetables, herbs and fruit study. The Scarborough Fair Study Protocol, Public Health2013, 13:23

35. Allgrove J. Physiology of calcium, phosphate, magnesium and vitamin D, Calcium and Bone Disorders in Children and Adolescent, 2nd, revised edition.

References: Muscle and Joints

1. Sayer A.A., Sarcopenia, Editorials BMJ 2010;341:c4097
2. NHS guidelines-Physical activity guidelines for adults.
3. NHS 'Could age-related muscle weakening be prevented?'
4. Argiles J.M. et al., Skeletal muscle Regulated Metabolism via Interorgan Crosstalk: Roles in Health and Disease, JAMDA, Vol 17, Issue 9, Sept 2016;789-796
5. So B. et al., Exercise-induced myokines in health and metabolic diseases, Integrative Medicine Research, 5.10.14
6. Cartee G.D. et al., Exercise Promotes Health Ageing of Skeletal Muscle, Cell Metabolism 23, June 14, 2016
7. Lamb S. et al., Better balance, fewer falls, Editorial BMJ 2015;351:h3930
8. 'Preserve your muscle mass' Harvard Health Publishing, Harvard Medical School
9. Celis_Morales C.A. et al., Associations of grip strength with cardiovascular, respiratory, and cancer outcomes and all cause mortality: prospective cohort study of half a million UK Biobank participants, BMJ 2018;361:k1651
10. 'Age-proof your knees' Harvard Health Publishing, Harvard Medical School
11. 'Avoiding Joint Pain: Protect Your Joints as You Age', Fisher-Titus Healthy Living Team
12. Zhang W. et al., Current research on pharmacologic and regenerative therapies for osteoarthritis, Bone Research volume 4, Article 15040(2016)
13. Arthritis Research UK
14. Lesley Alderman 'Caring for hips and knees to avoid artificial joints', The New York Times April 23, 2010
15. 'Exercise for stronger knees and hips', Harvard Health Publishing, Harvard Medical School
16. 'How the right exercise can keep your joints healthy', Cleveland Clinic

References: Food is Life, Gut Health, Blue Zones

1. Armstrong L.E. et al., Water Intake, Water Balance, and the Elusive Daily Water Requirement, Nutrients 2018, 10, 1928.
2. www.bda.uk.com Food Fact Sheet – Fluid
3. NHS guidelines 'Six to eight glasses of water still best'
4. British Nutrition Foundation, Healthy hydration for adults and teenagers
5. Eatwell Guide, Public Health England
6. GP delivered brief weight loss interventions, Albury C. et al., British Journal of General Practice, September 2018.
7. Pixie Turner and Laura Thomas, How 'Expert' is your 'Expert' Nutritionist, Really?, Huffington Post, 24.1.18 update
8. Messina M., Soy and Health Update: Evaluation of the Clinical and Epidemiologic Literature, Nutrients, 2016 Dec; 8(12): 754
9. Finnamore H.E., Top dietary iron sources in the UK, BR J Gen Pract, 2014 Apr; 64(621): 172-173
10. Whelan K. et al., Mechanisms of Action of Probiotics and the Gastrointestinal Microbiota on Gut Motility and Constipation, Adv Nutr. 2017 May; 8(3):484-494
11. Carabotti M. et al., The gut-brain axis: interactions between enteric microbiota, central and enteric nervous systems, annals of Gastroenterology, 2015 Apr-Jun; 28(2): 203-209
12. Escorihuela E., Public Guide: The Mediterranean Diet and Younger Living, www.youngerlives.com
13. Francis R. et al., Vitamin D and Bone Health: A Practical Guideline for Patient Management, ROS.org.uk
14. Consultation on fortifying flour starts next year, BMJ 2018;363:k4561
15. Lai H.T.M. et al., Omega 3 poyunsaturated fatty acids and healthy ageing, BMj 2018;363:k4
16. Cassidy et al., Associations between Diet, Lifestyle Factors, and Telomere Length in Women, American Journal of Clinical Nutrition 91, no.5 (May 2010): 1273-80
17. Work out for your body type, Julie Bawden-Davis www.fit.com
18. Liu J.J. et al., Coffee consumption is Positively Associated with Longer Leukocyte Telomere Length in the Nurses' Health Study, Journal of Nutrition 146, no. 7 (july 2016): 1373-78
19. www.fao.org/nutrition/education/food-based-dietary-guidelines/regions/countries/canada/fr/
20. Multidisciplinary workshop 'Instead of antibiotics... what healthy alternatives can we recommend' Chelsea Physic Garden 3.10.

21. Kim E.S. et al., Association between purpose in life and objective measures of physical function in older adults, JAMA Psychiatry 2017;74(10):1039-1045
22. Panagiotakos D.B. et al., Sociodemographic and Lifestyle Statistics of Oldest Old People (>80 Years) Living in Ikaria Island: The Ikaria Study, Cardiol. Res. Pract. 2011;2011:679187
23. Panagiotakos D.B. et al., Adherence to the Mediterranean food pattern predicts the prevalence of hypertension, hypercholesterolaemia, diabetes and obesity, among healthy adults; the accuracy of the MedDietScore, Preventive Medicine, Vol 44 issue 4, April 2007, 335-40
24. Rajpathak S.N. et al., Lifestyle Factors of People with Exceptional Longevity, J Am Geriatr Soc. 2011 Aug;59(8):1509-12
25. Dan Buettner and Sam Skemp, 'Blue Zones, lessons from the world's longest lived', Am J Lifestyle Med. 2016 Sep-Oct; 10(5): 318-321
26. Poulain M. et al., The Blue Zones: areas of exceptional longevity around the world, Vienna Yearbook of Population Research 2013 (Vol. 11), pp87-108
27. Poulain M. et al., Identification of a geographic area characterised by extreme longevity in the Sardinia island, Exp Ger, Elsevier, 2004, 39(9) pp 1423-1429
28. Fraser G.E. et al., Ten years of life: Is it a matter of choice? Arch Intern Med. 201 Jul 9; 161(13): 1645-52

References: Alcohol and the female form

1. Macdonald H., The case for calling alcohol a drug, BMJ 2018;363:k4370
2. Editorial, Kypri K.et al., Alcohol must be recognised as a drug BMJ 2018;362:k3944
3. www.drinkaware.co.uk
4. Rosenberg K. et al., The effect of alcohol on resting metabolic rate, Br.J.Nutr. (1978), 40, 293
5. Why You're not Losing Weight, Dr Sara Gottfried, Goop.com
6. Nutrients commonly depleted by alcohol, Healthy Drinker
7. Alcohol Alert, National Institute on Alcohol Abuse and Alcoholism No.22 PH 348 October 1993
8. Alcohol and its effects on metabolism, Medical weight loss clinic
9. Media distort findings of drinking study, Gabriel L. Van Duinen, BMJ 2018; 362:k3891
10. Defining alcohol related dementia, R. T. Rao, BMJ 2018; 362:k3894

References: Psychology of Fashion, body image and the female state

1. How jeans conquered the world, Stephanie Hegarty, BBC World Service, 28.2.12
2. Vogue magazine 1986 to present day
3. Facial Shift Adjusting to an altered appearance, Dawn Shaw 2016
4. The Beauty Myth, Naomi Wolf, Vintage 1990
5. Body Image, Sarah Grogan, Routledge 1999
6. The Psychology of Fashion, Carolyn Mair, Routledge 2019
7. Fashion, Culture and Identity, Fred Davis, The University of Chicago Press 1992
8. Body Image, A Handbook of Theory, Research and Clinical Practice, Edited by Thomas F. Cash and Thomas Pruzinsky The Guildford Press 2002
9. Female body shape, Somatotype and constitutional physiology, Wikipedia
10. The Heath-Carter Anthropometric Somatotype (www.somatotype.org)

References: Friendship amongst women

1. Shelley E. Taylor, Tend and Befriend Theory, University of California, Los Angeles, Theories of Social Psychology, Sage Publications.
2. Taylor S.E. et al., Behavioural Reponses to Stress in Females: Tend-and Befriend, Not Fight-or-Flight, Psychological Review 2000, Vol 107, No.3, 411-429
3. www.nurseshealthstudy.org
4. Candyce H. Kroenke et al., Postdiagnosis social networks and breast cancer mortality in the After Breast Cancer Pooling Project, cancer, 2017 Apr 1;123(7): 1228-1237
5. Science Daily, 'Women with more social connections have higher breast cancer survival, study shows'

6. The 2005 Australian Longitudinal Study of Ageing
7. Aukett R. et al., Gender differences in friendship patterns, Sex Roles, July 1988, volume 19. Issue 1-2, pp 57-66
8. Misra N. et al., Loneliness, depression and sociability in old age, Ind. Psychiatry J. 2009 Jan-Jun; 18(1):51-55
9. Debba Haupert 'The girlfriend instinct – the value of female friendships', ThoughtCo.
10. Jessica Wolf 'Are they friends or not? Just a second of laughter can reveal relationship status, UCLA study finds' newsroom.ucla.edu
11. Bryant G.A. et al., Detecting affiliation in colaughter across 24 societies, PNAS April 26, 2016 113 (17) 4682-4687
12. Science Daily, 'UCLA Researchers Identify Key Biobehavioral Pattern Used By Women To Manage Stress'
13. Sharon Greenthal 'Why Midlife Women Need Friends More Than Ever', Huffington Post

References: Sleep

1. Mandibular advancement appliances for snoring and obstructive sleep apnoea, patient information leaflet, Queen Victoria Hospital, East Grinstead.
2. How exposure to blue light affects your brain and body, AKAMAI products
3. Shukla M. et al., Mechanism of Melatonin in alleviating Alzheimer's Disease, Current Neuropharmacology, 2017 Oct; 15(7): 1010–1031.
4. The Sleep Disorder Centre by Peter Venn and Jonathan Ratoff, Queen Victoria NHS Foundation Trust
5. Irish L.A. et al., The role of sleep hygiene in promoting public health: a review of empirical evidence, Sleep Med. Rev. 2015 Aug; 22:23-36
6. Chung K. et al., Sleep hygiene education as a treatment of insomnia: a systematic review and meta-analysis, Family Practice, Volume 35, Issue 4, August 2018:365-375
7. American Sleep Association 'Sleep Hygiene Tips'
8. American Sleep Association 'Sleep Debt, signs, symptoms and treatments'
9. Tassia do Vale Cardoso Lopes et al., Eating late negatively affects sleep pattern and apnea severity in individuals with sleep apnea, J Clin Sleep Med. 2019; 15(3): 383-392
10. Xiao Tan et al., Association between self-reported sleep duration and body composition in middle-aged and older adults, J Clin Sleep Med. 2019; 15(3): 431-435
11. BMA guide 'Anticipating and managing fatigue associated with doctors' working pattern
12. Senturk A. et al., The effect of lavender oil application via inhalation pathway on haemodialysis patients' anxiety and sleep quality, Holistic Nurse Pract. 2018 Nov/Dec; 32(6):324-335
13. Healthy Sleep, Medline Plus, U.S. National Library of Medicine
14. Insomnia: Relaxation techniques and sleeping habits, Institute for Quality and Efficiency in Health Care, March 9.3.17
15. Akerstedt T. et al., Sleep duration, mortality and the influence of age, European Journal of Epidemiology, October 2017, Vol 32, Issue 10, pp 881-891
16. Soucise A. et al., Sleep quality, duration and breast cancer aggressiveness, Breast Cancer Research and Treatment, July 2017, Volume 164, Issue 1, pp 169-178
17. Tam T. et al., Short sleep duration increased metabolic impact in healthy adults: A population-based cohort study, Sleep, Volume 40, Issue 10, 1.10.17, zsx130
18. Burman D., Sleep Disorders: Circadian Rhythm Sleep-Wake Disorders, Family Physician Essentials, 460:33-36, 2017 Sep.
19. Burman D., Sleep Disorders: Restless Legs Syndrome, Family Physician Essentials, 460:29-32, 2017 Sep.
20. Chung M-H. et al., The mediating and moderating effects of sleep hygiene practice on anxiety and insomnia in hospital nurses, International Journal of Nursing Practice, Volume 21, Issue S2, Pages 9-18, May 2015

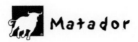